Anaesthesia Review

Anaesthesia Review 13
Edited by Leon Kaufman and Robert Ginsburg

ISBN 0443 04853 3
ISSN 0263-1512

Anaesthesia Review 14

Edited by

Leon Kaufman MD FRCA
Consulting Anaesthetist,
University College Hospital, and St Mark's Hospital, London;
Senior Lecturer,
Faculty of Clinical Sciences,
University College, London, UK

Robert Ginsburg MB BS BSc FRCA
Consultant Anaesthetist,
King's College Hospital,
London, UK

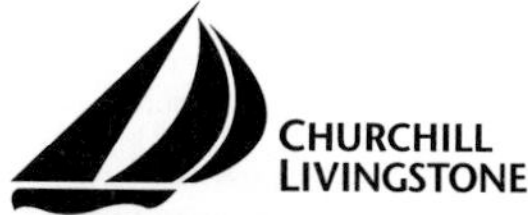

NEW YORK EDINBURGH LONDON MADRID MELBOURNE SAN FRANCISCO AND TOKYO 1998

CHURCHILL LIVINGSTONE
Medical Division of Pearson Professional Limited

Distributed in the United States of America by Churchill Livingstone Inc.,
650 Avenue of the Americas, New York, NY 10011, and by associated companies,
branches and representatives throughout the world.

First published 1998

ISBN 0-443-06018 5
ISSN 0263-1512

British Library Cataloguing in Publication Data
A catalogue record for this book is available from the British Library

Library of Congress Cataloging in Publication Data
A catalog record for this book is available from the Library of Congress

Medical knowledge is constantly changing. As new information becomes available, changes in treatment, procedures, equipment and the use of drugs become necessary. The editors and the publishers have, as far as possible, taken care to ensure that the information given in this text is accurate and up to date. However, readers are strongly advised to confirm that the information, especially with regard to drug usage, complies with current legislation and standards of practice.

For Churchill Livingstone:

Commmissioning Editor: Mike Parkinson
Project Editor: Kay Hunston
Designer: Sarah Cape

The publisher's policy is to use **paper manufactured from sustainable forests**

Typeset by B.A. & G.M. Haddock
Printed in Singapore

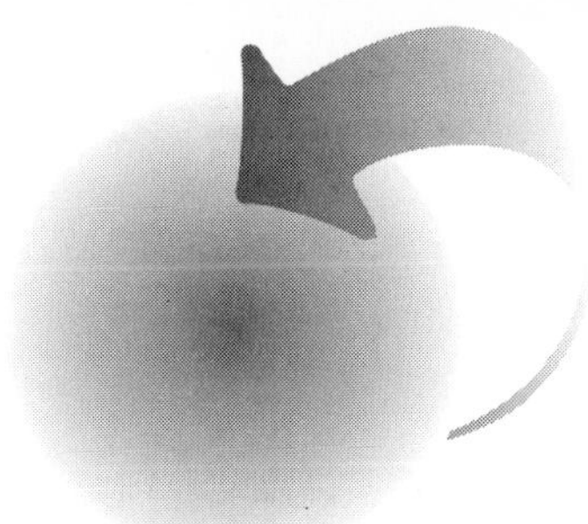

Contents

Preface

The review series still appears to be attractive as assessed by the response of its readers. It is gratifying to see that authors have updated their concepts of assessing patients. This applies in particular to Goldman who has modified his concept of multifactorial index of cardiac risks in view of the advances in technology.

The emphasis is again on medicine and pharmacology in relationship to anaesthesia. The therapeutic implications of hypertension and metabolic disorders are considered as well as advances in adult cardiac surgery. There is also a chapter on the management of the child with congenital heart disease undergoing non-cardiac surgery. Patients undergoing major surgery and cardiac surgery are nursed in intensive care and advances in mechanical ventilation are outlined. It is worthy of note that there is still no simple means of identifying patients likely to develop multiple organ failure.

The management of pain has not been completely resolved and there are chapters on the treatment of acute and chronic pain. Pain relief in obstetrics is also outlined, while pharmacology is represented by sections on the new neuromuscular blocking agents, imidazolines and the α_2-adrenoceptors, an area of potential interest to anaesthesia.

As usual there are update sections. The literature is expanding at a rapid rate and readers are advised to consult original papers to which only reference has been made.

It remains for us to thank our many contributors for the clarity and comprehensive coverage of their sections. Sylvia Wiggins has again dutifully collated the material, while the publishers are thanked for their harmonious co-operation.

145 Harley Street
London W1N 2DE, UK
1997

Leon Kaufman
Robert Ginsburg

Contributors

Helen Daly MB BCh BaO LRCS/PI FRCA
Senior Registrar, Anaesthetic Department, Guy's Hospital, London, UK

Simon R. Finfer MB BS MRCP FRCA
Senior Staff Specialist, Intensive Therapy Unit, Royal North Shore Hospital of Sydney, St Leonard's, New South Wales, Australia

Brian Glenville BSc MS FRCS
Consultant Cardiothoracic Surgeon, St Mary's Hospital, London, UK

Leonidas Hadjinikolaou MD
Senior Registrar in Cardiothoracic Surgery, St Mary's Hospital, London, UK

Jennifer M. Hunter MB ChB PhD FRCA
Reader in Anaesthesia, University of Liverpool and Honorary Consultant Anaesthetist, Royal Liverpool University Hospital, Liverpool, UK

Leon Kaufman, MD FRCA
Consulting Anaesthetist, University College Hospital and St Mark's Hospital, London; Honorary Senior Lecturer, Faculty of Clinical Sciences, University College London, London, UK

Franco Moscuzza MB BS FRCA
Senior Registrar, Anaesthetic Department, Guy's Hospital, London, UK

Rajesh Munglani DCH FRCA
Lecturer and Consultant in Anaesthesia and Chronic Pain, John Farman Professor at the Royal College of Anaesthetists, Addenbrooke's Hospital Cambridge, UK

Geraldine O'Sullivan MD FRCA
Consultant Anaesthetist, Department of Anaesthesia, St Thomas' Hospital, London, UK

Maurizio Renna MD
Consultant Anaesthetist, Department of Anaesthesia, Ealing Hospital NHS Trust, Southall, Middlesex, UK

Graeme Rocker MA DM MRCP FRCP(C)
Director of Intensive Care, Victoria General Hospital, and Assistant Professor, Department of Medicine (Respirology), Dalhousie University, Halifax, Nova Scotia, Canada

S Clare Stanford BSc DPhil
Senior Lecturer, Department of Pharmacology, University College London, London, UK

R. Zimlichman MD
Head Department of Medicine, Hypertension and the Donolo Institute of Physiological Hygiene, Wolfson Medical Center, Holon and Sackler School of Medicine, Tel Aviv University, Tel Aviv, Israel

Leon Kaufman

Medicine relevant to anaesthesia – 1

CARDIOVASCULAR SYSTEM

PRE-OPERATIVE ASSESSMENT

In 1977, Goldman et al (1977) produced a multifactorial index of cardiac risks in patients undergoing noncardiac surgical operations and this was revised in 1995 (Goldman). A further revision was effected by Mangano & Goldman (1995) to take into account the availability of new techniques and tests for assessing cardiac function. Initially, only two major risk factors were recognised, namely a recent myocardial infarction and current congestive cardiac failure. In an unselected series of cases, the risk of peri-operative myocardial infarction was found to be 2%. If patients with known cardiovascular disease were excluded, the risk of peri-operative death from cardiac causes was 1%. In patients with suspected coronary artery disease, the risk is 3–5 times higher than those selected for pre-operative thallium scintigraphy. However, in those patients with peripheral vascular or aortic disease, the risk of developing cardiovascular complications rises to 29%. The risks are also greater in patients having aortic surgery compared with those having cataract surgery.

Risks also need to be assessed on the patient's ability for exercise, such as climbing up stairs or carrying shopping, without cardiac symptoms, while those who can raise their heart rate with exercise have a lower risk of complications. Mangano & Goldman (1995) emphasise that no single parameter is a true reflection of the status of the patient. The place of pre-operative electrocardiogram and echocardiography are discussed, drawing attention to the fact that resting transthoracic or transoesophageal echocardiography adds much more information than that provided by routine clinical and ECG studies.

Leon Kaufman MD FRCA, 145 Harley Street, London W1N 2DE, UK

Determination of ejection fraction by radionuclide ventriculography does not appear to add more than pre-operative clinical examination. Thallium scintigraphy is of value in patients who cannot exercise.

Recommendations for pre-operative cardiac evaluation and management of patients for major non-cardiac surgery are set out. It is worthy of note that patients in class I or class II require no major pre-operative diagnostic testing except perhaps 12-lead electrocardiography and careful monitoring during operation, whereas those with coronary artery disease of either class III or IV rated index should be given aggressive medical treatment prior to operation (Class I–II = low cardiac risk: Class III–IV = high cardiac risk). The group most difficult to manage appear to be those whose functional cardiac status is unknown and they may require extensive pre-operative investigations, coronary angiography and possibly re-vascularisation.

Juste et al (1996) have drawn attention to an anomaly in assessing patients considered to be cardiac anaesthetic risks. Although attention has been drawn to cardiac assessment as set out by Goldman (1977) and recently updated (Goldman 1995, Mangano & Goldman 1995), acute myocardial infarction is not a major cause of death following major surgery. However, multiple organ failure (of which myocardial infarction is one cause) is a major cause of death in intensive care units following major surgery. There is no simple means of identifying patients likely to develop multiple organ failure (see also report of the Committee on Peri-operative Cardiovascular Evaluation for Non-cardiac Surgery 1996). Howell et al (1996) found that a pre-operative history of hypertension is associated with a small, but significant, increase in peri-operative cardiovascular death following surgery under general anaesthesia (see also Howell et al 1997).

Carson et al (1996) have studied the effects of anaemia and cardiovascular disease on surgical morbidity and mortality and found, as expected, that the mortality for patients with underlying cardiovascular disease was greater than those without, irrespective of the haemoglobin concentration. They also showed that the mortality increased as the patient's haemoglobin decreased and was evident even in mild anaemia. It would seem, therefore, that at operation, for patients who have cardiovascular disease, not only should blood loss be corrected, but attention should be paid to maintaining the haemoglobin concentration.

HEART FAILURE

The management of chronic heart failure has been reviewed by Cohn (1996) in which he emphasises that the management is no longer confined to relief of symptoms, but extends to improvement of left ventricular function. Reduced ejection fraction is prominent in chronic heart failure and there is related increase in the left ventricular volume (see also Robotham et al 1991). An ejection fraction of below 0.45 indicates left ventricular dysfunction. Even if the patient is symptomless an ejection fraction of less than 30% leads to a 30% risk of symptomatic heart failure within 3 years. Diastolic dysfunction is also important in heart failure, especially in elderly patients and those with hypertension. Treatment includes restriction of salt in the diet, while drug therapy involves the use of diuretics, vasodilators and digoxin.

Northridge (1996) has debated the merits of treatment with nitrates or frusemide and concluded that there were distinct disadvantages in the use of frusemide in the treatment of acute and chronic heart failure. Nitrates, on the other hand, are ideal for acute heart failure, relieving pulmonary congestion without affecting stroke volume or increasing myocardial oxygen demand.

Drugs that relax the arterial and venous smooth muscle include nitroprusside and nitroglycerine, hydralazine and isosorbide or ACE inhibitors. Other vasodilators include α-adrenergic antagonists such as prazosin. The therapeutic value of digoxin has recently been questioned, especially in patients with normal cardial rhythm.

Thromboembolism is a potential complication of heart failure and anticoagulation has also been recommended, either with warfarin or with aspirin.

Patients with chronic heart failure have increased levels of circulating catecholamines and this has led to the introduction of β-blockers in patients who are already receiving treatment with digoxin, diuretics and ACE inhibitors. Packer et al (1996a) have shown that carvedilol, a non-selective β-receptor antagonist (which also has α_1-receptor antagonist action and also is antioxidant), reduced the mortality risk as well as the need for hospitalisation (see also Pfeffer & Stevenson 1996). On the other hand, d-sotalol was associated with increased mortality due to arrhythmias (Waldo et al 1996).

A calcium channel blocker, amlodipine, appears to have a place in the management of severe chronic heart failure (Packer et al 1996b).

Persistent dry cough develops in about 25% of patients being treated with ACE inhibitors. It may improve with reducing the dose and, in many instances, the drug may have to be discontinued. Hargreaves & Benson (1995), however, found that inhalation of sodium cromoglycate was effective in treating ACE inhibitor cough.

Surprisingly, amiodarone, which is effective in reducing the incidence of ventricular arrhythmias and improving ventricular function, did not reduce the incidence of sudden death (Singh et al 1995).

Endothelin-1 (ET-1) may be involved in the pathogenesis of severe cardiovascular failure, due to its vasoconstrictor properties, and antagonists are being developed which may have therapeutic potential in man (Kaddoura & Poole-Wilson 1996)

MYOCARDIAL ISCHAEMIA

Prognosis of patients with myocardial ischaemia has been based on ECG abnormalities, serum creatine kinase MB (CK-MB) and now troponin T, a binding protein involved in the contractile apparatus of cardiac myocytes, has been found to be a sensitive marker of outcome (Ohman et al 1996, see Van de Werf 1996).

The term apoptosis, or programmed cell death, is a highly regulated and active process as opposed to necrosis and it has been suggested that it is involved in loss of myocardial cells (Mallat et al 1996). Narula et al (1996) have found that apoptosis leads to loss of myocytes in patients with end-stage cardiomyopathy and it may also contribute to progressive myocardial dysfunction (see also Colucci 1996).

Sudden death in children and young adults has been reviewed by Liberthson (1996). In the first year, most of the deaths are congenital and thereafter, until the age of 30, the commonest conditions of sudden death include myocarditis, hypertrophic cardiomyopathy, coronary artery disease, congenital coronary-artery abnormalities, conduction system abnormalities, mitral valve prolapse and aortic dissection.

Mitral regurgitation due to flail leaflet is associated with high morbidity and mortality and surgery is almost unavoidable within 10 years after diagnosis has been made (Ling et al 1996).

Pre-operatively it is often difficult to assess the severity of coronary artery stenosis as it can be difficult without sophisticated technology. It is estimated, from animal studies, there is no impairment of maximum blood flow in the coronary vessels until 75% of the cross-section area of the artery is obstructed (Wilson 1996). Resting flow does not decrease until over 90% of the arterial lumen is affected, although Pijls et al (1996) have found there was a correlation between the physiological assessment and non-invasive testing.

There is debate whether a patient should be subjected to myocardial revascularisation by bypass surgery or angioplasty (Simoons 1996). The technique of angioplasty has improved with balloon angioplasty, atherectomy and laser angioplasty, coronary artery stents as well as the use of thrombolytic agents (Bittl 1996). Peri-operative myocardial infarction or ischaemia may occur during operation and this is common in patients undergoing vascular surgery. Clinically silent myocardial infarction occurs in 30% of patients and it is fatal in 50%. A strong predictor of risk was angina, but previous infarction was not (Mamode et al 1996).

During endoscopic cholangio-pancreatography (ERCP) tachycardia frequently occurs and can lead to myocardial ischaemia. In a series studied by Rosenberg et al (1996), one patient had acute infarction and 10 others had signs of myocardial ischaemia during endoscopy and when the endoscope was removed the ST deviation disappeared. Metoprolol, by reducing the incidence of tachycardia, may reduce the risk of myocardial complications.

Yellon et al (1996) debate whether angina is protective in that brief periods of ischaemia with intermittent reperfusion protect the myocardium against a subsequent, longer insult.

Hyperkalaemia is a cause of cardiac arrest: one patient developed severe hyperkalaemia following operation and was found to have a serum potassium of 9.4 mmol/l. He was successfully treated by peritoneal dialysis. It was subsequently found that the patient had what appeared to be muscular dystrophy, with a high CPK (Jackson et al 1996). Hyperkalaemia has also been seen following bypass cardiac surgery. It was suggested that the reason for this was the postoperative use of noradrenaline as opposed to adrenaline which tends to lower serum potassium (Ganeshan & Bihari 1996).

The place of calcium channel blockers and ACE inhibitors in preventing myocardial infarction and stroke has not been extensively evaluated and only thiazide diuretics and β-blockers have been shown to prevent myocardial infarction and stroke in patients with hypertension (Beevers & Sleight 1996). There has also been a suggestion that there is an increase in gastrointestinal haemorrhage with calcium antagonists (Gordon 1996), while there also appears to be a possible increased risk of carcinoma: the organs being mostly affected are the uterus as well as the lymphatic and haemopoietic systems (Pahor et al 1996). It is suggested that inhibition of apoptosis is the explanation of the development of carcinoma (Dargie 1996).

CARDIAC ARRHYTHMIAS

The mechanisms of supraventricular tachycardia are outlined by Ganz & Friedman (1995). Originally, the term paroxysmal atrial tachycardia was used to described supraventricular tachycardia, but it became clear that many arrhythmias do not arise in the atrial muscles, but in the atrio-ventricular junction. The drug of choice in treatment is adenosine, an endogenous nucleoside that is capable of blocking atrio-ventricular nodal conduction (Camm & Garratt 1991).

The indications for cardiac pacing are discussed by Kusumoto & Godschlager (1996). These include sinus-node dysfunction (sick-sinus syndrome), heart block (second and third degree), fascicular block, neurocardiogenic syncope and cardiomyopathy. The types of pacemakers were discussed by Sutton (1989) in *Anaesthesia Review 6*.

RECEPTORS

Views on receptors involved in the cardiovascular system are being constantly updated. Current concepts on the adrenergic receptors are outlined by Insel (1996), angiotensin receptors by Goodfriend et al (1996) and calcium ion channels by Katz (1993) and Brown et al (1995) (see also Gibb 1997). It is now accepted there are nine types of adrenergic receptors, including α1A, α1B, and α1D, α2A, α2B, and α2C, β1, β2 and β3. Adrenergic receptors are linked to G proteins as are acetylcholine, dopamine, histamine, prostaglandin, vasopressin, oxytocin, angiotensin and other transmitters.

There are now two angiotensin II receptors, AT_1 and AT_2, recognised and it is the AT_1 receptor which is involved in intense vasoconstriction of angiotensin II. Angiotensin is one of the most powerful vasoconstrictors and also stimulates secretion of aldosterone. It inhibits the release of renin, increases tubular reabsorption of sodium, causes vasoconstriction of the efferent arterioles and promotes the release of AVP. The AT_2 receptor is seen in fetal brain and kidneys and the effect of ACE inhibitors on the developing fetus is unknown.

Calcium ions are essential for cell motility, cell division, hormone secretion, skeletal integrity and blood clotting. There are calcium ion sensors in cells and in response to hypercalcaemia, parathyroid cells secrete less parathyroid hormone, while the C cells of the thyroid secrete more calcitonin. The G protein is also involved in the receptor. An increase in extracellular calcium concentration decreases the glomerular filtration rate, leads to diuretic action in the proximal tubule and inhibits the action of ADH. Calcium is important in cardiac function and when depolarisation takes place, sodium and calcium passes through the ion selective channels. Calcium is also involved in neuromuscular conduction.

At least 16 vasoactive peptides have been identified, including natriuretic peptides A, B and C, endothelins 1–3, bradykinin, calcitonin gene related peptide (CGRP) and angiotensin. A more recent compound isolated from phaeochromocytoma tissue is adreomedullin (ADM). The ADM precursor has 185 amino acids and the active compounds are ADM and PAMP, both of which have hypotensive actions (see Sharp 1996).

PROSTHETIC HEART VALVES

Prosthetic heart valves have a life expectancy of 20–30 years, while 10–20% of homograft prothesis and 30% of heterograft prothesis fail within 10–15 years. Mechanical valves are preferred in patients who are young, who are likely to survive more than 10–20 years and who require anticoagulant therapy for other reasons such as atrial fibrillation. Bioprosthetic valves are reserved for patients who are elderly, whose life expectancy is less than 10–20 years and in whom anticoagulant therapy is contra-indicated. Prosthetic heart valves are likely to gather thrombi and require long-term anticoagulant therapy (Vonpatanasin et al 1996). The INR should be kept between 2.5 and 4.9. Some patients require warfarin and others can be controlled with aspirin, but patients with homograft bioprosthesis do not require anticoagulant therapy.

VENOUS THROMBOEMBOLISM

Patients who suffer major trauma are liable to develop thromboembolism and low-molecular-weight heparin appears to be more successful than low-dose heparin (Geerts et al 1996). Levine et al (1996) and Koopman et al (1996) felt that low-molecular-weight heparin could be administered safely at home. In a study involving total hip replacement, Bergqvist et al (1996) showed that enoxaparin was more effective in preventing thromboembolism if given for a full month after operation, compared to those who only received the drug during their stay in hospital. It is worthy of note that the initial dose was given 12 h prior to surgery and that the majority of patients received epidural-spinal analgesia without complication.

CARDIAC SURGERY

Fletcher et al (1996) have drawn attention to the fact that there are very few papers on the effects of cardiopulmonary bypass on the eye, although there have been some observations indicating that it increases intraocular pressure. Fletcher et al (1996) noted that cardiopulmonary bypass caused dilatation of the pupils and they believe this to be due to hypothalamic sympathetic nerve stimulation.

INTRAVASCULAR COAGULATION

This condition may be **acute** following infection, obstetric complications, trauma, transfusion of incompatible blood and liver disease; or **chronic** resulting from malignancy, retained fetal products, liver disease and localised intravascular coagulation. Diagnosis is made clinically and aided by the platelet count, prothrombin time, activated partial thromboplastin time, fibrinogen levels and estimation of fibrinogen degradation products. Treatment consists of treating the underlying condition, maintenance of blood volume and tissue perfusion and replacement of blood components, including platelets and coagulating factors as necessary. If the platelet count is below $50 \times 10^9/l$, one donor unit should be given for every 10 kg of body weight. Fresh frozen plasma (FFP) contains more fibrinogen than cryoprecipitate and should be given in the dose 15 ml/kg body weight. If FFP cannot maintain fibrinogen concentration above 0.5 g/l, then cryoprecipitate can be given. There is no evidence that heparin improves the morbidity or mortality and results with natural thrombin inhibitors have been disappointing. Plasma inhibitors such as tranexamic acid or aprotinin are generally contra-indicated (Baglin 1996). They can be used if there is evidence of fibrinolysis, to stop bleeding.

KIDNEY

The causes and pathophysiology of acute renal failure are discussed by Brady & Singer (1995) and Thadhani et al (1996). Prerenal failure accounts for approximately 70% of the cases in general practice and 40% in hospital. Persistent prerenal failure is the commonest cause of ischaemic induced tubular necrosis. In hospital, exposure to drugs such as aminoglycosides, radiocontrast material, especially in patients receiving angiotensin converting enzyme inhibitors, or treatment with NSAIDs can cause renal failure. In renal vascular disease, ACE inhibitors and diuretics can also cause renal failure. Postrenal causes are due to obstruction of the urinary tract, while intrinsic causes include damage to the tubules, interstitium vessels or the glomerulus.

Treatment may involve use of vasodilators. Dopamine dilates renal arterioles and increases renal blood flow and the glomerular filtration rate, but the efficacy of this drug is being questioned. Calcium-channel blockers also improve vascular tone, but may cause hypotension and decreased renal perfusion. Atrial natriuretic peptides (ANP) have vasodilator properties, but have not been shown to be useful. Although mannitol and frusemide apparently are effective against ischaemic injury in animals they have been ineffectual in man. Every effort should be made to prevent further kidney damage, and hyperkalaemia should be treated with glucose and insulin. Metabolic acidosis should be corrected and doses of any medication eliminated by the kidney adjusted. Anaemia may result from decreased production of erythropoietin, while uraemia causes platelet dysfunction and bleeding. Treatment may involve dialysis, haemofiltration, veno-venous and arterio-venous shunts. Mortality from acute renal tubular necrosis is about 50%. The prognosis depends on whether the oliguria is less than 400 ml/day at presentation, the creatinine is greater than 265 μmol/l, age and multi-organ failure. During recovery, there may be a marked diuresis (polyuric phase).

In chronic renal insufficiency, the ACE inhibitor benazepril appears to protect against progression of renal insufficiency (Maschino et al 1996). Hannedouche et al (1994) found that in hypertensive patients with chronic renal failure enalapril also delayed the progression towards end-stage renal failure and was more effective than β-blockers.

SUDDEN INFANT DEATH SYNDROME (SIDS)

There has been a decrease in the incidence of SIDS, but it still remains a major cause of infant mortality. The risk may be reduced by the supine sleeping position and avoiding the prone position and loose bedding which can slip over the baby's head (Fleming et al 1996). Blair et al (1996) further showed that maternal smoking during pregnancy and exposure to tobacco smoke increased the incidence of SIDS. It has been suggested that antimony was a cause, but this has not been found to be so (Fleming et al 1994). The pulmonary pathology indicates that there is a T lymphocyte-mediated pulmonary inflammatory response in SIDS and the products of eosinophil degranulation cause epithelial damage and pulmonary oedema leading to respiratory obstruction and hypoxaemia (Howat et al 1994).

Infants of mothers who smoke have been found to have reduced respiratory function and are likely to develop wheezing. It appears that a family history of asthma, maternal hypertension and *in utero* smoke exposure lead to reduced respiratory function in the neonate (Stick et al 1996).

HAEMORRHAGIC BRAIN INJURY

Premature babies are particularly prone to haemorrhage and ischaemic brain injury and the early use of FFP or increasing the intravascular volume had little effect on reducing the incidence of the condition (Northern Neonatal Nursing Initiative Trial Group 1996, Koppe 1996).

RESPIRATORY DISTRESS SYNDROME

Neonatal respiratory distress syndrome is associated with prematurity and deficiency of surfactant. Schwartz et al (1994) have shown that surfactant decreased mortality and morbidity in low birth weight infants, while Verder et al (1994) found that in infants with moderate to severe respiratory distress syndrome treated with nasal continuous positive airway pressure, a single dose of surfactant reduced the need for subsequent mechanical ventilation. It appears to be more effective in white children as compared with black children (Hamvas et al 1996). New techniques of treating severe respiratory distress syndrome involve the use of endotracheal perfluorocarbon liquid during IPPR (partial liquid ventilation). This led to clinical improvement and survival in some infants who were not expected to survive (Lowe Leach et al 1996, Merritt & Heldt 1996).

Other new techniques include extracorporeal membrane oxygenation (ECMO), but this technique is expensive and involves complex technology. ECMO reduced the risk of death or severe disability (UK Collaborative ECMO Trial Group 1996, Soll 1996).

The guidelines for paediatric life support are outlined by the Paediatric Life Support Working Party of the European Resuscitation Council (1994). The aim of neonatal intensive care is not only to avoid serious disability or prolong survival, but to preserve normal function (Bion 1995). For home resuscitation, Tonkin et al (1995) recommends that mothers should be taught how to ventilate the infant by the nasal route.

TRACHEOSTOMY

Tracheostomy in children is a hazardous procedure and was formerly performed for epiglottitis and acute laryngotracheobronchitis, but today the main indication is subglottic stenosis in infants following prolonged intubation for respiratory distress syndrome and prematurity (Shinkwin & Gibbin 1996).

ANAESTHESIA

Anaesthesia, including the physiology and pharmacology of drugs for the young child, has been considered by Darowski (1994). Techniques and management are also outlined and in particular reference is made to postoperative pain, which has been poorly treated in children.

Managing acute pain in children is detailed in the *Drug and Therapeutics Bulletin* (1995). Reference is made to anticipating and preventing pain with adequate and regular dosing. Intramuscular injections should be avoided and drugs should be given orally, rectally or by infusion. Analgesics include paracetamol, in an oral suspension, in the dose of 15 mg/kg up to a maximum of 60 mg/kg/day. Aspirin should be avoided, but ibuprofen (20 mg/kg/day in divided doses) is available as well as diclofenac. NSAIDs should be avoided in children with a history of gastrointestinal bleeding and also those with possible renal impairment. Opioids recommended are codeine (0.5–1 mg/kg every 4–6 h), either alone or with paracetamol. Morphine is recommended for acute, severe pain and can be given by mouth in the dose 200–500 μg/kg but, after major surgery, the drug should be given intravenously or subcutaneously. A loading dose of 50–100 μg/kg is infused over 30 min and, thereafter, analgesia maintained at the rate of 5–40 μg/kg/h. The respiratory rate should be monitored and the rate not allowed to fall below 20 min^{-1} in children under 5 years of age. Patient-controlled analgesia (PCA) in general is not suitable for children under 5 years. Extradural morphine can be administered either through a catheter into the epidural space or more commonly through the caudal route. EMLA cream enables pain-free venepuncture to be performed, but it must be applied for at least 60 min before the injection. Regional analgesia is often undertaken when the child is already under general anaesthesia and can provide prolonged control of severe pain.

De Lima et al (1996) have confirmed that there have been changes of attitude and practice amongst anaesthetists following publications indicating that operations on neonates are not painless.This has prompted debate on whether the fetus feels pain (Derbyshire & Furedi 1996). In fact it has been shown that there is an endocrine response of the fetus to invasive procedures (Giannakoulopoulos et al 1994), although this has been debated by Clark (1994) who postulates there may be stress without distress (see also Derbyshire 1994, Bennett 1994).

Wolf (1994) suggests that neonatal sedation is more an art than a science. The management of newborn babies with respiratory distress syndrome differs from that used postoperatively, in that the former group do not require the same degree of pain relief as those having surgery. Propofol is contra-indicated as it can result in metabolic acidosis. Chloral hydrate is also inadvisable for long-term sedation. Jacqz-Aigrain et al (1994) reported favourably on the use of midazolam for sedation of newborn babies who are being ventilated.

After major trauma resuscitation is the first line of treatment and analgesia should be administered by slow intravenous injection. Inhalation of entonox is of value, particular in the management of burns.

Vallance (1996) has indicated that drugs can cause fetal death or damage at any stage of pregnancy. Anti-cancer drugs cause embryonic death at 0–16 days, while later in pregnancy, during the second and third trimester, β-blockers can cause retardation of growth. ACE inhibitors cause abnormalities of renal function and scalp development. Fetal well-being can be affected by prostaglandins during induction of uterine contractions: however, the period of greatest risk for malformation is 17–60 days.

Drugs that affect fetal development taken by the father and excreted in the semen may also cause problems. Low doses of 5-α reductase inhibitors during pregnancy cause abnormalities of external genitalia of the male offspring. Griseofulvin also appears in the semen and should be avoided for 6 months prior to fertilisation.

OPEN HEART SURGERY

Bellinger et al (1995) have compared results of heart surgery performed with circulatory arrest with surgery with low-flow bypass and found that the circulatory arrest had a higher risk of delayed motor development and neurological abnormalities in children under 1 year.

ASTHMA

Martinez et al (1995) found that wheezing in infants was generally a transient condition with diminished airway function at birth, but this did not necessarily lead to predisposition to asthma. However, in some children, there are already increased levels of IgE and these children are more likely to develop asthma (see Silverman 1995). Roosevelt et al (1996) found there was no place for the use of dexamethasone in the treatment of bronchiolitis in the first 12 months of life, as the condition is commonly due to respiratory syncytial virus.

Infants with chronic neonatal lung disease have arousal mechanisms which reduce the incidence of oxygen desaturation, but they also disrupt sleep (Harris & Sullivan 1995).

MISCELLANEOUS

COCAINE

Molecular mechanisms of cocaine addiction indicate the importance of the central dopamine re-uptake transport system to which cocaine binds strongly. Dopamine remains at high concentrations in the synapse, which may account for the psychological stimulatory effects of the drug (Leshner 1996).

The management of cocaine abuse and dependence is outlined by Mendelson & Mello (1996). Psychotherapy is indicated, as well as antidepressant drugs and, possibly, bromocriptine which decreases the craving for cocaine. Buprenorphine significantly decreases cocaine use, as does carbamazepine.

Myocardial infarction may be associated with cocaine and it is important to differentiate between this and myocardial infarction not influenced by cocaine. The treatment is different and cocaine-associated myocardial infarction should be treated with benzodiazepines to decrease central adrenergic stimulation, aspirin to reduce thrombus formation and nitroglycerine to reverse coronary vasoconstriction. Prolonged ischaemia can be treated with low doses of phentolamine or verapamil. Beta-adrenergic agonists are contra-indicated as they enhance the coronary vasoconstriction (Hollander 1996).

ITCHING

Greaves & Wall (1996) have reviewed the pathophysiology of itching and have concluded that the nerve pathways and the relationship to pain are still not understood. Histamine appears to play a major role in itching as well as substance P and interleukin-2. Opioid μ-receptors are involved in the central nervous system and regulate the extent and quality of itch. Histamine itch is made worse with pretreatment with low concentration of opioids. Curiously, intravenous naloxone inhibits itching of cholestasis. Apparently scratching of skin generates inhibitory activity which suppresses itch excitation (see also Kam & Tan 1996).

References

For references see end of Medicine Relevant to Anaesthesia - 2

Leon Kaufman

Medicine relevant to anaesthesia – 2

RESPIRATION

SMOKING

The tracheo-bronchial tract of chronic smokers is known to be hyper-irritable, but little is known of the upper airway reflex sensitivity. Erskine et al (1994) found that reflex sensitivity was increased in chronic cigarette smokers and this was unaltered in those who stopped smoking for 24 h. After this period the sensitivity decreased.

Smoking is associated with increased levels of F_2-isoprostanes, which are involved in oxidative damage by free radicals (Morrow et al 1995). The polyunsaturated acids of the n-3 variety are present in fish and have anti-inflammatory actions. A high dietary intake of n-3 fatty acids may protect cigarette smokers against chronic obstructive airways disease (Shahar et al 1994).

Hole et al (1996) strongly advised smokers with reduced FEV_1 to stop smoking. In adolescents, especially girls, cigarette smoking is associated with evidence of mild airway obstruction and slow development of lung function (Gold et al 1996). Active and even passive smoking are associated with impairment of the endothelium-dependent dilatation of blood vessels in healthy young adults, possibly suggesting early arterial deterioration (Celermajer et al 1996). During induction of anaesthesia, there are increased concentrations of carboxyhaemoglobin, while oxygen desaturation readily ensues (Dennis et al 1994).

ASTHMA

Asthma is still a major hazard in the community, the admission rate in England and Wales rising from 20 000 a year in the 1960s to about 100 000 a year in the

Leon Kaufman MD FRCA, 145 Harley Street, London W1N 2DE, UK

1980s while death rates are still cause for concern. An attack requires immediate care (du Bois 1995, McFadden & Hejal 1995). In a study from the US, asthma was given as a cause of death in 4% of patients, but in patients over 35 years, who had asthma associated with chronic obstructive pulmonary disease (COPD), the outlook was less favourable (Silverstein et al 1994). It was found that reduced chemosensitivity to hypoxia and reduced perception of dyspnoea could predispose to fatal attacks of asthma (Kikuchi et al 1994). Other studies have also shown there is a relationship between coronary disease and chronic respiratory infections. Jousilahti et al (1996) have found that symptoms of chronic bronchitis predict the risk of coronary artery disease independently from known major cardiovascular risk factors.

Asthma may also be exercise-induced, associated with changes in heat and water that occur during the exchange of large volumes of air (McFadden & Gilbert 1994). About 250 agents have been known to cause occupational asthma and isocyanates, which are used in industry, appear to be responsible for 10% of these cases (Chan-Yeung & Malo 1995).

Barnes (1996) has reviewed the pathophysiology of asthma, indicating that many inflammatory cells, including mast cells, macrophages and eosinophils, are involved and that cytokines are important mediators amplifying and perpetuating the inflammatory process. The epithelial cells in the airway are an important source of cytokines as well as nitric oxide and endothelin. Not only is there bronchoconstriction in asthma, but there is also exudation of plasma, the involvement of neural mechanisms (adrenergic, cholinergic and non-adrenergic, non-cholinergic (NANC)), secretion of mucus and finally leading to an increase in the resistance of the airway smooth muscle and also fibrosis which is irreversible. It also now becoming apparent that many of the inflammatory proteins are induced by transcription factors affecting selected target genes.

In addition to histamine, prostaglandins, thromboxane and leukotrienes can constrict smooth muscle. Several cells in the bronchial airway can generate leukotrienes via 5-lipoxygenase. McGill & Busse (1996) have reported on the use of a 5-lipoxygenase inhibitor, namely zileuton, which has anti-inflammatory and bronchodilator properties. In mild to moderate asthma its effect is modest and it does not appear to be the first line of treatment.

Asthma-like symptoms may occur in extrathoracic airway dysfunction, particularly in chronic illness of the upper respiratory tract (Bucca et al 1995).

Treatment

For mild asthma symptoms there is no need to prescribe β_2 agonists on a regular basis and they can be used when needed (Drazen et al 1996, O'Byrne & Kerstjens 1996). On the other hand, Chapman et al (1994) found with salbutamol that the drug regularly administered was more effective and was associated with less frequent symptoms of asthma. Haahtela et al (1994) recommended maintenance doses of budesonide, but discontinuing the treatment resulted in exacerbation of the condition. It is worthy of note that salbutamol is said to have little effect on the pulmonary vasculature (Kiely et al 1995).

Nelson (1995) has also reviewed the place of β-adrenergic bronchodilators in asthma and drawn attention to the fact that high doses and repeated exposure to the β_2-adrenergic agonist results in desensitisation. Prolonged exposure reduces the number of receptors, but up-regulation can be stimulated by glucocorticoids and thyroid hormone. The principal side effects of β-adrenergic agonists include tremor, increased heart rate and palpitations, vasodilation and reflex tachycardia and decreased arterial oxygen tension. Acute metabolic responses include hyperglycaemia, hypokalaemia and hypomagnesaemia, but these diminish and are not important in long-term therapy. Long-term administration may result in tolerance, bronchial hyper-responsiveness (when the drug is discontinued) and incidences of bronchospasm have been reported (see also *Drug and Therapeutics Bulletin* 1997).

Grove & Lipworth (1995) have reassessed the use of β-adrenergic agonists in the treatment of asthma. There is no evidence to suggest that tolerance to these drugs results in deleterious effects with their regular use. Tolerance does not appear to develop to the bronchodilator effects of short-acting β-adrenoceptor agonists, but does occur in relationship to the anti-bronchoconstrictor effects. However, with long-acting β_2-adrenergic agonists, there is evidence that tolerance does develop to both the anti-bronchoconstrictor and bronchodilator effects. Tolerance can be prevented and reversed by systemic corticosteroids, but there is less evidence for the effect of inhaled steroids.

Others have studied β-adrenoceptor genotypes and there is down-regulation of the receptor after long standing exposure to agonists (Hall et al 1995). Prostaglandin E_2 (PGE_2) has considerable broncho-protective effects in patients with asthma (Pavord & Tattersfield 1995), while inhaled nitrogen dioxide and sulphur dioxide alter the airway response of asthmatic patients to inhalation of allergens (Devalia et al 1994, Tunnicliffe et al 1994). Sulphur dioxide and nitrogen dioxide are found in high concentrations in heavy traffic and nitrogen dioxide can even be encountered in the home environment.

The inhalation of β_2 agonists has been reported to increase the mortality in New Zealand (Blauw & Westendorp 1995). It may well be that there is an increase in bronchial reactivity in patients who are already hyper-reactive. On the other hand, it is often difficult to distinguish between the side effect of a drug and death from the underlying cause (Tattersfield 1994, Buist & Vollmer 1994).

Barnes (1995) has reviewed the effects of inhaled glucocorticoids in the treatment of asthma and was concerned about systemic side effects, particularly in children. However, studies on the pituitary-adrenal function in patients on inhaled glucocorticoids have been inconclusive. Other regimes had been tried, including low-dose salmeterol, but Greening et al (1994) found no difference between increasing the dose of steroids and low-dose steroids with β-adrenoceptor agonists.

Topical timolol, a non-selective β-antagonist, used in the treatment of glaucoma may impair respiratory function and exercise tolerance in elderly patients, even when there is no history of reversible airways disease. The eye drops drain down the nasolacrimal duct and are absorbed from the nasopharyngeal mucosa into the systemic circulation (Diggory et al 1995).

Theophylline is also used in the management of asthma and, although classified as a bronchodilator, it also modulates the immune response, is anti-inflammatory and broncho-protective. It is a phosphodiesterase inhibitor, and clinical trials of more effective inhibitors are in progress. Theophylline does have a place in the management of chronic asthma, but has a narrow therapeutic index (Weinberger & Hendels 1996).

THE ACUTE RESPIRATORY DISTRESS SYNDROME

The acute respiratory distress syndrome has been reviewed by Kollef & Schuster (1995). It is usually associated with abdominal sepsis or lung infection. The definition of **acute lung injury** is a condition in which there is impaired oxygenation, that is the ratio of partial pressure of arterial oxygen (mmHg PaO_2) to the fraction of inspired oxygen (FiO_2) is less than 300, the detection of bilateral pulmonary infiltrates, pulmonary artery occlusion (wedge) pressure less than 18 mmHg, with no clinical evidence of elevated left atrial pressure. The criteria for **ARDS** is the same, except that the PaO_2 to FiO_2 must be less than 200 and this is irrespective of the level of PEEP. Predisposing factors include direct lung injury (e.g. aspiration), or indirect injury (bacterial sepsis or pancreatitis). Overall mortality is greater than 50%.

ARDS appears to develop as a result of endothelial injury mediated by inflammatory cells in the alveoli with leakage of protein exudate. The neutrophils are involved in this process and selectins appear to aid the neutrophil adhesion. Plasma selectins were lower in those patients who progressed to ARDS and they reflect the possible sequestration of selectin in binding to the endothelium microvascular beds (Donnelly et al 1994). Prophospholipase A_2 is raised in acute lung injury (Rae et al 1994).

The anatomy, physiology and fluid mechanics of the airways are outlined in detail by Burwell & Jones (1996a) as well as the pathophysiology (Burwell & Jones 1996b).

Treatment

Treatment includes ventilation with PEEP and extracorporeal respiratory support has been advocated, but appears to have little advantage. The prone position appears to improve oxygenation and enhances removal of secretions (Ryan & Pelosi 1996). Fluids are usually restricted to diminish the incidence of pulmonary oedema. Surfactant has been recommended, but appears to have no significant effect (Anzueto et al 1996). Other drugs include corticosteroids, antioxidants, which appear to have no beneficial effect, ketoconazole (an inhibitor of thromboxane synthesis), nitric oxide, which is a selective pulmonary vasodilator, but caution is still advised in its use as rebound pulmonary hypertension can develop when the dose is reduced (Warren & Higenbottam 1996). Non-steroidal anti-inflammatory drugs, such as ibuprofen and indomethacin, inhibit prostaglandin synthesis, but clinical trials have failed to demonstrate any improvement. Vasodilator agents improve cardiac performance, but may interfere with gas exchange. Phosphodiesterase inhibitors have also been advocated, but have not reduced overall mortality. Antibiotics are recommended in the early stage of the disease, but prolonged administration of antibiotics without infection may lead to antibiotic-resistant bacteria. Most patients who die of ARDS do so within the first 14 days and tracheostomy may be required in the survivors. Multi-organ dysfunction often develops and there are also complications with the management, including barotrauma, nosocomial pneumonia and 'stress'-related gastrointestinal bleeding.

Mechanical ventilation

Details of mechanical ventilation were considered in *Anaesthesia Review 12* (Tobin 1994). One of the main difficulties is weaning patients from mechanical ventilation. Esteban et al (1995) have compared four methods and found that a once daily trial of spontaneous respiration led to extubation 3 times more quickly than intermittent mandatory ventilation and twice as quickly as pressure-support ventilation. Brochard et al (1995) have shown that non-invasive ventilation for acute exacerbation of chronic pulmonary disease reduces the need for intubation, the length of stay in hospital and the mortality rate (see Elliott 1995). This study suggests that non-invasive ventilation should be the first line of treatment of certain patients with acute exacerbations of COPD. The exercise tolerance and quality of life can be improved by extensive rehabilitation by improving diaphragmatic and pursed-lip breathing and various exercises (Goldstein et al 1994). Unfortunately, nasal ventilation was of little value in Duchenne muscular dystrophy in patients whose FVC was below 20 and 50% of predicted values (Raphael et al 1994).

DYSPNOEA

Manning & Schwartzstein (1995) have discussed the pathophysiology of dyspnoea, drawing attention to the fact that many of the studies have been done in young healthy adults and that in patients with COPD, using chemical stimuli and adding respiratory loads, they indicate that caution is advised in extrapolating this information to other disorders with dyspnoea. 'Dyspnoea is a sense of muscular effort in the conscious awareness of voluntary activation of skeletal muscles.' Afferent and efferent signals contribute to the sensation of dyspnoea, but there is also involvement of chemoreceptors, hypercapnia and hypoxia, mechanoreceptors in the upper airway and in the lung and chest wall. There is a view that there is a mismatch between the outgoing motor activity to the respiratory muscles and incoming afferent stimuli.

Lacasse et al (1996) have shown that respiratory rehabilitation relieves the dyspnoea of chronic obstructive airways disease, although the value in relationship to exercise is not clear (see Clark 1996).

Incentive spirometry is also of value in preventing the pulmonary complications associated with acute chest syndrome in patients with sickle cell disease (Bellet et al 1995).

GENERAL ANAESTHESIA

Rothen et al (1995) have investigated the cause of atelectasis during general anaesthesia. They compared two groups of patients: those who were administered 30% oxygen and those who were given 100%, and following induction of anaesthesia there was a significantly greater increase in the amount of atelectasis in the latter group. As anaesthesia progressed the atelectasis increased. During the course of anaesthesia, in the patients given 30% oxygen, the shunt increased to 2.7% of cardiac output, whereas in those given 100% oxygen it reached 5.7% of cardiac output. They felt that atelectasis could be avoided by only administering 30% oxygen to patients during the course of anaesthesia.

In another study, Reber et al (1996), using spiral computed tomography to assess the formation of atelectasis by volumetric analysis, found that the induction of anaesthesia resulted in atelectasis in the dependent regions of the lung, but there was also a non-gravitational effect from the apex to the base of the lung. Atelectasis comprised 10% of the lung tissue with a further 8–10% being poorly ventilated above the atelectatic area.

INTENSIVE CARE

Attempts have been made in intensive care units to improve the haemodynamic parameters by raising the cardiac index and increasing mixed venous oxygen saturation in critically ill patients (Gattinoni et al 1995). A similar study undertaken by Hayes et al (1994) using dobutamine failed to improve cardiac index and systemic oxygen delivery. In fact they found their aggressive therapy was detrimental, while Gattinoni et al (1995) only found that there was no improvement (see also Hinds & Watson 1995). Atkinson et al (1994) have developed an algorithm which would indicate which patients were likely to survive intensive care therapy.

OXYGEN THERAPY

Long-term oxygen therapy has been reviewed by Tarpy & Celli (1995). 'In patients with hypoxaemia, oxygen supplementation improves survival, pulmonary haemodynamics, exercise capacity and neuropsychological performance. It may also decrease the oxygen cost of breathing and improve the quality of sleep.' They also maintain there is no place for administration of short courses of oxygen.

Reactive oxygen species (ROS) are involved in many disorders including pneumoconiosis, adult respiratory distress syndrome, asthma, cystic fibrosis and HIV. In all conditions, nitric oxide interacts with superoxide anion and protects the lungs against oxygen radicals. The use of superoxide dismutase has been singularly disappointing (Cross et al 1994).

The physiological effects of hyperbaric-oxygen therapy are set out by Tibbles & Edelsberg (1996). Indications for hyperbaric-oxygen include carbon monoxide poisoning, decompression sickness, arterial gas embolism, radiation-induced tissue therapy, clostridial myonecrosis, necrotising fascilitis, refractory osteomyelitis, acute traumatic ischaemic injury, compromised skin grafts and flaps and even exceptional blood loss. Thermal burns appear to heal quicker given hyperbaric-oxygen, but a controlled trial did not confirm this. Side effects include reversible myopia, rupture of the middle ear, barotrauma and generalised seizures.

PULMONARY EMPHYSEMA

There are two pathological types of pulmonary emphysema – in one the large air spaces are in the centre of the acinus close to the terminal bronchioles, usually in the upper part of the lung, while in the panacinar form the whole acinus is affected involving either the whole lung or the lower zones. There is an association between pulmonary emphysema and a hereditary deficiency of

α_1-proteinase inhibitor, which inhibits the enzymes which effect elastin in the lung. In smokers there is an increase in the neutrophils and macrophages which release proteolytic enzymes. Treatment with bronchodilators only moderately improves lung function, but stopping smoking is of great value. Treatment may involve the use of α_1-proteinase inhibitor, but it does not affect the existing damage (Hutchison 1994).

CYSTIC FIBROSIS

Patients with pulmonary disease in cystic fibrosis develop bronchiectasis and obstructive pulmonary disease. Therapy is directed to reduction in the viscoelasticity of the sputum, antibiotics, which may be given by inhalation, and anti-inflammatory therapy (Ramsey 1996).

DIABETES

Some aspects of diabetes have been reviewed in previous editions (see *Anaesthesia Review 13*). Tests for diabetes are still being reviewed and McCance et al (1994) found that glycated haemoglobin (HbA) and fasting plasma glucose concentrations were reasonable alternatives to measurement of glucose concentration following a challenge with glucose. There are problems with glycated haemoglobin and large differences exist between HbA_1 and HbA_{1c} regarding control of diabetic patients. HbA_{1c} appears to suggest a high risk of long term diabetic complications (Kilpatrick et al 1994). The β_3-adrenergic-receptor appears to be involved in the control of visceral adipose tissue and contributes to the resting metabolic rate. There is evidence to suggest that mutations of the gene for the β_3-adrenergic-receptor will lead to obesity and NIDDM (Walston et al 1995, see also Arner 1995).

The psychological care of patients with diabetes is described by Jacobson (1996). The onset of the disease may cause immense psychological problems to patients and they find the care and attention to use of insulin can be restrictive to their lifestyle. They also suffer from depression, anxiety and eating disorders.

INSULIN

The *Drug and Therapeutics Bulletin* (1996) indicates there are more than 30 insulin preparations on the market and the duplication of the preparations is unnecessary. Most preparations are given by standard syringe, although there are now pens and cartridges, some of which are preloaded and disposable. In addition, it is suggested that only 10 preparations are necessary, including, one short-acting insulin of human pork and beef type, one intermediate-acting insulin of each species, a single long-acting insulin and three biphasic insulins. Of the human insulins available, the following are short-acting: human actrapid, human velosulin and humulin S. The human intermediate insulins include human insulatard, human monotard, humulin Zn, humulin I and humulin lente. The long-acting insulin is represented by human ultratard, while the biphasic ones consist of human mixtard and humulin with varying proportions of soluble and isophane insulin. In the UK, 40% of all insulin prescribed is in the premixed biphasic form, mostly in a mixture 30% soluble and 70% isophane insulin. Human insulin is either made by enzymatic modification of porcine insulin or biosynthetically by bacteria or yeast.

INSULIN RESISTANCE

Insulin resistance is known to occur and high fasting insulin concentrations appears to be a predictor of ischaemic heart disease in men (Despres et al 1996). Insulin resistance occurs in obesity, hypertension, hyperlipaemia and hyperuricaemia. The secretion of insulin is 4–5 times higher than normal, but curiously enough, the majority of those with insulin resistance do not become diabetic. There appears to be a genetic failure in the beta cell in the pancreas (Polonsky et al 1996, Godsland & Stevenson 1995). Diabetics who have suffered acute myocardial infarction may be improved with insulin infusion (Davey & McKeigue 1996).

There are molecular changes at the active site of the insulin receptor which are genetically determined and a single amino acid alteration at the insulin binding site has been shown to be one of the causes of insulin resistance (Williams 1994, Tong et al 1995, Taylor 1996, see also Devnyck 1995). Insulin resistance and compensatory hyperinsulinaemia are involved in the regulation of blood pressure and probably result in hypertension in susceptible patients (Reaven et al 1996).

Hypoglycaemia

Hypoglycaemia is usually associated with overdose of insulin, but Bruce et al (1995) found repeated episodes of hypoglycaemia in two patients with spinal muscular atrophy due to reduced gluconeogenesis: the muscle mass in the patients was reduced to 10% of body weight (normal 30–40%). Bruce et al (1995) uttered a warning that the condition was often confused with respiratory insufficiency.

One of the dangers of human insulin has been unawareness of hypoglycaemia. During episodes of hypoglycaemia, the uptake of glucose in the brain is preserved, which reduces the response of hormones which attempt to maintain the normal blood sugar (Boyle et al 1995, see also Bolli & Fanelli 1995). However, Deary & Frier (1996) found that the link between severe hypoglycaemia and awareness was not proven.

Debrah et al (1996) have suggested that caffeine might be beneficial in that it enhances the sympathoadrenal and symptomatic response to moderate hypoglycaemia.

Hyperglycaemia

Hyperglycaemia was associated with a marked increase in postsurgical infection, even in non-diabetic patients (Larkin 1996).

NON-INSULIN DEPENDENT DIABETES MELLITUS (NIDDM)

Initial treatment of NIDDM, if diet measures failed, was with phenformin which tended to produce lactic acidosis. Metformin lowers fasting blood glucose concentration and glycosylated haemoglobin values. The major effects of metformin are to inhibit gluconeogenesis, reduce the glucose output from the liver and lower fasting blood glucose concentrations. It does not increase plasma insulin concentrations or cause hypoglycaemia (Crofford 1995, Bailey & Turner 1996)

Surgical operations

Eldridge and Sear (1996) have reviewed the peri-operative management of insulin-dependent diabetic patients in the Oxford region and found that the regime advocated by Alberti & Thomas (1979) has been replaced by a simpler regime. Alberti & Thomas (1979) advocated an infusion of glucose which also contained insulin and potassium, whereas current practice in the region is to use separate infusions of insulin and glucose. The ease with which it is possible to measure blood glucose levels has altered the need for complicated regimes and the most important complication associated with the management of diabetics at operation is hypoglycaemia. The classical signs of hypoglycaemia due to sympathetic stimulation may not be readily seen with use of human insulin and nor for that matter in the presence of adrenergic blocking agents. For patients with well controlled NIDDM, Raucoules-Aime et al (1996) recommended a no insulin, no glucose regime even for major surgical procedures, provided the blood glucose was measured frequently and insulin administered as necessary.

CNS

BRAIN INJURY

The mechanisms of secondary brain injury are discussed in detail by Siesjo & Siesjo (1996). There is an increase in the calcium concentration within the cell, overloading the mitochondria and a decrease in protein synthesis resulting in increase in enzyme activity. McIntosh et al (1996) reported on recent studies involving pharmacological manipulation of neurotransmitters which might possibly diminish neurone damage and improve function activity following traumatic brain injury. Calcium channel blockers have been advocated, but no clinical benefit has been derived following nicardipine and nimodipine. Calpain, a cysteine protease, is activated when the calcium concentrations are increased and this results in neuronal damage. The use of calpain inhibitors appears to be a promising area for further study.

Plasma noradrenaline, adrenaline and dopamine are said to be increased following severe brain injury and may be useful markers predicting likelihood of recovery. Low magnesium may interfere with NMDA neurotransmission, which again may play a part in brain injury. Other transmitters include ANP/KA and EAA which are involved in glutamate release. Riluzole inhibits the glutamate release presynaptically and appears to have a protective action following experimental brain injury. Other treatments involve the use of inhibitors of free radicals and inhibitors of lipid peroxidation. Endogenous growth factors, inhibitors of inflammation as well as hypothermia are also discussed by McIntosh et al (1996).

SLEEP APNOEA

It is estimated that 2–4% of the middle-aged population suffer from sleep apnoea, defined as repeated episodes of obstructive apnoea and hypopnoea during sleep, together with day-time sleepiness and alterations in cardiopulmonary function. The obstructive type is upper airway resistance leading to arousal without necessarily giving rise to apnoea or hypopnoea. They are usually heavy snorers. Closure of the upper airway usually occurs during REM sleep, because of poor tone of the upper airway muscles during this stage of sleep. The size of the upper airway is also determined by the soft tissues as there may be increased adipose tissue in fat patients and fatty infiltration into the pharyngeal tissues. There may be tonsil hypertrophy or skeletal abnormalities of the face. Genetic and environmental factors also affect the airway (see also Douglas & Polo 1994, Simonds 1994).

Hoffstein (1994) has analysed the relationship between snoring and blood pressure, the implications being that in snoring there is sleep apnoea. However, he found that in the absence of sleep apnoea, snoring was not associated with raised blood pressure.

Sleep apnoea leads to risks of nocturnal dysarrhythmias, pulmonary hypertension, right and left ventricular failure, myocardial infarction and stroke. Motor vehicle accidents are common in sleep apnoea patients and it is reported that they are 7 times more frequent than in the general population. The diagnosis may be made on history and on sleep studies. Behavioural treatment consists of weight reduction and avoidance of alcohol. Medical treatment involves positive airway pressure via a mask and use of oral appliances and thyroxine in patients with hypothyroidism. Protriptyline and fluoxetine have proved disappointing. Surgical treatment involves tracheostomy, palatal surgery and maxillofacial surgery (Strollo & Rogers 1996).

Nocturnal angina pectoris has also been found to be associated with sleep apnoea and the angina decreased during treatment with continuous positive airway pressure (Franklin et al 1995). Oral theophylline appears to reduce the number of periods of apnoea, hypopnoea and duration of arterial oxyhaemoglobin desaturation during sleep (Javaheri et al 1996).

EPILEPSY

For partial seizures, carbamazepine, phenytoin, valproic acid, phenobarbitone and primidone are all effective, carbamazepine and phenytoin being the drugs of choice. For tonic-clonic seizures, valproic acid, phenytoin and carbamazepine are all effective with valproic acid being the preferred drug. Ethosuximide is of value when there are no seizures, while carbamazepine is recommended for refractory seizures. There is an increase in the number of fetal deformities in pregnant women being treated with antiepileptic drugs, especially valproic acid and carbamazepine and it was felt that folic acid is of value in preventing these (Brodie & Dichter 1996).

Dichter & Brodie (1996) have also reviewed the anti-epileptic drugs recently introduced in the United States, including gabapentin, lamotrigine, felbamate. Those introduced into Europe include clobazam, vigabatrin, oxcarbarzepine, zonisamide, tiagabine and topiramate. It is suggested that gabapentin and lamotrigine may be the drugs of choice for newly diagnosed epileptics and lamotrigine was better tolerated than carbamazepine (Brodie et al 1995). All these drugs have side effects, so much so that Perucca (1996) suggests that new drugs cannot be recommended as a first line treatment. It must be emphasised that control and prompt treatment of seizures is essential as there is a high incidence of sudden death in epileptic patients (Nashef & Brown 1996).

MYOPATHY

Patients in intensive care units develop weakness and paralysis and it is suggested they either have a neuropathy or myopathy. Most patients have muscle wasting and biochemical signs of malnourishment and had prolonged sepsis and multi-organ dysfunction. Most of the patients who survived fully recovered, but only 4–7 months after the onset of paralysis (Latronico et al 1996).

There has been little effective treatment for motor neurone disease until the advent of riluzole. It appears to act presynaptically by affecting glutamate transmission. It has a variety of side effects including somnolence, vertigo and causes a dose-related rise in serum aminotransferases (Wokke 1996). Chronic fatigue has attracted much attention, but Wessely et al (1995) found there was no evidence that it was related to a viral infection.

MIGRAINE

The diagnosis of migraine is based on history of attacks to distinguish it from other types of headache. Woods et al (1994) were able to show that it appears to be related to cerebral hypoperfusion. At the onset of an attack, 5-HT is released and, on the basis of this, sumatriptan was developed which binds to receptors for 5-HT_{1D} and, to a lesser extent, to 5-HT_{1A} and 5-HT_{1F} (Olesen 1994). Stimulation of the trigeminal ganglion releases a powerful vasodilator neuropeptide related to calcitonin and it is believed that this causes the headache. Sumatriptan, which relieves the attack of migraine quickly and reliably, is believed to act presynaptically at the trigeminal nerve ending. A possible side effect of sumatriptan is coronary vasoconstriction (Goadsby & Olesen 1996).

PARKINSONISM

The diagnosis of Parkinson's disease is entirely clinical and depends on the presence of akinesia, rigidity and usually tremor. The condition may be misdiagnosed due to essential tremor or arteriosclerotic pseudoParkinsonism. Parkinsonism may be drug-induced by drugs which deplete presynaptic stores of dopamine, e.g. reserpine or, more commonly, neuroleptic drugs such as chlorpromazine, haloperidol, flupenthixol and sulpiride (Quinn 1995a). The treatment of Parkinson's disease involves anticholinergic agents, amantadine, levodopa, dopamine agonists, such as pergolide, which stimulates D_1 and D_2 dopamine receptors and selegiline, which is a selective inhibitor of monoamine oxidase type B (Quinn 1995b).

Dystonia involves the delivery of dopamine, but the condition results from the loss of production of tetrahydrobiopterin, which is a co-factor for tyrosine hydroxylase and is involved in the synthesis of dopamine (Williams 1995).

PSYCHIATRIC CONDITIONS

SCHIZOPHRENIA

It is believed that antipsychotic drugs block the D_2 subtype of dopamine receptor in the mesolimbic dopamine system and that atypical neuroleptic drugs, such as clozapine, have antipsychotic activity without producing the extra pyramidal symptoms (Pickar 1995, Kane 1996). The other recently introduced drug, risperidone, has dopamine 2 receptor and 5-HT_2 receptor blocking properties. A side effect of clozapine is agranulocytosis.

ANXIETY AND DEPRESSION

The treatment of anxiety has been reviewed by Lader (1994) and a variety of drugs have been used including benzodiazepines, buspirone, β-adrenergic blockers, tricyclic antidepressants, selective serotonin reuptake inhibitors, monoamine oxidase inhibitors, antipsychotic drugs and antihistamines. A recent selective inhibitor of 5-HT reuptake is fluoxetine (prozac). Cytochrome P-450 (CYP2D6), which is responsible for the destruction of tricyclic antidepressants, is inhibited by fluoxetine and there are, therefore, interactions between the two types of compounds. The main indication for fluoxetine is depression. It also causes an interaction with MAOIs resulting in anxiety, restlessness, confusion, inco-ordination and insomnia and it has been known to be fatal (serotonin syndrome). This may also occur with lithium or carbamazepine (Gram 1994).

The reason for the clinical effectiveness of lithium is unknown and appears to relieve both mania and depression. Increased dopamine function in mania is thought to be due to dopamine, and lithium attenuates dopamine function. Brain 5-HT is diminished in patients with depression and lithium increases synthesis and turnover of 5-HT. Noradrenaline has also been implicated as a cause of depression, but has little effect on β-adrenoceptor binding. Lithium has a narrow therapeutic index and side effects include tremor, lethargy, memory impairment, excessive thirst and polyuria. It also elevates serum thyrotropin, indicating mild thyroid deficiency. Plasma lithium levels are increased with thiazides, NSAIDs and ACE inhibitors, while the levels are decreased with bronchodilators such as aminophylline. It is said to prolong neuromuscular blocking agents and increases the risk of neuroleptic malignant syndrome and the extrapyramidal signs of Parkinsonism (Price & Heninger 1994).

Drug reactions with MAOIs have been known for many years, resulting in hypertension, in the presence of sympathomimetic amines or coma following the administration of pethidine. There are now known to be two types of MAO – MAO-A, which preferentially oxidises noradrenaline and 5-HT, while MAO-B oxidises phenylethylamine. The MAOI selegiline selectively inhibits MAO-B and is thought less likely to cause a hypertensive crisis (Livingston 1995).

CARCINOID

Anaesthetic management of patients suffering from carcinoid tumour has been simplified by the introduction of octreotide given preoperatively 50–500 μg, 3 times a day. Induction of anaesthesia should be designed to minimise haemodynamic fluctuations and avoidance of histamine release. Reilly (1996) advocates the use of etomidate, fentanyl and vecuronium for induction, followed by fentanyl and isoflurane as maintenance agents. Arterial and central venous pressure lines should be set up prior to induction of anaesthesia. Hypotension at operation is treated with incremental doses of octreotide (10 μg i.v.), while hypertension and tachycardia can be attenuated by increasing the depth of anaesthesia, by the administration of short-acting β-blockers, such as esmolol, or the 5-HT antagonist, ketanserin. Postoperative morphine should be avoided and instead PCA should consist of fentanyl or pethidine and epidural infusion of fentanyl and bupivacaine have also been administered.

MISCELLANEOUS

ANTI-EMETICS

Ondansetron was one of the earliest $5HT_3$ receptor antagonists and more recently granisetron has also been advocated for the treatment of nausea and vomiting following chemotherapy. Wilson et al (1996) have reported its use in postoperative nausea and vomiting and found that 1 mg was well tolerated. Granisetron is believed to produce an irreversible block of the receptors which may account for its long duration of action.

The combination of dexamethasone and ondansetron have proved successful in the management of nausea and vomiting following chemotherapy. Lopez-Olaondo et al (1996) have shown that this combination was equally effective in the prevention of postoperative nausea and vomiting.

Omeprazole may have a place in the prevention of aspiration of gastric contents by its effect in reducing gastric acid secretion and pH (Levack et al 1996).

GOUT

Treatment of gout has historically been with colchicine, but its onset of action is slow and the effective dose is similar to that which causes gastrointestinal symptoms. In the acute attack non-steroidal anti-inflammatory drugs are the first choice, including indomethacin. If the attack affects only one joint then intra-articular injection of steroids is often effective. Prophylaxis against acute attacks are with small doses of colchicine or NSAIDs. The use of uricosuric drugs include probenecid and sulfinpyrazone. Allopurinol, a xanthine oxidase inhibitor, is also advocated (Emmerson 1996).

References

Alberti K G M M, Thomas D J B 1979 The management of diabetes during surgery. Br J Anaesth 51: 693–710
Anzueto A, Baughman R P, Guntupalli K K et al 1996 Aerosolized surfactant in adults with sepsis-induced acute respiratory distress syndrome. N Engl J Med 334: 1417–1421
Arner P 1995 The bbb$_3$-adrenergic receptor – a cause and cure of obesity? N Engl J Med 333: 382–383
Atkinson S, Bihari D, Smithies M et al 1994 Identification of futility in intensive care. Lancet 344: 1203–1206
Baglin T 1996 Disseminated intravascular coagulation: diagnosis and treatment. BMJ 312: 683–687
Bailey C J, Turner R C 1996 Metformin. N Engl J Med 334: 574–579
Barnes P J 1995 Inhaled glucocorticoids for asthma. N Engl J Med 332: 868–875
Barnes P J 1996 Pathophysiology of asthma. Br J Clin Pharmacol 42: 3–10
Beevers D G, Sleight P 1996 Short acting dihydropyridine (vasodilating) calcium channel blockers for hypertension: is there a risk? BMJ 312: 1143–1145
Bellet P S, Kalinyak K A, Shukla R et al 1995 Incentive spirometry to prevent acute pulmonary complications in sickle cell diseases. N Engl J Med 333: 699–703
Bellinger D C, Jonas R A, Rapport L A et al 1995 Developmental and neurologic status of children after heart attack surgery with hypothermic circulatory arrest or low-flow cardiopulmonary bypass. N Engl J Med 332: 549–555
Bennett P 1994 Fetal stress response. Lancet 344: 615
Bergqvist D, Benoni G, Bjorgell O et al 1996 Low-molecular-weight heparin (enoxaparin) as prophylaxis against thromboembolism after total hip replacement. N Engl J Med 335: 696–700
Bittl J A 1996 Advances in coronary angioplasty. N Engl J Med 335: 1290–1302
Blair P S, Fleming P J, Bensley D et al 1996 Smoking and the sudden infant death syndrome: results from 1993–5 case-control study for confidential injury into stillbirths and deaths in infancy. BMJ 313: 195–198
Blauw G J, Westendorp R G J 1995 Asthma deaths in New Zealand: whodunnit? Lancet 345: 2–3
Bion J 1995 The outcomes of neonatal intensive care. BMJ 310: 681–683
Bolli G B, Fanelli C G 1995 Unawareness of hypoglycaemia. N Engl J Med 333: 1771–1772
Boyle P J, Kempers S F, O'Connor A M, Nagy R J 1995 Brain glucose uptake and unawareness of hypoglycemia in patients with insulin-dependent diabetes mellitus. N Engl J Med 333: 1726–1731
Brady H R, Singer G G 1995 Acute renal failure. Lancet 346: 1533–1540
Brochard L, Mancebo J, Wysocki M et al 1995 Noninvasive ventilation for acute exacerbations of chronic obstructive pulmonary disease. N Engl J Med 333: 817–822
Brodie M J, Richens A R, Yuen A W C 1995 Double-blind comparison of lamotrigine and carbamazepine in newly diagnosed epilepsy. Lancet 345: 476–479
Brodie M J, Dichter M A 1996 Antiepileptic drugs. N Engl J Med 334: 168–175
Brown E M, Pollak M, Seiddman C E et al 1995 Calcium-ion-sensing cell-surface receptors. N Engl J Med 333: 234–240
Bruce A K, Jacobsen E, Dossing H, Kondrup J 1995 Hypoglycaemia in spinal muscular atrophy. Lancet 346: 609–610
Bucca C, Rolla G, Brussino L et al 1995 Are asthma-like symptoms due to bronchial or extrathoracic airway dysfunction? Lancet 346: 791–795
Buist A S, Vollmer W M 1994 Preventing deaths from asthma. N Engl J Med 331: 1584–1585
Burwell D R, Jones J G 1996a The airways and anaesthesia – I. Anatomy, physiology and fluid mechanics. Anaesthesia 51: 849–857
Burwell D R, Jones J G 1996b The airways and anaesthesia – II. Pathophysiology. Anaesthesia 51: 943–954
Camm A J, Garratt C J 1991 Adenosine and supraventricular tachycardia. N Engl J Med 325: 1621–1629
Carson J L, Duff A, Poses R M et al 1996 Effect of anaemia and cardiovascular disease on surgical mortality and morbidity. Lancet 348: 1055–1060

Celermajer D S, Adams M R, Clarkson P et al 1996 Passive smoking and impaired endothelium-dependent arterial dilatation in healthy young adults. N Engl J Med 334: 150–154
Chan-Yeung M, Malo J-L 1995 Occupational asthma. N Engl J Med 333: 107–112
Chapman K R, Kesten S, Szalai J P 1994 Regular vs as-needed inhaled salbutamol in asthma control. Lancet 343: 1379–1382
Clark D A 1994 Stress without distress: the intrauterine perspective. Lancet 344: 73–74
Clark C J 1996 Is pulmonary rehabilitation effective for patients with COPD? Lancet 348: 1111
Cohn J N 1996 The management of chronic heart failure. N Engl J Med 335: 490–498
Colucci W S 1996 Apoptosis in the heart. N Engl J Med 335: 1224–1226
Committee on Perioperative Cardiovascular evaluation for non-cardiac surgery 1996 Executive summary of the ACC/AHA task force report: guidelines for perioperative cardiovascular evaluation for non-cardiac surgery. Anesth Analg 82: 854–860
Crofford O B 1995 Metformin. N Engl J Med 333: 588–589
Cross C E, van der Vliet A, O'Neill C A, Eiserich J P 1994 Reactive oxygen species and the lung. Lancet 344: 930–933
Dargie H J 1996 Calcium-channel blockers: managing uncertainty. Lancet 348: 487–489
Darowski M J 1994 Anaesthesia for the young child. Hosp Update 20: 259–266
Davey G, McKeigue P 1996 Insulin infusion in diabetic patients with acute myocardial infarction. BMJ 313: 639–640
Deary I J, Frier B M 1996 Severe hypoglycaemia and cognitive impairment in diabetes. BMJ 313: 767–768
Debrah K, Sherwin R S, Murphy J, Derr D 1996 Effect of caffeine on recognition and of physiological responses to hypoglycaemia in insulin-dependent diabetes. Lancet 347: 19–24
De Lima J, Lloyd-Thomas A R, Howard R F et al 1996 Infant and neonatal pain: anaesthetists' perceptions and prescribing patterns. BMJ 313: 787
Derbyshire S W G 1994 Fetal stress response. Lancet 344: 615
Derbyshire S W G, Furedi A 1996 Do fetuses feel pain? BMJ 313: 795–797
Despres J-P, Lamarche B, Mauriege P et al 1996 Hyperinsulinemia as an independent risk factor for ischemic heart disease. N Engl J Med 334: 952–957
Devalia J L, Rusznak C, Herdman M J et al 1994 Effect of nitrogen dioxide and sulphur dioxide on airway response of mild asthmatic patients to allergen inhalation. Lancet 344: 1668–1671
Devynck M-A 1995 Do cell membrane dynamics participate in insulin resistance? Lancet 345: 336–337
Dennis A, Curran J, Sherriff J, Kinnear W 1994 Effects of passive and active smoking on induction of anaesthesia. Br J Anaesth 73: 450–452
Dichter M A, Brodie M J 1996 New antiepileptic drugs. N Engl J Med 334: 1583–1588
Diggory P, Cassels-Brown A, Vail A et al 1995 Avoiding unsuspected respiratory side-effects of topical timolol with cardioselective or sympathomimetic agents. Lancet 345: 1604–1606
Donnelly S C, Haslett C, Dransfield I et al 1994 Role of selectins in development of adult respiratory distress syndrome. Lancet 344: 215–219
Douglas N J, Polo O 1994 Pathogenesis of obstructive sleep apnoea/hypopnoea syndrome. Lancet 344: 653–655
Drazen J M, Israel E, Boushey H A et al 1996 Comparison of regularly scheduled with as-needed use of albuterol in mild asthma. N Engl J Med 335: 841–847
Drug and Therapeutics Bulletin 1995 Managing acute pain in children. Drug Ther Bull 33: 41–44
Drug and Therapeutics Bulletin 1996 Insulin preparations – time to rationalise. Drug Ther Bull 34: 11–14
Drug and Therapeutics Bulletin 1997 Using bbb$_2$-stimulants in asthma. Drug Ther Bull 35: 1–3
du Bois R M 1995 Respiratory medicine. BMJ 310: 1594–1597
Eldridge A J, Sear J W 1996 Peri-operative management of diabetic patients. Any changes for the better since 1985? Anaesthesia 51: 45–51
Elliott M W 1995 Noninvasive ventilation in chronic obstructive pulmonary disease. N Engl J Med 333: 870–871

Emmerson B T 1996 The management of gout. N Engl J Med 334: 445–451
Erskine R J, Murphy P J, Langton J A 1994 Sensitivity of upper airway reflexes in cigarette smokers: effect of abstinence. Br J Anaesth 73: 298–302
Esteban A, Frutos F, Tobin M J et al 1995 A comparison of four methods of weaning patients from mechanical ventilation. N Engl J Med 332: 345–350
Fleming P J, Cooke M, Chantler S M, Golding J 1995 fire retardants, biocides, plasticisers, and sudden infant deaths. BMJ 309: 1994–1996
Fleming P J, Blair P S, Bacon C et al 1996 Environment of infants during sleep and risk of the sudden infant death syndrome: result of 1993–5 case-control study for confidential inquiry into stillbirths and deaths in infancy. BMJ 313: 191–195
Fletcher G C, Asbury A J, Brown J H 1996 Pupil changes during cardiopulmonary bypass. Br J Anaesth 76: 20–22
Franklin K A, Nilsson J B, Sahlin C, Naslund U 1995 Sleep apnoea and nocturnal angina. Lancet 345: 1085–1087
Ganeshan N, Bihari D 1996 Life-threatening hyperkalaemia after cardiac surgery. Lancet 348: 755
Ganz L I, Friedman P L 1995 Supraventricular tachycardia. N Engl J Med 332: 162–173
Gattinoni L, Brazzi L, Pelosi P et al 1995 A trial of goal-oriented hemodynamic therapy in critically ill patients. N Engl J Med 333: 1025–1032
Geerts W H, Jay R M, Code K I et al 1996 A comparison of low-dose heparin with low-molecular-weight heparin as prophylaxis against venous thromboembolism after major trauma. N Engl J Med 335: 701–707
Giannakoulopoulos X, Sepulveda W, Kourtis P et al 1994 Fetal plasma cortisol and bbb-endorphin response to intrauterine needling. Lancet 344: 77–81
Gibb A J 1997 Structure and function of ion channel receptors. In: Kaufman L, Ginsburg R (eds). Anaesthesia Review 13. Edinburgh: Churchill Livingstone, 85–102
Goadsby P J, Olesen J 1996 Diagnosis and management of migraine. BMJ 312: 1279–1283
Godsland I F, Stevenson J C 1995 Insulin resistance: syndrome or tendency? Lancet 346: 100–103
Gold D R, Wang X, Wypij D et al 1996 Effects of cigarette smoking on lung function in adolescent boys and girls. N Engl J Med 335: 931–937
Goldman L, Caldera D L, Nussbaum S R et al 1977 Multifactorial index of cardiac risk in noncardiac surgical procedures. N Engl J Med 297: 845–850
Goldman L 1995 Cardiac risk in noncardiac surgery: an update. Anesth Analg 80: 810–820
Goldstein R S, Gort E H, Stubbing D et al 1994 Randomised controlled trial of respiratory rehabilitation. Lancet 344: 1394–1397
Goodfriend T L, Elliott M E, Catt K J 1996 Angiotensin receptors and their antagonists. N Engl J Med 334: 1649–1654
Gordon R D 1996 Calcium antagonists and gastrointestinal haemorrhage: the balancing act. Lancet 347: 1056
Gram L F Fluoxetine. N Engl J Med 331: 1354–1361
Greaves M W, Wall P D 1996 Pathophysiology of itching. Lancet 348: 938–940
Greening A P, Ind P W, Northfield M et al 1994 Added salmeterol versus higher-dose corticosteroid in asthma patients with symptoms on existing inhaled corticosteroid. Lancet 344: 219–224
Grove A, Lipworth B J 1995 Tolerance with bbb_2-adrenoceptor agonists: time for reappraisal. Br J Clin Pharmacol 39: 109–118
Haahtela T, Jarvinen M, Kava T et al 1994 Effects of reducing or discontinuing inhaled budesonide in patients with mild asthma. N Engl J Med 331: 700–705
Hall I P, Wheatley A, Wilding P, Liggett S B 1995 Association of Glu 27 bbb_2-adrenoceptor polymorphism with lower airway reactivity in asthmatic subjects. Lancet 345: 1213–1214
Hamvas A, Wise P H, Robert M P H et al 1996 The influence of the wider use of surfactant therapy on neonatal mortality among blacks and whites. N Engl J Med 334: 1636–1640
Hannedouche T, Landais P, Goldfarb B et al 1994 Randomised controlled trial of enalapril and bbb blockers in non-diabetic chronic renal failure. BMJ 309: 833–837
Hargreaves M R, Benson M K 1995 Inhaled sodium cromoglycate in angiotensin-converting enzyme inhibitor cough. Lancet 345: 13–16
Harris M-A, Sullivan C E 1995 Sleep pattern and supplementary oxygen requirements in infants with chronic neonatal lung disease. Lancet 345: 831–832

Hayes M A, Timmins A C, Yau E H S et al 1994 Elevation of systemic oxygen delivery in the treatment of critically ill patients. N Engl J Med 330: 1717–1722
Hinds C, Watson D 1995 Manipulating hemodynamics and oxygen transport in critically ill patients. N Engl J Med 333: 1074–1075
Hoffstein V 1994 Blood pressure, snoring, obesity and nocturnal hypoxaemia. Lancet 344: 643–645
Hole D J, Watt G C M, Davey-Smith G et al 1996 Impaired lung function and mortality risk in men and women: findings from the Renfrew and Paisley prospective population study. BMJ 313: 711–715
Hollander J E 1996 Cocaine-associated myocardial infarction. J R Soc Med 89: 443–447
Howat W J, Moore I E, Judd M, Roche W R 1994 Pulmonary immunopathology of sudden infant death syndrome. Lancet 343: 1390–1392
Howell S J, Sear Y M, Yeates D et al 1996 Hypertension, admission blood pressure and perioperative cardiovascular risk. Anaesthesia 51: 1000–1004
Howell S J, Hemming A E, Allman K G et al 1997 Predictors of postoperative myocardial ischaemia. The role of intercurrent arterial hypertension and other cardiovascular risk factors. Anaesthesia 52; 107–111
Hutchison D C S 1994 Pulmonary emphysema. BMJ 309: 1244–1245
Insel P A 1996 Adrenergic receptors – evolving concepts and clinical implications. N Engl J Med 334: 580–585
Jacqz-Aigrain E, Daoud P, Burtin P et al 1994 Placebo-controlled trial of midazolam sedation in mechanically ventilated newborn babies. Lancet 344: 646–650
Javaheri S, Parker T J, Wexler L et al 1996 Effect of theophylline on sleep-disordered breathing in heart failure. N Engl J Med 335: 562–567
Jackson M A, Lodwick R, Hutchinson S G 1996 Hyperkalaemic cardiac arrest successfully treated with peritoneal dialysis. BMJ 312: 1289–1290
Jacobson A M 1996 The psychological care of patients with insulin-dependent diabetes mellitus. N Engl J Med 334: 1249–1253
Jousilahti P, Vartiainen E, Tuomilehto J, Puska P 1996 Symptoms of chronic bronchitis and the risk of coronary disease. Lancet 348: 567–572
Juste R N, Lawson A D, Soni N 1996 Minimising cardiac anaesthetic risk: the tortoise or the hare? Anaesthesia 51: 255–262
Kaddoura S, Poole-Wilson 1996 Endothelin-1 in heart failure: a new therapeutic target? Lancet 348: 418–419
Kam P C A, Tan K H 1996 Pruritus – itching for a cause and relief? Anaesthesia 51: 1133–1138
Kane J M 1996 Schizophrenia. N Engl J Med 334: 34–41
Katz A M 1993 Cardiac ion channels. N Engl J Med 328: 1244–1251
Kiely D G, Cargill R I, Lipworth B J 1995 Cardiopulmonary interactions of salbutamol and hypoxaemia in healthy young volunteers. Br J Clin Pharmacol 40: 313–318
Kirkuchi Y, Okabe S, Tamura G et al 1994 Chemosensitivity and perception of dyspnea in patients with a history of near-fatal asthma. N Engl J Med 330: 1329–1334
Kilpatrick E S, Rumley A G, Dominiczak M H, Small M 1994 Glycated haemoglobin values: problems in assessing blood glucose controlling diabetes mellitus. BMJ 309: 983–986
Kollef M H, Schuster D P 1995 The acute respiratory distress syndrome. N Engl J Med 332: 27–37
Koopman M M W, Prandoni P, Piovella F et al 1996 Treatment of venous thrombosis with intravenous unfractionated heparin administered in the hospital as compared with subcutaneous low-molecular-weight heparin administered at home. N Engl J Med 334: 682–687
Koppe J G 199 Prevention of brain haemorrhage and ischaemic injury in premature babies. Lancet 348: 208–209
Kusumoto F M, Goldschlager N 1996 Cardiac pacing. N Engl J Med 334: 89–98
Lacasse Y, Wong E, Guyatt G H et al 1996 Meta-analysis of respiratory rehabilitation in chronic obstructive pulmonary disease. Lancet 348: 1115–1119
Lader M 1994 Treatment of anxiety. BMJ 309: 321–324
Larkin M 1996 Hyperglycemia increases postsurgical infection. Lancet 348: 1158
Latronico N, Fenzi F, Recupero D et al 1996 Critical illness myopathy and neuropathy. Lancet 347: 1579–1582

Leshner A I 1996 Molecular mechanisms of cocaine addiction. N Engl J Med 335: 128–129

Levack I D, Bowie R A, Braid D P et al 1996 Comparison of the effect of two dose schedules of oral omeprazole with oral ranitidine on gastric aspirate pH and volume in patients undergoing elective surgery. Br J Anaesth 76: 567–569

Levine M, Gent M, Hirsh J et al 1996 A comparison of low-molecular-weight heparin administered primarily at home with unfractionated heparin administered in the hospital for proximal deep-vein thrombosis. N Engl J Med 334: 677–681

Liberthson R R 1996 Sudden death from cardiac causes in children and young adults. N Engl J Med 334: 1039–1044

Ling L H, Enriquez-Sarano M, Seward J B et al 1996 Clinical outcome of mitral regurgitation due to flail leaflet. N Engl J Med 335: 1417–1423

Livingston M G 1995 Interactions with selective MAOIs. Lancet 345: 533–534

Lopez-Olaondo L, Carrascosa F, Pueyo F J et al 1996 Combination of ondansetron and dexamethasone in the prophylaxis of postoperative nausea and vomiting. Br J Anaesth 76: 835–840

Lowe Leach C, Greenspan J S, Rubenstein D et al 1996 Partial liquid ventilation with perflubron in premature infants with severe respiratory distress syndrome. N Engl J Med 335: 761–767

Mangano D T, Goldman L 1995 Preoperative assessment of patients with known or suspected coronary disease. N Engl J Med 333: 1750–1756

Mallat Z, Tedgui A, Fontaliran F et al 1996 Evidence of apoptosis in arrhythmogenic right ventricular dysplasia. N Engl J Med 35: 1190–1196

Mamode N, Scott R N, McLaughlin S C et al 1996 Perioperative myocardial infarction in peripheral vascular surgery. BMJ 312: 1396–1397

Manning H L, Schwartzstein R M 1995 Pathophysiology of dyspnea. N Engl J Med 333: 1547–1553

Martinez F D, Wright A L, Taussig L M et al 1995 Asthma and wheezing in the first six years of life. N Engl J Med 332: 133–138

Maschino G, Alberti D, Janin G et al 1996 Effect of the angiotensin-converting-enzyme inhibitor benazepril on the progression of chronic renal insufficiency. N Engl J Med 334: 939–945

McCance D R, Hanson R L, Charles M-A et al 1994 Comparison of tests for glycated haemoglobin and fasting and two hour plasma glucose concentrations as diagnostic methods for diabetes. BMJ 308: 1323–1328

McFadden E R, Gilbert I A 1994 Exercise-induced asthma. N Engl J Med 330: 1362–1367

McFadden E R, Hejal R 1995 Asthma. Lancet 345: 1215–1220

McGill K A, Busse W W 1996 Zileuton. Lancet 348: 519–524

McIntosh T K, Smith D H, Garde E 1996 Therapeutic approaches for the prevention of secondary brain injury. Eur J Anaesthesiol 13: 291–309

Mendelson J H, Mello N K 1996 Management of cocaine abuse and dependence. N Engl J Med 334: 965–972

Merritt T A, Heldt G P 1996 Partial liquid ventilation – the future is now. N Engl J Med 335: 814–815

Morrow J D, Frei B, Longmire A W et al 1995 Increase in circulating products of lipid peroxidation (F_2-isoprostanes) in smokers. N Engl J Med 332: 1198–1203

Narula J, Haider N, Virmani R et al 1996 Apoptosis in myocytes in end-stage heart failure. N Engl J Med 335: 1182–1189

Nashef L, Brown S 1996 Epilepsy and sudden death. Lancet 348: 1324–1325

Nelson H S 1995 bbb-adrenergic bronchodilators. N Engl J Med 333: 499–606

Northern Neonatal Nursing Initiative Trial Group 1996 Randomised trial of prophylactic early fresh-frozen plasma or gelatin or glucose in preterm babies: outcome at 2 years. Lancet 348: 229–232

Northridge D 1996 Frusemide or nitrates for acute heart failure? Lancet 347: 667–668

O'Byrne P M, Kerstjens H A M 1996 Inhaled bbb$_2$-agonists in the treatment of asthma. N Engl J Med 335: 886–887

Ohman E M, Armstrong P W, Christenson R H et al 1996 Cardiac troponin T levels for risk stratification in acute myocardial ischaemia. N Engl J Med 335: 1333–1341

Olesen J 1994 Understanding the biologic basis of migraine. N Engl J Med 331: 1714–1714

Packer M, Bristow M R, Cohn J N et al 1996a The effect of carvedilol on morbidity and mortality in patients with chronic heart failure. N Engl J Med 334: 1349–1355
Packer M, O'Connor C M, Ghali J K et al 1996b Effect of amlodipine on morbidity and mortality in severe chronic heart failure. N Engl J Med 335: 1107–1114
Paediatric Life Support Working Party of the European Resuscitation Council 1994 Guidelines for paediatric life support. BMJ 308: 349–355
Pahor M, Guralnik J M, Ferrucci L et al 1996 Calcium-channel blockade and incidence of cancer in aged populations. Lancet 348: 493–497
Pavord I D, Tattersfield A E 1995 Bronchoprotective role for endogenous prostaglandin E_2. Lancet 345: 436–438
Perucca E 1996 The new generation of antiepileptic drugs: advantages and disadvantages. Br J Clin Pharmacol 42: 531–544
Pfeffer M A, Stevenson L W 1996 bbb-adrenergic blockers and survival in heart failure. N Engl J Med 334: 1396–1397
Pickar D 1995 Prospects for pharmacotherapy of schizophrenia. Lancet 345: 557–562
Pijls N H J, de Bruyne B, Peels K et al 1996 Measurement of fractional flow reserve to assess the functional severity of coronary-artery stenoses. N Engl J Med 334: 1703–1708
Polonsky K S, Sturis J, Bell G I 1996 Non-insulin-dependent diabetes mellitus – a genetically programmed failure of the beta cell to compensate for insulin resistance. N Engl J Med 1996: 334: 777–783
Price L H, Heninger G R 1994 Lithium in the treatment of mood disorders. N Engl J Med 331: 591–598
Quinn N 1995a Parkinsonism – recognition and differential diagnosis. BMJ 310: 447–452
Quinn N 1995b Drug treatment of Parkinson's disease. BMJ 310: 575–579
Rae D, Porter J, Beechey-Newman N et al 1994 Type 1 prophospholipase A_2 propeptide in acute lung injury. Lancet 344: 1472–1474
Ramsey B W 1996 Management of pulmonary disease in patients with cystic fibrosis. N Engl J Med 335: 170–188
Raphael J-C, Chevret S, Chastang C et al 1994 Randomised trial of preventive nasal ventilation in Duchenne muscular dystrophy. Lancet 343: 1600–1604
Raucoules-Aime, Labib Y, Levraut J et al 1996 Use of i.v. insulin in well-controlled non-insulin-dependent diabetics undergoing major surgery. Br J Anaesth 76: 198–202
Reaven G M, Lithell H, Landsberg L 1996 Hypertension and associated metabolic abnormalities – the role of insulin resistance and the sympathoadrenal system. N Engl J Med 334: 374–381
Reber A, Engberg G, Sporre B, et al 1996 Volumetric analysis of aeration in the lungs during general anaesthesia. Br J Anaesth 76: 760–766
Reilly C S 1996 Anaesthesia for carcinoid syndrome. J R Soc Med 89: 279P
Robotham J L, Takata M, Berman M, Harasawa Y 1991 Ejection fraction revisited. Anesthesiology 74: 172–183
Roosevelt G, Sheehan K, Grupp-Phelan J et al 1996 Dexamethasone in bronchiolitis: a randomised controlled trial. Lancet 348: 292–295
Rosenberg J, Overgaard H, Andersen M et al 1996 Double blind randomised controlled trial of effect of metoprolol on myocardial ischaemia during endoscopic cholangiopancreatography. BMJ 313: 258–261
Rothen H U, Sporre B, Engberg G et al 1995 Prevention of atelectasis during general anaesthesia. Lancet 345: 1387–1391
Ryan D W, Pelosi P 1996 The prone position in acute respiratory distress syndrome. BMJ 321: 860–861
Schwartz R M, Luby A M, Scanlon J W, Kellogg R J 1994 Effect of surfactant on morbidity, mortality and resource use in newborn infants weighing 500 to 1500 g. N Engl J Med 330: 1476–1480
Shahar E, Folsom A, Melnick S L et al 1994 Dietry n-3 polyunsaturated fatty acids and smoking-related chronic obstructive pulmonary disease. N Engl J Med 331: 228–244
Sharp D 1996 Adrenomedullin: hypertension-control contender? Lancet 348: 47
Shinkwin C A, Gibbin K P 1996 Tracheostomy in children. J R Soc Med 89: 188–192
Siesjo B K, Siesjo P 1996 Mechanisms of secondary brain injury. Eur J Anaesthesiol 13: 247–268

Silverman M 1995 Asthma and wheezing in young children. N Engl J Med 332: 181–182
Silverstein M D, Reed C E, O'Connell E J et al 1994 Long-term survival of a cohort of community residents with asthma. N Engl J Med 331: 1537–1541
Simonds A K 1994 Sleep studies of respiratory function and home respiratory support. BMJ 309: 35–40
Simoons M L 1996 Myocardial revascularization – bypass surgery or angioplasty? N Engl J Med 335: 275–276
Singh S N, Fletcher R D, Fisher S G et al 1995 Amiodarone in patients with congestive heart failure and asymptomatic ventricular arrhythmia. N Engl J Med 333: 77–82
Soll R F 1996 Neonatal extracorporeal membrane oxygenation – a bridging technique. Lancet 348: 70
Stick S M, Burton P R, Gurrin L et al 1996 Effects of maternal smoking during pregnancy and a family history of asthma on respiratory function in newborn infants. Lancet 348: 1060–1064
Strollo P J, Rogers R M 1996 Obstructive sleep apnea. N Engl J Med 334: 99–104
Sutton R 1989 Anaesthesia in pacemaker surgery. In: Kaufman L (ed). Anaesthesia Review 6. Edinburgh: Churchill Livingstone, 57–73
Tarpy S P, Celli B R 1995 Long-term oxygen therapy. N Engl J Med 333: 710–714
Tattersfield A E 1994 Use of bbb_2 agonists in asthma: much ado about nothing? BMJ 309: 794–796
Taylor R 1996 Insulin resistance: circumventing nature's blocks. lancet 348: 1045–1046
Thadhani R, Pascual M, Bonventre J V 1996 Acute renal failure. N Engl J Med 334: 1448–1460
Tibbles P M, Edelsberg J S 1996 Hyperbaric-oxygen therapy. N Engl J Med 334: 1642–1648
Tobin M J 1994 Mechanical ventilation. N Engl J Med 330: 1056–1061
Tong P, Thomas T, Berrish T et al 1995 Cell membrane dynamics and insulin resistance in non-insulin-dependent diabetes mellitus. Lancet 345: 357–358
Tonkin S L, Davis S L, Gunn T R 1995 Nasal route for infant resuscitation by mothers. Lancet 345: 1353–1354
Tunnicliffe W S, Burge P S, Ayres J G 1994 Effect of domestic concentrations of nitrogen dioxide on airway responses to inhaled allergen in asthmatic patients. Lancet 344: 1733–1736
UK Collaborative ECMO Trial Group 1996 UK collaborative randomised trial of neonatal extracorporeal membrane oxygenation. Lancet 348: 75–82
Vallance P 1996 Drugs and the fetus. BMJ 312: 1053–1054
Van der Werf F 1996 Cardiac troponins in acute coronary syndromes. N Engl J Med 335: 1388–1390
Verder H, Robertson B, Greisen G et al 1994 Surfactant therapy and nasal continuous positive airway pressure for newborns with respiratory distress syndrome. N Engl J Med 331: 1051–1055
Vongpatanasin W, Hillis D, Lange R A 1996 Prosthetic heart valves. N Engl J Med 335: 407–416
Waldo A L, Camm A J, deRuyter H et al 1996 Effect of d-sotalol on mortality in patients with left ventricular dysfunction after recent and remote myocardial infarction. Lancet 348: 7–12
Walston J, Silver K, Bogardus C et al 1995 Time of onset of non-insulin-dependent diabetes mellitus and genetic variation in the bbb_3-adrenergic-receptor gene. N Engl J Med 333: 343–347
Warren J B, Higenbottam T 1996 Caution with use of inhaled nitric oxide. Lancet 348: 629
Weinberger M, Hendeles L 1996 Theophylline in asthma. N Engl J Med 334: 1380–1388
Wessely S, Chalder T, Hirsch S et al 1995 Postinfectious fatigue: prospective cohort study in primary care. Lancet 345: 1333–1338
Williams B 1994 Insulin resistance: the shape of things to come. Lancet 344: 521–524
Williams A C 1995 Dopamine, dystonia and the deficient co-factor. Lancet 345: 1130
Wilson R F 1995 Assessing the severity of coronary-artery stenoses. N Engl J Med 334: 1735
Wilson A J, Diemunsch P, Lindeque B G et al 1996 Single dose i.v. granisetron in the prevention of postoperative nausea and vomiting. Br J Anaesth 76: 515–518
Wokke J 1996 Riluzole. Lancet 348: 795–799
Wolf A R 1994 Neonatal sedation: more art than science. Lancet 344: 628–629
Woods R P, Iacoboni M, Mazziotta J C 1994 Bilateral spreading cerebral hypoperfusion during spontaneous migraine headache. N Engl J Med 331: 1689–1692
Yellon D M, Baxter G F, Marber M S 1996 Angina reassessed: pain or protector? Lancet 347: 1059–1062

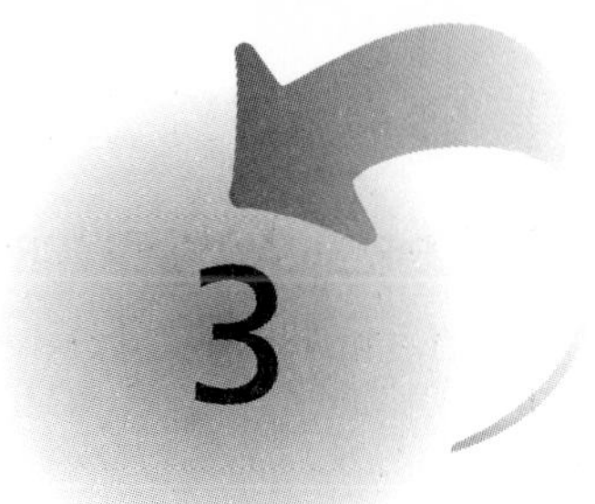

Leonidas Hadjinikolaou   Brian Glenville

New advances in adult cardiac surgery

INTRODUCTION

The 1970s and 1980s saw remarkable advances in the treatment of coronary artery, valvular diseases and heart failure. Coronary artery bypass grafting, with the use of internal thoracic arteries and vein grafts, became one of the most common operations in the Western world. Extensive use of allograft (human), xenograft (porcine) and sophisticated mechanical valves provided good results in the current treatment of various types of cardiac valvular diseases. Finally, the good long term results of heart transplantation established this method as the treatment of choice for the end-stage heart failure. Rapid development in cardiopulmonary bypass technology and cardiac assist devices, as well as in the intensive care treatment, significantly contributed to these advances.

In the 1990s, the accumulation of experience resulted in an expansion of cardiac surgery into older and more seriously ill patients. Also, logistic problems have generally turned the tide of cardiac surgery towards methods that have shortened the hospital stay and minimised the use of intensive care beds. Fast-track programmes, minimally invasive cardiac procedures and use of laser techniques reflect these tendencies. Furthermore, a combination of logistic and organ availability problems has pushed cardiac surgery into developing methods such as a bridge to transplantation and alternative methods for treating end-stage heart failure, such as cardiomyoplasty, aorto-myoplasty and heart volume reduction. Other advances include the use of stentless xenograft and autologous pericardial valves, the Ross operation for the treatment of aortic valve disease and surgery for atrial arrhythmias.

Leonidas Hadjinikolaou MD, Senior Registrar in Cardiothoracic Surgery, St Mary's Hospital, Praed Street, London W2 1NY, UK

Brian Glenville FRCS MS, Consultant Cardiothoracic Surgeon, St Mary's Hospital, Praed Street, London W2 1NY, UK

CORONARY ARTERY BYPASS GRAFTING IN ELDERLY PATIENTS

The number of elderly patients undergoing coronary artery bypass grafting (CABG) continues to increase, not only because there are more elderly in the population with symptomatic heart disease, but also because CABG appears to be generally beneficial in the elderly (CASS Investigators 1985). Elderly patients are classified as those older than 70–75 years of age, and they seem to comprise approximately 10–20% of the CABG population in recent series (Tuman et al 1992, He et al 1994).

The indications and the surgical technique to perform CABG in the elderly do not differ markedly from those in younger patients. The use of left internal mammary artery along with vein grafts has resulted in lower mortality and superior patency rates than those with vein grafts only (Gardner et al 1990). However, operative mortality and morbidity in elderly patients undergoing isolated CABG are persistently higher than those in younger patients (Tuman et al 1992, Edmunds et al 1988, Horneffer et al 1987). Table 3.1 shows a comparison of CABG morbidity and mortality in patients in different age groups. The most common causes of death are low cardiac output state, neurological events, major infection, prolonged intubation, reoperation for bleeding and perioperative myocardial infarction. Among the early postoperative complications, neurological deficits are strongly associated with age. The incidence of postoperative neurological events in patients > 75 years (8.9%) is more than twice that of patients 65–74 (3.6%) and 9 times larger than in patients < 65 (0.9%). Preoperative neurological abnormality, recent myocardial infarction (< 30 days) and duration of cardiopulmonary bypass are additional risk factors for postoperative neurological events (Tuman et al 1992).

MINIMALLY INVASIVE DIRECT CORONARY ARTERY BYPASS

Adaptation of laparoscopic and thoracoscopic techniques used in the treatment of intra-abdominal and intra-thoracic disease has allowed the development of a minimally invasive approach to cardiac operations that in the past were only amenable to open surgical intervention. Minimally invasive coronary artery bypass (MIDCAB) employs short incisions in the chest wall and may be divided into those operations performed with cardiopulmonary bypass (CPB) and those without CPB.

The major advantages of MIDCAB over the traditional CABG, performed through a median sternotomy and CPB with global heart ischaemia, include the avoidance of morbidity and mortality of the median sternotomy incision, especially in the context of infection. Furthermore, MIDCAB without CPB may avoid the damaging effects of CPB (Kirklin et al 1983, Blauth et al 1988). Both approaches may result in a substantial cost reduction (Benetti 1991).

At present single vessel coronary artery disease involving the left anterior descending artery (LAD) and/or right coronary artery (RCA) remains the primary indication. Usually the patient has recurrent angina following angioplasty and/or stenting or a lesion unsuitable for angioplasty (ostial lesion and complex multiple lesions in the LAD or RCA). The gastroepiploic

Table 3.1 Postoperative morbidity and mortality after coronary artery surgery in elderly patients

	Age (years)		
	< 65	65–74	≥75
Mortality (%)	3.9	5.5	7.3
Morbidity			
CK-MB > 40 IU/l (%)	6.3	6.3	7.7
ECG ischaemia (%)	27.2	27.3	29.7
Perioperative MI (%)	4.8	4.9	6.1
Postop IABP (%)	5.9	7.7	7.7
Low CO state (%)	2.8*	5.6	4.9
Major infection (%)	2.1*	4.7[†]	10.2[‡]
Pulmonary morbidity (%)	3.5*	8.2[†]	13.8[‡]
Renal insufficiency (%)	2.7	4.7[†]	11.4[‡]
Neurologic event (%)	0.9*	3.6[†]	8.9[‡]

CK-MB, creatine kinase myocardial band; ECG, electrocardiographic; CO, cardiac output; MI, myocardial infarction; IABP, intra-aortic balloon pump. Differences were accounted statistically significant at the probability level of < 0.05 (Tuman et al 1992).
* < 65 years different from 65–74 years.
[†] 65–74 years different from ≥ 75 years.
[‡] < 65 years different from ≥ 75 years.

artery has been used for grafting the posterior descending artery (PDA). Patients considered to be at high risk from conventional CABG because of associated diseases (i.e. renal failure, chronic obstructive airways disease, diffuse cerebrovascular disease) and redo surgery are also candidates for MIDCAB. Patients in these categories may have multivessel disease and may be approached by a combination of MIDCAB and angioplasty with or without stenting, at the same time or as part of a staged procedure (Angelini et al 1996). Evidence of small, heavily calcified or intramyocardial LAD at angiography are current contraindications for MIDCAB.

The surgical technique of MIDCAB without CPB include endotracheal intubation, haemodynamic monitoring and external defibrillator pads. The skin incision ranges from a parasternal vertical incision over the 3rd and 4th costal cartilages for the LAD and 4th and 5th costal cartilages for the RCA (Stanbridge et al 1996) to a horizontal incision over the 4th intercostal space (Robinson et al 1995, Calafiore et al 1996). The left internal mammary artery (LIMA) is harvested through the same incision with or without the use of a thoracoscope. For thoracoscopic dissection a double lumen endotracheal intubation is required to facilitate dissection (Robinson et al 1995, Acuff et al 1996). Positioning the patient in a 30° right lateral decubitus position will assist in the dissection of the LIMA. One or more costal cartilages may be resected to achieve better visualisation and dissection of the full length of the LIMA. Before division of the LIMA the patient is heparinised (1 mg/kg), and diluted papaverine is injected onto the pedicle or into the LIMA. The role of ischaemic preconditioning before the occlusion of the vessel by a preliminary occlusion followed by reperfusion prior to reocclusion for the anastomosis remains to be identified. During the anastomosis ECG changes are monitored (ST-segment analysis) and trans-oesophageal echocardiography can monitor any wall motion changes. Such changes in wall motion are rare, as are arrhythmias including ventricular fibrillation. Pharmacological intervention can improve anastomotic conditions and short acting β-blockers to slow the heart rate are sometimes used. The postoperative course is short and early extubation either in the operating room or soon after is a common practice.

The largest experience to date with MIDCAB was recently reported by Califiore and colleagues (1996). They operated on 155 patients anastomosing LIMA to LAD via a MIDCAB approach. The mean LAD occlusion time was 23.3 ± 5.8 min. (range 16–39 min) with a mortality rate of 0.6% (1/155). Two patients (1.2%) were reopened for bleeding, both from intercostal branches. Mean intensive care unit stay was 4.2 ±6 h, and 77% were discharged from the hospital on the second postoperative day. In the follow-up early after the operation, 94.2% of the LIMAs were found patent. Nine patients (5.8%) underwent early reoperation for graft failure. A further two patients underwent late reoperation for graft failure, raising the reoperation rate to 7% (11/155). At mean follow-up 5.6 months, 143 patients were alive and free of symptoms (92.2%). Stenoses at the anastomotic sites and the sites of the stay sutures, steal syndrome from the 1st intercostal artery and postoperative pain are the major drawbacks for MIDCAB today. Strategies such as infiltration of local anaesthetic and administering aliquots via an intrapleural drain (Cohen et al 1996), along with non-steroidal anti-inflammatory drugs and opioids have succeeded in reducing this problem. In some centres, placement of thoracic epidural catheters with low dose local anaesthetic and opioid mixture in boluses has improved pain relief without causing cardiovascular instability (Rodriguez et al 1997).

TRANSMYOCARDIAL LASER REVASCULARIZATION

Several observations have led to the conclusion that the myocardium may be directly supplied by ventricular blood. A review of comparative anatomy reveals that the reptilian heart consists of multiple channels radiating out from a myocardial cavity. On the basis of this finding, Sen et al (1965, 1968) performed the 'snake heart' operation and reported improved survival and diminished infarct size in animals with ischaemic areas treated with transmyocardial acupuncture. Likewise, it has been shown embryologically that, initially, the developing myocardium is directly supplied by ventricular blood through an extensive capillary network. As the coronary arteries develop, these capillaries usually regress. In some patients with congenital heart abnormalities this microvascular pattern persists, and there is evidence of systolic flow through them (O'Connor et al 1982). A veritable network of vessels is also found in the normal myocardium and, in the setting of coronary occlusion, may increase by forming collateral vessels. The rational for transmyocardial revascularization (TMR) builds on these observations.

Theoretically, it has been stated that it is impossible for blood to flow from the ventricle into the myocardium during either systole or diastole (Piffarre et al 1968, 1969). Studies of intramyocardial pressure have demonstrated a pressure gradient across the myocardium (Nematzadeh et al 1984). The pressure in the myocardium approaches left ventricular pressure during systole but decreases across the myocardium to the epicardium. This gradient would, therefore, permit flow, and this flow may be enhanced by increased left ventricular pressure or diminished tissue pressure due to ischaemia (Horvath et al 1995).

The operation is performed on the beating heart through a left thoracotomy, with a high-energy CO_2 laser which drills transmural channels (1 mm in diameter) into the left ventricle. Each high-energy laser pulse is delivered during end diastole and transects the heart within 10–60 ms.

Cooley et al (1994) found that although after TMR reactive fibrous scar tissue had caused narrowing of the original laser tract, the channels had endothelialized and they contained red blood cells. These findings suggest that the laser channels may be functional. There is accumulating evidence that TMR prevents acute regional ischaemia (Mirohseini et al 1993, Horvath et al 1995). However, this method needs to be clinically evaluated on a long-term basis.

VALVULAR SURGERY

NEW VALVES

Surgical treatment of valvular heart disease is a field of constant clinical and experimental research. Recently, much attention has been devoted to the improvement of valve repair techniques. These improvements include aortic and mitral valve extension procedures using autologous pericardium, new physiological mitral annuloplasty rings, techniques to repair the mitral and tricuspid subvalvular apparatus, and the use of artificial chordae. Duran et al (1991) performed aortic valve repair (annulus and leaflet plasties) in 69 cases and cusp extension with glutaraldehyde-treated pericardium in 38 cases, with 30 months reoperation freedom 77% and 93%, respectively. Sarsam et al (1993) described the remodelling of the aortic annulus for annuloaortic ectasia. Mitral valve repair for mitral regurgitation due to degenerative disease has an actuarial freedom of reoperation 95% at 8 years (David et al 1993). Advanced myxomatous change in the leaflets was the only significant factor associated with higher risk of reoperation. Mitral valve repair has been shown to be the treatment of choice in ischaemic mitral insufficiency, where annulus dilatation is present in all cases and the sole mechanism of regurgitation in 50% of the cases (Dion 1993). Mitral valve repair may also be indicated in patients undergoing surgery for endomyocardial fibrosis (Souza et al 1992). Conventional techniques for the repair of mitral insufficiency caused by leaflet prolapse due to chordal rupture have been shown to have certain limitations. In such situations, artificial chordae implantation can expand the indications for mitral (David et al 1991) and tricuspid repair (Bortolotti et al 1993). However, chordae transposition technically remains the first choice in the repair of chordal rupture. In the young, rheumatic patients with triple-valve disease, the clinical outcome of valve repair does not appear to be as good as in other patients (Prabhakar et al 1993).

The use of aortic homografts has been widely applied as a treatment for infective endocarditis. Mitral homografts are currently under investigation, and experimental studies (Revuelta et al 1992) and clinical applications (Agar et al 1994) have demonstrated interesting results. The mitral valve can be used entirely or as a partial homograft, implanted in either the mitral or tricuspid position (Pomar et al 1993).

New biological valves have also come into use. The Carpentier-Edwards pericardial valve (Baxter Healthcare Corp., Edwards Division, Irvine, CA, USA) implanted in the aortic position shows minimal calcification without structural deterioration at 7 years follow-up (Frater et al 1992). The results are less encouraging with the Mitroflow valve (Mitroflow International, Richmond, British Columbia, Canada; Loisance et al 1993). Intraoperative creation of a cardiac bioprosthesis using glutaraldehyde-treated autologous pericardium is an attractive surgical innovation. The valve can be mounted using a semi-automated procedure. The advantage of this technique is the use of autologous tissue, without activation of the immunological cascade reaction (Love et al 1992). The Autogenics version of this valve type is being currently redesigned after early problems.

Stentless bioprostheses have also been under investigation, in particular, to evaluate their haemodynamic and clinical characteristics. Stentless bioprostheses are emerging as a new surgical option in both aortic (David et al 1992, Gasabona et al 1992) and mitral (Vrandecic et al 1992) valve replacement. The operative time for surgical implantation of stentless bioprostheses is longer than that for mounted bioprostheses, consequently requiring a longer period of aortic cross-clamping. Potential advantages of the unstented valve over its stented counterpart are improved haemodynamic performance and durability.

Ross et al (1992) used the patients own living pulmonary valve for aortic valve replacement in a series of 339 patients. No form of anticoagulation was used and there were no thromboembolic complications. After 20 years of follow-up, freedom of reoperation was 85% and the actuarial survival was 80%. There has been no evidence of primary tissue degeneration. The potential growth of this autograft makes this technique an interesting alternative to valve replacement in the paediatric population.

MINIMALLY INVASIVE VALVE SURGERY

Cosgrove et al (Navia & Cosgrove 1996, Cosgrove 1996) have described a minimal approach to the mitral valve using a small parasternal incision. Concomitant coronary artery disease and pectus excavatum are contra-indications for this procedure. The incision is similar to the vertical parasternal MIDCAB approach to the RCA, but slightly longer (10 cm). The right internal mammary artery is mobilised and ligated to improve exposure and ensure haemostasis. Venous cannulation is performed directly to the right atrium, or superior and inferior vena cavae with arterial return via the ascending aorta. Alternatively, femoro-femoral cannulation can be performed. The aorta is cross-clamped and antegrade cardioplegia administered through the aortic root. The mitral valve is approached via an incision in the intra-atrial septum after a right atriotomy. Retrograde cardioplegia is also possible with this exposure. De-airing of the heart is accomplished by gentle suction on the cardioplegia cannula. In a series of 49 patients, the mortality was 0% and the morbidity included 4% cerebrovascular accidents, 2% myocardial infarction and 0% reopening for bleeding. There was 7% decrease in direct costs and the mean hospital stay was 5.8 days. The transeptal approach to the mitral valve may be associated with transient junctional rhythm, due to the injury of interatrial conduction pathways. None of the patients in this series developed this complication.

Pompili et al (1996) have developed a method of mitral valve replacement with port-access technology. This complicated method has been successfully applied to 15 dogs. It is worth noting that the shape of the dog's thoracic cage results in the heart being closer to the lateral chest wall. The motivation behind this approach is the potential to decrease the postoperative discomfort, morbidity and overall cost. However, de-airing the heart after the completion of the operation may be more difficult and the length of the operation too long.

Cosgrove (1996) has also described a minimal approach to the aortic valve, through a 10 cm transverse incision over the second intercostal space. Both internal mammary arteries are identified and divided. The aorta is cannulated directly, while the right atrial cannula may be passed via a separate lateral stab incision later used for one of the drainage tubes. Patient selection should exclude those with risk factors for ischaemic heart disease, especially those with young age, since both internal mammary arteries are sacrificed. In a series of 50 patients, the mortality was 2% and the morbidity included reoperation for bleeding (4%), cerebrovascular accidents (2%) and myocardial infarction (2%). There was a 19% cost saving and the mean hospital stay was 5.5 days. Our own initial experience with this approach is encouraging.

SURGERY FOR CONGESTIVE HEART FAILURE

DYNAMIC CARDIOMYOPLASTY

Ventricular assistance with autologous muscle tissue is an attractive potential adjunct therapy for heart failure. The disadvantages of mechanical circulatory assistance, such as thromboembolism and infection, and the shortcomings of cardiac transplantation, such as donor availability and immunosuppression, are avoided. Patients due for cardiomyoplasty are selected from the population referred for management of congestive heart failure. They usually have progression of heart failure despite maximal medical therapy and are not suitable for transplantation because of advanced age and/or associated medical problems. Indications for dynamic cardiomyoplasty (DCM) include idiopathic or ischaemic cardiomyopathy, left ventricular aneurysms and Chagas's disease. Previous left thoracotomy, complex or intractable arrhythmias, major pulmonary dysfunction, renal failure and hepatic failure have been reasons for exclusion in some series (Furnary et al 1992). The need for intravenous inotropic support or a mechanical assist device were also exclusion criteria. Persistent NYHA functional Class IV has also recently been defined as a contraindication (Furnary et al 1992, Grandjean et al 1991, Carpentier et al 1993). Severe dilatation of the heart (cardiothoracic ratio > 0.6 mm, left ventricular end-diastolic diameter > 75 mm), mitral regurgitation or left ventricular wall calcification are conditions that may reduce the benefits of cardiomyoplasty (Chachques et al 1992).

The surgical technique usually includes two separate incisions. A lateral approach for muscle flap dissection and a subsequent median sternotomy for cardiac access. The latissimus dorsi muscle is dissected, transported into the intrapleural space after removal of 5 cm lateral portion of the 2nd or 3rd rib, and wrapped around the ventricles. The procedure can be undertaken with or without cardiopulmonary bypass, depending on the need for additional procedures, like coronary grafting, valve replacement or left ventricular aneurysmectomy (Moreira et al 1995). Two intramuscular pacing electrodes are implanted into the proximal portion of the latissimus dorsi muscle and an intramyocardial sensing lead placed in either the right or left ventricle. The latter is used for synchronization of muscle stimulation with ventricular contraction. Skeletal muscle stimulation is started 2 weeks after the operation (Carpentier et al 1991). After a 6 week muscle-conditioning protocol, the muscle fibres are transformed from glycolytic fast-twitch morphology (type II) to the nonfatigueable oxidative slow-twitch (type I) variety (Eisenberg & Salmons 1981).

Operative mortality varies widely – 0% (Moreira et al 1995), 16% (Magovern et al 1993) and 27% (Furnary et al 1992). The two major causes of death are biventricular heart failure and sudden ventricular dysrhythmia. As expected, early postoperative morbidity is significant, including transient need for inotropic support and IABP, renal failure, mesenteric ischaemia, atrial fibrillation and pulmonary complications. Long term survival is significantly lower than that obtained by heart transplantation. Magovern et al (1993) compared the operative mortality and one year survival between patients operated on for congestive heart failure. Operative mortality was 7%, 4% and 16% for heart transplantation, coronary artery bypass grafting and DCM, respectively. The corresponding one year survival was 94%, 91% and 65%. Moreira et al (1995) have reported a 5 year survival of 42.5% and Carpentier (1993) a 7 year survival of 70.4%. Preoperative NYHA functional class IV and elevated PVR have been associated with poorer late survival. The functional status has been shown to improve. Left ventricular ejection fraction increases approximately 4–6% and most patients with NYHA functional class III–IV improve into NYHA class I–II. There is also a significant improvement in cardiac index. In conclusion, DCM improves functional class and left ventricular function in patients with severe cardiomyopathy. However, the long-term survival after this surgical procedure may be limited by the patients' condition before the operation.

DYNAMIC AORTOMYOPLASTY

Dynamic aortomyoplasty (DAM) consists of wrapping the latissimus dorsi muscle around the aorta and electrostimulating it during diastole. Its principle resembles that of the intra-aortic balloon counterpulsation and its use to date has been exclusively experimental. Potential candidates for DAM may be patients with end-stage heart failure with severe dilatation of the heart, mitral regurgitation or left ventricular wall calcification, conditions that reduce the benefits of cardiomyoplasty. Technical contraindications may include a calcified aorta, aortic valve regurgitation and Marfan's disease (Chachques et al 1994).

The surgical dissection and preconditioning of the dorsalis latissimus muscle resembles that of cardiomyoplasty. There are two major techniques to wrap the muscle around the aorta. Chachques et al (1994) wrap the muscle around the ascending aorta after enlarging the aorta with the use of autologous pericardium. Others (Constance et al 1993, Lazzara et al 1994) have experimented with wrapping the muscle around the descending aorta after dividing three sets of intercostal arteries. The disadvantages of the first method include the risk of aortic dissection, aortic rupture, aneurysm formation and thromboembolic events. The disadvantages of the second method include counterpulsation away from the vicinity of the coronary ostia, at a relatively smaller diameter aortic segment and the risk of paraplegia (Pattison et al 1991). None of these complications have been encountered in the experimental models to date.

Although there is no clinical experience with DAM, experimental data have provided evidence that it decreases the left ventricular afterload (Chachques et al 1994, Cabrera Fisher et al 1991) and improves indices of systolic and diastolic ventricular function. The exact mechanism of these effects is not clearly understood. Coronary blood flow would not be expected to improve left ventricular function in the absence of myocardial ischaemia. Also, the reduction of the afterload during diastole would not be expected to be as significant as with IABP. An alternative explanation for these changes may be an increase in the sympathetic tone to the heart mediated through the central nervous system as a result of burst stimulation of the skeletal muscle (Lazzara et al 1994). Clinical results are awaited.

PARTIAL LEFT VENTRICULECTOMY (BATISTA OPERATION)

According to Laplace's law, reducing the left ventricular diameter decreases wall tension. An operation has been developed by Randas Batista (Curitiba, Brazil) to remove left ventricular muscle and, therefore, to reduce the left ventricular radius. The operation was designed for patients with end-stage heart disease with left ventricular dilatation. In May 1996, the technique was adopted by Cleveland clinic for patients with idiopathic dilated cardiomyopathy with left ventricular end diastolic diameter greater than 7 cm, candidates for heart transplantation. Patients with ischaemic cardiomyopathy, cardiac fibrosis and active myocarditis have been excluded. In an anecdotal report (McCarthy 1997), 23 patients were described as having undergone the procedure. Eighteen had an additional Cosgrove-Edwards ring, 12 tricuspid valve annuloplasty, one mitral valve replacement and one CABG. There was only one death, 3 months after the operation, due to cardiac arrest. Two patients had LVAD and one with persistent need for inotropic support are awaiting transplantation. One was found to suffer myocarditis, one suffered rhabdomyolysis, coagulopathy and acute renal failure, one prosthetic mitral valve thrombosis and one ventricular tachycardia and received an implantable cardiovertor defibrillator. Nineteen out of 22 surviving patients have been deactivated from transplantation. In early follow-up, 68% are subjectively NYHA functional class I or II. The others are class III in various phases of postoperative recovery. Further clinical evaluation of this technique is awaited.

IMPLANTABLE LEFT VENTRICULAR ASSIST DEVICE

The implantable left ventricular assist device (LVAD) is currently being used as a bridge to heart transplantation. Univentricular support with an LVAD has been shown to be feasible for many patients awaiting transplantation (McCarthy et al 1991, Kormos et al 1990), with generally better results than those obtained with a total artificial heart (McCarthy et al 1994, Johnson et al 1992). The major disadvantage of univentricular support is that good right ventricular function is important to obtain optimal results. Co-existence of right ventricular failure occurs in approximately 15% of these patients and they need, at least temporarily, right ventricular mechanical support (McCarthy et al 1995). Unfortunately, it is to date not possible to predict which patients are at risk for early right heart failure. Patients are usually in severe cardiogenic shock on cardiopulmonary bypass, receiving inotropic support and/or IABP. An LVAD is used before weaning from cardiopulmonary bypass and ECMO is occasionally needed in addition to the LVAD.

The Heart mate 1000 IP (Thermo Cardiosystems, Inc., Woburn, MA, USA) is a widely known pneumatically-driven pusher plate LVAD, with a remarkably low risk of thromboemboli. It has a pump inflow from the left ventricular apex and pump outflow to the ascending aorta. It is usually implanted in the upper quadrant of the abdominal wall underneath the left rectus muscle and on the top of the posterior rectus fascia. In a recent series, the mortality rate after LVAD implantation was 24%, mainly due to multiple organ failure; specifically, the combination of renal and hepatic failure. Pretransplantation duration of support averaged 76 days (22–153 days). All survivors presented a significant haemodynamic improvement, received a donor heart and were discharged (100% survival after transplantation). Both renal and liver function returned to normal before transplantation, enforcing the view that rising blood urea nitrogen levels should not be considered as a contraindication to LVAD insertion (McCarthy et al 1995, Farrar 1994). Other devices such as the Novacor electrical system (Baxter Healthcare) are also providing encouraging results.

The ultimate goal of the implantable LVAD may be its use as an alternative to medical therapy for patients with end-stage heart disease who are not candidates for transplantation or other surgical therapy.

SURGERY FOR ATRIAL ARRHYTHMIAS

COX MAZE OPERATION

During the past several years, the maze procedure has become an important method of treating patients with medically refractory atrial fibrillation and atrial flutter (Cox et al 1995). The procedure has undergone 3 modifications (maze procedure I, II and III). Maze I procedure was complicated with an inability to generate an appropriate sinus tachycardia in response to maximum exercise and occasional postoperative left atrial dysfunction. Maze II was extremely difficult to perform technically. Maze III, although still a complicated surgical procedure with multiple cuts in the atria, has been proved safe and effective. The results reported by Cox et al (1995) are summarised as follows. Operative mortality was approximately 2.5%. Perioperative morbidity included mainly atrial arrhythmias (60%), fluid retention (10%) and pancreatitis (5%). Recurrent arrhythmia occurred in 6% but it converted to sinus rhythm with medical therapy. In a follow-up ranging from 3 to 81 months, 75% of the patients were in sinus rhythm and 25% atrially paced. The chronotropic response to maximal exercise was entirely normal in more than 87% of patients. Inappropriate sinus tachycardia sometimes occurred several months after the maze III procedure, but this is a minor clinical problem that is easily controlled. To date, the maze procedure has been widely used, alone or in combination with mitral valve or other procedures (atrial septal defect closure, tricuspid valve operations, aortic valve replacement, etc.), with highly successful restoration of sinus rhythm and improvement in exercise capacity (Tamai et al 1995, Blitz et al 1992, McCarthy et al 1993, Hioki et al 1993).

FAST-TRACKING PATIENTS AFTER CARDIAC SURGERY

Early extubation after cardiac surgery is not a new concept. In the 1970s, Prakash et al (1977) showed that it is possible to extubate cardiac surgical patients in less than an hour after surgery. However, the postoperative cardiorespiratory complications were not uncommon in view of the myocardial protection and surgical techniques at the time. Concurrently, opioid-based anaesthesia began to gain popularity due to its ability to ensure haemodynamic stability, even in patients with marginal cardiac reserve (Lowenstein et al 1969, Stanley et al 1976). As a result of high dose narcotic anaesthesia, it was necessary to continue postoperative ventilatory support for 12–24 h in cardiac patients. Thus, the practice of prolonged sedation and ventilatory support became widely accepted for the management of postoperative cardiac surgical patients in the 1980s.

The renewed interest of early extubation in cardiac patients is mainly related to cost-containment and efficient resource utilization. Early extubation is now feasible because of improvements in anaesthesia management coupled with the advancement in surgical techniques, myocardial protection and postoperative haemostasis. The concept of balanced anaesthesia for cardiac surgery was re-established in the late 1980s when large outcome studies demonstrated the safety of different anaesthetic techniques (Slogoff et al 1989, Tuman et al 1989). Inhalation anaesthetics, such as isoflurane, were confirmed to not cause clinically significant coronary steal (Leung et al 1991, Cheng et al 1992). Postoperative sedative medication, such as propofol, was found to provide shorter postoperative sedation and shorter time to extubation with a lower incidence of hypertension (McMurray et al 1990).

The preoperative status does not necessarily predict the postoperative course and, therefore, prolonged mechanical ventilation following cardiac surgery should not be uncritically considered as routine. The fast-track selection criteria vary significantly among different centres. Table 3.2 presents the selection criteria implemented at the Royal Brompton and National Heart Hospital. Notably, mitral valve surgery is excluded due to the unacceptably high number of these patients that required unplanned intensive care

Table 3.2 Fast-track selection criteria (Howard 1995)

- Parsonnet score < 10
- Age up to 74 years old
- Absence of serious lung disease or condition that compromise postoperative respiratory function
- Less than 30% overweight by standard body mass index
- Hypertension, if present, must be controlled
- Controlled blood sugar if diabetic
- Left ventricular ejection fraction recorded > 30%, or > 50% if myocardial infarction within the last month
- Surgery must be for
    - First time CABG
    - First time aortic valve surgery with or without CABG
    - Simple congenital repair
    - Simple other surgery, e.g. atrial myxoma, pericardial window
- Aspirin must have been stopped 7 days preoperatively or platelets preordered to be given postoperatively
- Neurologically intact
- Absence of other systemic condition that may compromise a rapid recovery from surgery

CABG = coronary artery bypass grafting.

management. Of the patients due for adult cardiac operations, 33% met the fast-track criteria (409/1245) (Howard 1995). In the John Radcliffe Hospital (Oxford, UK) 1000 consecutive patients who underwent open heart surgery were fast-tracked, including 690 coronary artery bypass grafting (CABG) operations, 182 aortic valve replacement (AVR) with or without CABG, 88 mitral valve replacement (MVR) with or without CABG and 18 double valve replacement with or without CABG (Westaby et al 1993). During the period of study, only 45 patients (4.3%) were scheduled to be admitted directly to the intensive care unit (ICU). They included patients with pre-existing renal or respiratory failure, those who were originally brought to the operating theatre from the ICU, and others after repair of postinfarction ventricular septal rupture who required prolonged intra-aortic balloon pump support. Patients undergoing hypothermic circulatory arrest for thoracic aortic surgery were also recovered in the ICU. Only in 10 patients (1%) did attempts at early extubation fail or were abandoned because of specific complications (6 CABG, 2 AVR, 1 MVR and 1 double valve replacement). The reasons for fast-track failure were prolonged inotropic support for left ventricular failure (4 patients), chronic obstructive airways disease (3 patients), perioperative myocardial infarction (one patient), aspiration (one patient) and chest infection (one patient). In St Mary's Hospital, fast-track failure has been 7.3% (10/137) and the two most frequent causes of failure were perioperative myocardial infarction (3/10) and bleeding (2/10). Cheng et al (1996) have reported 15% (9/60) fast-failure, due to resternotomy for bleeding, low cardiac output syndrome, stroke and inadequate arterial blood gases.

The major advantages of fast-tracking patients following cardiac surgery are the shortened postoperative length of stay, the reduction in the numbers of cases cancelled and improvements in intrapulmonary shunt fractions (Engelman et al 1994). Interestingly, the myocardial ischaemia burden has been shown to be higher on the 2nd postoperative day in patients with early extubation (Cheng et al 1996).

The surgical management has not been dramatically modified to allow for fast-tracking. It is worth noting, however, that the shorter the operation and the cardiopulmonary bypass time, the earlier the extubation. A core temperature of about 32°C during cardiopulmonary bypass may also play an optimal role in the success of fast-tracking cardiac patients, than the traditional 28°C. Engelman et al (1994) have established a new protocol for fast-tracking cardiac patients which includes methylprednisolone sodium succinate before cardiopulmonary bypass followed by dexamethasone for 24 h postoperatively, prophylactic digitalization, metoclopramide HCl, docusate sodium and ranitidine.

Randomised studies have shown that the operative and late (1–24 months) mortality, as well as the operative morbidity (resternotomy for bleeding, low cardiac output syndrome, inadequate arterial blood gases, stroke, mediastinal, sternal or leg wound infections) and the 30 day hospital readmission do not seem to differ between fast-track and non-fast-track CABG patients (Engelman et al 1994, Cheng et al 1996). Westaby et al (1993) have reported a mortality rate of 1.4% (14/1000). The mortality was 1% (7/690) in CABG, 2.2% (4/182) in AVR ± CABG and 3.4% (3/88) in MVR ± CABG. None of the deaths was related to the time of extubation. The two most common causes of death were perioperative myocardial infarction and left ventricular failure.

References

Acuff T E, Landreneau R J, Bartley G P et al 1996 Minimally invasive coronary artery bypass grafting. Ann Thorac Surg 61: 135–137

Agar C, Farge A, Ramsheyi A et al 1994 Mitral valve replacement using a cryopreserved mitral homograft. Ann Thorac Surg 58: 128-134

Angelini G D, Wilde P, Salerno T A et al 1996 Integrated left anterior small thoracotomy and angioplasty for multivessel coronary artery revascularization. Lancet 347: 757–758

Benetti F J 1991 Coronary artery bypass surgery without extracorporeal circulation versus percutaneous transluminal angioplasty. Comparison of costs. J Thorac Cardiovasc Surg 102: 802–803

Blauth C L, Arnold J V, Schulenberg W E et al 1988 Cerebral microembolism during cardiopulmonary bypass. J Thorac Cardiovasc Surg 96: 668–676

Blitz A, McLoughlin D, Gross J et al 1992 Combined maze procedure and septal myectomy in a septuagenarian. Ann Thorac Surg 54; 364–365

Bortolotti U, Tursi V, Fasoli G et al 1993 Tricuspid valve endocarditis: repair with the use of artificial chordae. J Heart Valve Dis 2: 567–570

Cabrera Fisher E I, Chachques J C, Garcia A et al 1991 Temporary mechanical circulatory support for severe cardiac failure: experimental study. Int J Artif Organs 14: 466–472

Calafiore A M, Giammarco G D, Teodori G et al 1996 Left anterior descending coronary artery grafting via left anterior small thoracotomy without cardiopulmonary bypass. Ann Thorac Surg 61: 1658–1665

Carpentier A, Chachques J C, Grandjean P A eds 1991 Cardiomyoplasty. Mount Kisco, NY: Futura

Carpentier A, Chachques J C, Acar C et al Dynamic cardiomyoplasty at seven years. J Thorac Cardiovasc Surg 106: 42–53

Chachques J C, Acar C, Portoghese M et al 1992 Dynamic cardiomyoplasty for long term assist. Eur J Cardiothorac Surg 6: 642–648

Chachques J C, Haab F, Cron C C et al 1994 Long term effects of dynamic cardiomyoplasty. Ann Thorac Surg 58: 128–134

Cheng D C H, Moyers J R, Knutson B et al 1992 Dose-response relationship of isoflurane and halothane versus coronary perfusion pressures: effects on flow redistribution in a collateralized chronic swine model. Anesthesiology 76: 113–122

Cheng D C H, Karski J, Peniston C et al 1996 Morbidity outcome in early versus conventional tracheal extubation after coronary artery bypass grafting: a prospective randomized controlled trial. J Thorac Cardiovasc 112: 755–764

Cohen A S, Hadjinikolaou L, Sogliani F et al 1996 Mini-sternotomy for coronary artery bypass grafting. Ann Thorac Surg 62: 1884–1885

Constance C G, Sbini G, Turi G K et al 1993 Descending thoracic aortomyoplasty: effect of chronically conditioned muscle on heart failure. Cardiovasc Surg 1: 291–295

Cooley D A, Frazier O H, Kadipasaoglu K A et al 1994 Transmyocardial laser revascularization. Anatomic evidence of long-term channel patency. Tex Heart Inst J 21: 220–224

Coronary Artery Surgery Study (CASS) Investigators 1985 Comparison of coronary artery bypass surgery and medical treatment in patients 65 years of age or older. N Engl J Med 313: 217–224

Cosgrove D M 1996 Minimally invasive valve replacement techniques: Teleconference from the Cleveland clinic

Cox J L, Boineau J P, Schuessler R B et al 1995 Modification of the maze procedure for atrial flutter and fibrillation. J Thorac Cardiovasc Surg 110: 473–484

David T E, Bos J, Rakowski H 1991 Mitral valve repair by replacement of chordae tendinae with polytetrafluoroethylene sutures. J Thorac Cardiovasc Surg 101: 495-501

David T E, Bos J, Rakowski H 1992 Aortic valve replacement with Toronto SPV bioprosthesis . J Heart Valve Dis 1: 244–248

David T E, Armstrong S, Sun Z et al 1993 Late results of mitral valve repair for mitral regurgitation due to degenerative disease. Ann Thorac Surg 56: 7–14

Dion R 1993 Ischaemic mitral regurgitation: when and how should it be corrected? J Heart Valve Dis 2: 536–543

Duran C, Kumar N, Gometza B et al 1991 Indications and limitations of aortic valve reconstruction. Ann Thorac Surg 52: 447–454

Edmunds L H, Stephenson L W, Edie R N et al 1988 Open-heart surgery in octogenarians. N Engl J Med 319: 131–136

Eisenberg B R, Salmons S 1981 The reorganization of subcellular structure in muscle undergoing fast-to-slow type transformation. A stereological study. Cell Tissue Res 220: 449–471

Engelman R M, Rousou J A, Flack J E et al 1994 Fast-track recovery of the coronary bypass patient. Ann Thorac Surg 58: 1742–1746

Frater R W M, Salomon N W, Rainer W G et al 1992 The Carpentier-Edwards pericardial aortic valve: intermediate results. Ann Thorac Surg 53: 764–771

Gardner T J, Greene P S, Rykiel M F et al 1990 Routine use of left internal mammary artery graft in the elderly. Ann Thorac Surg 49: 188–194

Gasabona R, De Paulis R, Zattera G F et al 1992 Stentless porcine and pericardial valve in aortic position. Ann Thorac Surg 54: 681–685

Grandjean P P, Austin L, Chan S et al 1991 Dynamic cardiomyoplasty: clinical follow-up results. J Cardiac Surg 6 (Suppl): 80–88

Howard C 1995 Fast-track care after cardiac surgery. Br J Nurs 4: 1112–1117

Farrar D J 1994 Preoperative predictors of survival in patients with Thoratec ventricular assist devices as a bridge to heart transplantation. J Heart Lung Transplant 13: 93–101

Furnary A P, Magovern J A, Christlied I Y 1992 Clinical cardiomyoplasty: preoperative factors associated with outcome. Ann Thorac Surg 54: 1139–1143

He G-W, Acuff T E, Ryan W H et al 1994 Determinants of operative mortality in elderly patients undergoing coronary artery bypass grafting. J Thorac Cardiovasc Surg 108: 73–81

Hioki M, Ikeshita M, Iedokoro Y et al 1993 Successful combined operation for mitral stenosis and atrial fibrillation. Ann Thorac Surg 55: 776–778

Horneffer P J, Gardner T J, Manolio T A et al 1987 The effect of age on outcome after coronary bypass surgery. Circulation 76 (Suppl): V6

Horvath K A, Smith W J, Laurence R G et al 1995 Recovery and viability of an acute myocardial infarct after transmyocardial laser revascularization J Am Coll Cardiol 25: 258–263

Johnson K E, Prieto M, Joyce L D et al 1992 Summary of the clinical use of the Symbion total artificial heart: a registry report. J Heart Lung Transplant 11: 103–116

Kirklin J K, Westaby S, Blackstone E H et al 1983 Complement and damaging effects of cardiopulmonary bypass. J Thorac Cardiovasc Surg 86: 845–857

Kormos R L, Borovetz H S, Gasior T et al 1990 Experience with univentricular support in mortality ill cardiac transplant candidates. Ann Thorac Surg 49: 261-271

Lazzara R R, Trumble D R, Magovern J A 1994 Autogenous cardiac assist with chronic descending thoracic aortomyoplasty. Ann Thorac Surg 57: 1540–1544

Leung J M, Goehner P, O'Kelly B F et al 1991 Isoflurane anesthesia and myocardial ischemia: comparative risk versus sufentanil anesthesia in patients undergoing coronary artery bypass graft surgery. Anesthesiology 74: 838–847

Loisance D Y, Mazzucotelli J P, Bertrand P C 1993 Mitroflow pericardial valve: long-term durability. Ann Thorac Surg 56: 131–136

Love J W, Schoen F J, Breznock E M 1992 Experimental evaluation of an autologous tissue heart valve. J Heart Valve Dis 1: 232–241

Lowenstein E, Hollowell P, Levine F H et al 1969 Cardiovascular response to large doses of intravenous morphine in man. N Engl J Med 281: 1389–1393

Magovern J A, Magovern G J, Maher T D et al 1993 Operation for congestive heart failure: transplantation, coronary artery bypass, and cardiomyoplasty. Ann Thorac Surg 56: 418–425

McCarthy P M, Portner P M, Tobler H G 1991 Clinical experience with the Novacor ventricular assist system. J Thorac Cardiovasc Surg 102: 578–587

McCarthy P M, Cosgrove III D M, Castle L W et al 1993 Combined treatment of mitral regurgitation and atrial fibrillation with valvuloplasty and the maze procedure. Am J Cardiol 71: 483–486

McCarthy P M, Sabik J F 1994 Implantable circulatory support devices as a bridge to heart transplantation. Semin Thorac Surg 6: 174–180

McCarthy P M, Savage R M, Fraser C D et al 1995 Cardiopulmonary bypass, myocardial management, and support technique. J Thorac Cardiovasc Surg 109: 409–418

McCarthy P M 1997 Partial left ventriculectomy as an alternative to cardiac transplantation: the Cleveland clinic experience. Cleveland Clinic Foundation, Unpublished data

McMurray T J, Collier P S, Carson I W et al 1990 Propofol sedation after heart surgery: a clinical and pharmacokinetic study. Anesthesia 45: 322–326

Mirohseini M, Shelgikar S, Cayton M M 1993 Transmyocardial laser revascularization of the myocardium, a review. J Clin Laser Med Surg 11: 15–19

Moreira L F P, Bocchi E A, Bacal F et al 1995 Present trends in clinical experience with dynamic cardiomyoplasty. Artif Organs 19: 211–215

Navia J L, Cosgrove III D M 1996 Minimally invasive mitral valve operations. Ann Thorac Surg 62: 1542–1544

Nematzadeh D, Rose J C, Schryver T H et al 1984 Analysis of methodology for intramyocardial pressure. Basic Res Cardiol 79: 86–97

O'Connor W N, Cash J B, Cotrill C M et al 1982 Ventriculocoronary connections in hypoplastic left hearts, an autopsy microscopy study. Circulation 665: 1078–1086

Pattison C W, Cumming D V E, Williamson A et al 1991 Aortic counterpulsation for up to 28 days with autologous latissimus dorsi in sheep. J Thorac Cardiovasc Surg 102: 766–773

Piffarre R 1968 Intramyocardial pressure during systole and diastole. Ann Thorac Surg 168: 871–875

Piffarre R, Jasuia M L, Lynch R D et al 1969 Myocardial revascularization by transmyocardial acupuncture. J Thorac Cardiovasc Surg 58: 424–431

Pomar J L, Mestres C A 1993 Tricuspid valvȩ replacement using a mitral homograft. Surgical technique and initial results. J Heart Valve Dis 2: 125–128

Pompili M F, Stevens J H, Burdon T A et al 1996 Port access mitral valve replacement in dogs. J Thorac Cardiovasc Surg 112: 1268–1274

Prabhakar G, Kumar N, Gometza B et al 1993 Triple-valve operations in the young rheumatic patient. Ann Thorac Surg 55: 1492–1496

Prakash O, Jonson B, Meij S et al 1977 Criteria for early extubation after intra-cardiac surgery in adults. Anesth Analg 56: 703–708

Revuelta J M, Cagigas J C, Bernal J M et al 1992 Partial replacement of mitral valve by homograft: an experimental study. J Thorac Cardiovasc Surg 194: 1274–1279

Robinson M C, Gross D R, Zeman W et al 1995 Minimally invasive coronary artery bypass grafting: a new method using an anterior mediastinotomy. J Cardiovasc Surg 10: 529–536

Rodriguez C R, Khan S, Platt M W et al 1997 Anaesthesia for minimally invasive coronary artery bypass grafting. Br J Intensive Care In press

Ross D N, Jackson M, Davies J 1992 The pulmonary autograft: a permanent aortic valve. Eur J Cardiothorac Surg 6: 113–117

Sarsam M A I, Yacoub M 1993 Remodeling of aortic valve annulus. J Thorac Cardiovasc Surg 105: 435–438

Sen P K, Udwadia T E, Kinare S G et al 1965 Transmyocardial acupuncture, a new approach to myocardial revascularization. J Thorac Cardiovasc Surg 50: 181–189

Sen P K, Daulatram J, Kinare S G et al 1968 Further studies in multiple transmyocardial acupuncture as a method of myocardial revascularization. Surgery 64: 861–870

Slogoff S, Keats A S 1989 Randomized trial of primary anesthetic agents on outcome of coronary artery bypass operations. Anesthesiology 70: 179–188

Stanbridge R De L, Cohen A, Hadjinikolaou L et al 1996 Early experience with minimal invasive coronary artery bypass grafting. Heart 75 (Suppl): 69

Stanley T H, Webster L R 1976 Anesthetic requirements and cardiovascular effects of fentanyl-oxygen and fentanyl-diazepam-oxygen anesthesia in man. Anesth Analg 57: 411–416

Souza U V A, Jebara V, Acar C et al 1992 Mitral valve repair in patients with endomyocardial fibrosis. Ann Thorac Surg 54: 89–92

Tamai J, Kosakai Y, Yoshioka T et al 1995 Delayed improvement in exercise capacity with restoration of sinoatrial node response in patients after combined treatment with surgical repair for organic heart disease and maze procedure for atrial fibrillation. Circulation 91: 2392–2399

Tuman K J, McCarthy R J, Pharm D et al 1992 Differential effects of advanced age on neurologic and cardiac risks of coronary artery operations. J Thorac Cardiovasc Surg 104: 1510–1517

Tuman K J, McCarthy R J, Spiess B D et al 1989 Does choice of anesthetic agent significantly affect outcome after coronary artery surgery? Anesthesiology 70: 189–198

Vrandecic M, Gontijo B F, Fantini F A et al 1992 Anatomically complete heterograft mitral valve substitute. J Heart Valve Dis 1: 254–259

Westaby S, Pillai R, Parry A et al 1993 Does modern cardiac surgery require conventional intensive care? Eur J Cardiothorac Surg 7: 313–318

R. Zimlichman

New concepts in understanding the hypertensive syndrome – therapeutic implications

During recent years, major changes in understanding the mechanisms and pathogenesis of hypertension have evolved. This major change in concept had major influence on changes in the therapeutic approach of hypertension as dictated by the new pathogenetic mechanisms.

The origin of the need to search for a new pathogenetic mechanisms for development of hypertension rose when data from big studies were reviewed and the reduction of stroke was found to be as expected (MacMahon et al 1986), but disappointing results were found regarding reduction of coronary artery disease which was roughly half the predicted (Samuelsson et al 1987). In the Multiple Risk Factor Intervention Trial (1986) (MRFIT), no benefit to coronary artery disease was seen at all and this became significant only 10.5 years after the beginning of the study. In the meta-analysis performed by MacMahon, the reduction in diastolic blood pressure was found to be only 5.7 mmHg during an average follow up of 5.6 years (MacMahon et al 1986).

The suggested explanations for this lack of expected decrease in coronary artery disease included: aggravation of other risk factors such as glucose metabolism, adverse effect on lipid profile, diuretic effect on rhythm disturbances, etc. It was also suggested that the blood pressure reduction was too small and that the length of the studies (more than 5 years in most studies), too short. This was a problematic explanation, since significant decrease in coronary artery disease was seen within one year of lipid lowering studies (European Working Party on High Blood Pressure in the Elderly 1985).

Another suggested explanation was that as hypertension is a non homogenous group and that partial 'resistance' to treatment in a specific subgroup of hypertensive patients renders the disease partially responsive, thus 'diluting' the beneficial effects of treatment to far beyond the expected coronary artery disease risk reduction. Some of these subgroups, like patients

Prof. R. Zimlichman MD, The E. Wolfson Medical Center, PO Box 5, Holon 58100, Israel

without metabolic syndrome may benefit from 'simple' blood pressure reduction, while other patients with additional risk factors require treatment of multiple risk factors necessitating a totally different therapeutic approach.

It was accepted for many years that hypertension is a non homogenous disease which includes groups of patients with elevated blood pressure but with various clinical presentations. It was clear that the obese bradycardic patient with mainly diastolic hypertension represents a different spectrum of the hypertensive syndrome than the lean tachycardic patient with mainly systolic hypertension. Reduction of the coronary risk in the subgroups by a specific medication will not necessarily have a similar effect regarding other risk factors in other subgroups of the broad clinical spectrum of the hypertensive syndrome. During recent years, the concept of clustering of risk factors gained growing attention. The association between hypertension, hyperinsulinemia impaired glucose metabolism and obesity was shown to be present at far too high a frequency, suggesting a common pathogenetic mechanism. In several epidemiological studies, obesity was found in most hypertensive patients (Lauer et al 1975). Glucose intolerance, independent of obesity, was found to be associated tightly with hypertension (Modan et al 1985). The San Antonio Heart Study demonstrated overlap among hypertension diabetes and obesity (Ferrannini et al 1990). It has been estimated that by 50 years of age, 85% of diabetic patients are hypertensive and obese, 80% of obese subjects have abnormal glucose tolerance and are hypertensive and 67% of hypertensive subjects are both diabetic and obese (MacMahon 1984, Ferrannini et al 1990). Numerous studies have shown that insulin resistance is a common finding shared by hypertension obesity and diabetes (MacMahon 1984, Ferrannini et al 1987).

It is becoming evident that insulin resistance and the resultant hyperinsulinemia may be the key metabolic abnormality of, or even may be causally related with, the metabolic syndrome, leading to hypertension but being associated with dyslipidemia and obesity.

It has been shown, in animal studies, that exogenous hyperinsulinemia further increases blood pressure in genetically predisposed hypertensive rats, but not in normotensive Wisto-Kyoto rats (Zimlichman et al 1995a), and induces vascular and myocardial structural damage especially in hypertensive rats but also to a lesser extent in normotensive Wisto-Kyoto rats (Zimlichman et al 1995b). We found that exogenous hyperinsulinemia induced severe medial proliferation in coronary arterioles of genetically predisposed hypertensive rats to an extent that 50% of the rats developed myocardial infarction (Zimlichman et al 1997). In another study, we have shown that sucrose feeding to Sprague-Dawley rats caused hyperinsulinemia and a significant increase in blood pressure, which returned to normal following correction of hyperinsulinemia by administration of the α-glucosidase inhibitor, acarbose (Madar et al 1997).

Numerous reports have shown close association between blood pressure and plasma insulin levels in both obese and non-obese human subjects (Modan et al 1985, Ferrannini et al 1987, Swislocki et al 1989, Rocchini et al 1987, 1991).

It should be stressed that plasma insulin levels reflect secretion, distribution, degradation and response to dietary load. Thus more standardized methods for estimation of insulin sensitivity were developed, such as insulin glucose ratio, post glucose load insulin measurement and, the most accurate but not simple to perform, especially in large groups of patients, the euglycemic hyperinsulinemic clamp technique. Significant linear correlation has been shown using these methods to correlate blood pressure and insulin sensitivity.

It has also been shown that factors known to improve insulin resistance, such as weight loss and exercise, are associated with blood pressure reduction (Rocchini et al 1987, 1989). Based on current data, it appears that hypertension and insulin resistance are causally related, at least in subjects with genetic predisposition for hypertension. The fact that in certain species, like dogs, hyperinsulinemia failed to increase blood pressure, may lead to the conclusion that genetic or other factors may play a role in the development of hypertension (Hall et al 1990).

MECHANISMS OF HYPERTENSION DEVELOPMENT

It is believed that the key issue in the metabolic syndrome is the selective insulin resistance, i.e. only part of insulin actions are impaired. This develops due to genetic factors, obesity or other environmental factors. Insulin, being secreted in excess leads to altered transmembrane ion flux, sodium retention, increased sympathetic nervous system activity and altered vascular function. But the most important result of hyperinsulinemia is its action as a growth factor inducing vascular smooth muscle cell hyperplasia and hypertrophy of cardiomyocytes. The vascular changes are typical of the tissue damage that is seen in progression to atherosclerosis. It is clear today that insulin and insulin growth like factors are mitogens that are capable of stimulating smooth muscle proliferation (Stout et al 1975, Eliahou et al 1995) leading to hypertrophy and hyperplasia and tissue changes that will progress to atherosclerosis.

In summary, although it is still possible that hyperinsulinemia is a simple marker of hypertension, numerous animal and human studies imply that hyperinsulinemia is directly and causally related to hypertension and to structural tissue change.

ATHEROGENIC EFFECTS OF METABOLIC HYPERTENSION

Hyperinsulinemia and insulin resistance affect lipid metabolism increasing low density lipoproteins and very low density lipoproteins with a substantial decrease in high density lipoproteins (Samuelsson et al 1987), are associated with collagen synthesis and content in arterial wall (Gilligan & Spector 1984), increased permeability (Wu et al 1990), vascular smooth muscle cell proliferation (Dzau 1990) and abnormal clotting factors (Laakso et al 1989).

INSULIN RESISTANCE AND CORONARY HEART DISEASE

Insulin infusions have been shown to accelerate atherosclerosis in a perfused human artery; they were shown to induce DNA synthesis and proliferation of vascular smooth muscle cells by way of the IGF-1 receptor (Banskota et al 1989, Foster 1989).

Further discussion in depth into this topic is beyond the scope of this review and can be found elsewhere (MacMahon et al 1984, Pool 1993). However, from the new concepts of causal association between hypertension, insulin resistance and other cardiovascular risk factors, a new understanding of hypertension resulted. Hypertension is considered today as one of the symptoms of the metabolic syndrome, i.e. no longer as a separate disease but as one of the presentations of a set of symptoms that together create the metabolic syndrome. We did not totally cancel the old concept of hypertension. We can still find, rarely, the lean hypertensive with normal insulin sensitivity, however, this patient represents a minority of the wide spectrum of hypertension.

THE METABOLIC SYNDROME

Thus, from the traditional definition of hypertensive subgroups, we create a new modern approach which defines the metabolic syndrome – as a group that comprises approximately 70–80% of all hypertensive subjects. This group should be classified as secondary hypertension, since we understand the mechanisms of development of hypertension in this syndrome but not its cause (genetic?) or cure. The second small group of secondary hypertension comprises the traditional 5–10% of hypertensive patients and represents patients with renovascular, endocrine and other causes of secondary hypertension.

Therefore the new group of essential hypertension includes patients with metabolic syndrome and with other diseases that induce secondary hypertension. It should be stressed that the transfer of the metabolic syndrome as a new major group from essential to secondary hypertension is somewhat semantic but, still, the change in the modern concept signifies definition of a major group of metabolic syndrome which comprises 70–80% of all patients with hypertension. If we accept the concept that hyperinsulinemia stands in the centre of the metabolic syndrome and that additional metabolic derangements, like dyslipidemia and obesity, are also a part of the syndrome, we will be able to understand the basic properties of the metabolic syndrome and its therapeutic significance.

We can now understand: (i) how loss of weight will improve dyslipidemia, insulin resistance and also lower blood pressure; and (ii) how, what in the past seemed to be separate unassociated diseases (hypertension, insulin resistance, hyperinsulinemia, non-insulin dependent diabetes mellitus (NIDDM) and dyslipidemia) can improve with a single treatment – weight loss. This is only possible if these diseases are not separate but are various expressions of one common problem – the metabolic syndrome.

MODERN APPROACH TO TREATMENT

Also we can now easily understand how, in humans, treatment with troglitazone, seemingly an oral antidiabetic, induces not only improvement in glycemia levels, but also reduces blood pressure. This is possible only if troglitazone acts through improvement of insulin sensitivity and with abstention from alcohol (Sowers et al 1991). It has been also clearly shown that most of the non-pharmacological treatments like low sodium, low calorie diet with weight loss exercise, and abstention from alcohol, that are so strongly recommended for hypertensive patients, act through correction of insulin sensitivity and other metabolic derangements associated with the metabolic syndrome (Pool 1993). From understanding the new concept of the metabolic syndrome, a major change in therapeutic considerations must arise. We should primarily examine the metabolic effects of antihypertensive medications relating to their effect on insulin resistance and other metabolic cardiovascular risk factors. How we can comply with the 'uneasy' or disturbing recommendations of the Joint National Committee regarding the choice of antihypertensive medications, bearing in mind the concept of metabolic syndrome. We can easily find a drawback in the recommendations of the Joint National Committee considering special groups of hypertensives with other cardiovascular risk factors, such as patients with diabetes, dyslipidemia, etc. In these, diuretics and β blockers are not advisable, but ACE inhibitors, calcium blockers and α blockers are highly recommended. The major change regarding this point is that this special therapeutic approach recommended for special small groups, should be applied to 80% of the hypertensive population, since these belong to the metabolic syndrome.

The modern approach to the treatment of hypertension is based upon the consensus that treatment should aim at lowering the total risk to an individual and not simply treat a certain value of blood pressure, glucose or lipids (Pyorala et al 1994). Thus, the understanding that certain antihypertensive medications can worsen metabolic cardiovascular risk factors is of the utmost importance. Some large outcome trials published in the 1980s gave poor results regarding cardiovascular morbidity and mortality (MacMahon et al 1986). In other studies, β blockers were not found to be as effective in primary prevention as in secondary prevention. It is known that β blockers lower high density lipoprotein concentrations and increase triglyceride and very low density lipoprotein levels (Ames 1986a). Diuretics are also known to alter the lipoprotein pattern increasing both low density lipoproteins, cholesterol, triglycerides and very low density lipoproteins, a lipoprotein pattern associated with increased cardiovascular risk (Ames 1986b). The changes in lipoprotein levels in this way probably increase cardiovascular risk to levels that counteract any benefit of blood pressure lowering. It has been shown that treatment with diuretics and β blockers is generally associated with an increase in insulin resistance (Pollare et al 1989a, 1989b, 1989c, Hanni et al 1994). These results are contrary to the results seen with calcium channel blockers (Pollare et al 1989b, Lind et al 1994, 1995, Reneland et al 1994), ACE-inhibitors (Ferrannini et al 1987, Skarfors et al 1989, Swislocki et al 1989, Zimlichman et al 1995a) and α blockers. Generally, it can be said that, regarding insulin resistance, β blockers and diuretics reduce insulin sensitivity, calcium channel blockers are neutral, while ACE-inhibitors are associated with mild, and α_1 blockers with significant, improvement. In addition, hypertensives treated for 10 years with a combination of a diuretic, β blockers and hydralazine developed overt diabetes more often than normotensive men matched for basal metabolic index, cholesterol, triglycerides and intravenous glucose tolerance test (Skarfors et al 1989). It should be stressed, however, that the rationale for minimizing all cardiovascular risk factors is strongly supported, but is still a somewhat hypothetical issue. Several big studies are being performed now and the data should be available soon.

Regarding the evidence presented in this review, it appears logical that patients with hypertension and the metabolic syndrome, i.e. insulin resistance and dyslipidemia, should be treated with medication that will not aggravate their cardiovascular risk factors. The close co-location of the atherosclerosis susceptibility gene (ATHS) and the insulin receptor gene (INR) may suggest a common genotype (Nishina et al 1992). This gene may be modified by physical activity, diet, drugs and other factors.

In treating essential hypertension, when the patient suffers from metabolic abnormalities, lowering the blood pressure alone will not achieve optimal results. The failure to recognize metabolic hypertension means that concomitant treatment of insulin resistance, dyslipidemia and other risk factors are overlooked. Modern treatment of hypertension and of metabolic factors is considered as the optimal treatment, aimed not only for the correction of blood pressure, but also of other metabolic factors for the prevention of atherosclerosis.

References

Ames R P 1986a The effects of antihypertensive drugs on serum lipids and lipoproteins II. Non-diuretic drugs. Drugs 32: 335–357

Ames R P 1986b The effects of antihypertensive drugs on serum lipids and lipoproteins. I. Diuretic drugs. Drugs 32: 260–278

Banskota N K, Taub R, Zellner K et al 1989 Insulin, insulin-like growth factor I and platelet-derived growth factor interact additively in the induction of the protooncogene c-myc cellular proliferation in cultured bovine aortic smooth muscle cells. Mol Endocrinol 3: 1183–1190

Dzau V J 1990 Atherosclerosis and hypertension: mechanisms and interrelationships. J Cardiovasc Pharmacol 15 (Suppl 5): S59–S64

Eliahou H E, Zeidel L, Gefel D et al 1995 Insulin increases arteriolar wall thickness in SHR and WKY rats independently of blood pressure. In: Cardionephrology, Il cuore nelle nefropatie e nella dialisi. Cosenza, Italy: Editoriale Bios, 65–68

European Working Party on High Blood Pressure in the Elderly 1985 Mortality and morbidity results from the European working party on High Blood Pressure in the Elderly trial. Lancet i: 1349–1354

Ferrannini E, Buzzigoli G, Bonadonna R et al 1987 Insulin resistance in essential hypertension. N Engl J Med 317: 350–357

Ferrannini E, Haffner S M, Stern M P 1990 Essential hypertension: an insulin-resistance state. J Cardiovasc Pharmacol 15 (Suppl 5): S18–S25

Foster D W: Insulin resistance – a secret killer [editorial]? 1989 N Engl J Med 320: 733–734

Gilligan J P, Spector S 1984 Synthesis of collagen in cardiac and vascular walls. Hypertension 6 (Suppl 3): III-44–III-49

Hall J E, Brands M W, Kivligh S D, Mizelle H L, Hidebrandt D A, Gaillard C A 1990 Chronic hyperinsulinemia and blood pressure: interaction with catecholamines? Hypertension 15: 519–527

Hanni A, Andersson P E, Lind L, Lithell H 1994 Electrolyte changes and metabolic effects of lisinopril/bendrofluazide treatment. Results from a randomized, double-blind study with parallel groups. Am J Hypertens 7: 615–622

Laakso M, Sarlund H, Mykkanen L 1989 Essential hypertension and insulin resistance in non-insulin-dependent diabetes. Eur J Clin Invest 19: 518–526

Lauer R M, Connor W E, Leaverton P E, Reiter M A, Clarke W R 1975 Coronary heart disease risk factors in school children: the Muscatine study. J Pediatr 86: 697–708

Lind L, Berne C, Pollare T, Lithell H 1994 Metabolic effects of isradipine as monotherapy or in combination with pindolol during long-term antihypertensive treatment. J Intern Med 236: 37–42

Lind L, Berne C, Pollare T, Lithell H 1995 Metabolic effects of anti-hypertensive treatment with nifedipine or furosemide: a double-blind, cross-over study. J Hum Hypertens 9: 137–141

MacMahon S W, Blacket R B, MacDonald G I, Hall W 1984 Obesity, alcohol consumption and blood pressure in Australian men and women: the National Heart Foundation of Australia Risk Factor Prevalence Study. J Hypertens 2: 85–91

MacMahon S W, Cutler J A, Furberg C D, Payne G H 1986 The effects of drug treatment for hypertension on morbidity and mortality from cardiovascular disease: a review of randomized controlled trials. Prog Cardiovasc Dis 3 (Suppl 1): 99–118

Madar Z, Cohen Melamed E, Zimlichman R 1987 Acarbose: reduces blood pressure and improves insulin sensitivity in sucrose-induced hypertension in rats. Isr J Med Sci In press

Modan M, Halkin H, Almog S et al 1985 Hyperinsulinemia: a link between hypertension, obesity and glucose intolerance. J Clin Invest 75: 809–817

Multiple Risk Factor Intervention Trial Research Group 1986 Coronary heart disease, death, nonfatal acute myocardial infarction and other clinical outcomes in the Multiple Risk Factor Intervention trial. Am J Cardiol 58: 1–13

Nishina P M, Johnson J P, Naggert J K et al 1992 Linkage of atherogenic lipoprotein phenotype to the low density lipoprotein receptor locus on the short arm of chromosome 19. Proc Natl Acad Sci USA 89: 708–712

Pollare T, Lithell H, Selinus I, Berne C 1989a Sensitivity to insulin during treatment with atenolol and metoprolol: a randomized, double blind study of effects on carbohydrate and lipoprotein metabolism in hypertensive patients. BMJ 298: 1152–1157

Pollare T, Lithell H, Morlin C et al 1989b Metabolic effects of diltiazem and atenolol: results from a randomized, double-blind study with parallel groups. J Hypertens 7: 551–559

Pollare T, Lithell H, Berne C 1989c A comparison of the effects of hydrochlorothiazide and captopril on glucose and lipid metabolism in patients with hypertension. N Engl J Med 321: 868–873

Pool P E 1993 The case for metabolic hypertension: is it time to restructure the hypertension paradigm? Prog Cardiovasc Dis 36: 1–38

Pyorala K, De Backer G, Graham I, et al on behalf of the Task Force: Prevention of Coronary Heart Disease in Clinical Practice 1994 Recommendations of the Task Force of the European Society of Cardiology, European Atherosclerosis Society and European Society of hypertension. Eur Heart J 15: 1300–1331

Reneland R, Andersson P-E, Hanni A, Lithell H 1994 Metabolic effects of long-term angiotensin-converting enzyme inhibition with fosinopril in patients with essential hypertension: relationship to angiotensin-converting enzyme inhibition. Eur J Clin Pharmacol 46: 431–436

Rocchini A P 1991 Insulin resistance and blood pressure regulation in obese and nonobese subjects. Hypertension 17: 837–842

Rocchini A P, Katch V, Schork A, Kelch R P 1987 Insulin's role in blood pressure regulation during weight loss in obese adolescents. Hypertension 10: 267–273

Rocchini A P, Key J, Bondie D et al 1989 The effect of weight loss on the sensitivity of blood pressure to sodium in obese adolescents. N Engl J Med 321: 580–585

Samuelsson O G, Wihelmsen L W, Svardsudd K F 1987 Mortality and morbidity in relation to systolic blood pressure in two populations with different management of hypertension: the study of men born in 1913 and the multifactorial primary prevention trial. J Hypertens 5: 57–66

Skarfors E T, Lithell H O, Selnus I et al 1989 Do antihypertensive drugs precipitate diabetes in predisposed men? BMJ 298: 1147–1152

Sowers J R, Standly P R, Ram J L, Zemel M B, Resnick L M 1991 Insulin resistance, carbohydrate metabolism and hypertension. Am J Hypertens 4: 466–472

Stout R W, Bierman E, Ross R 1975 Effect of insulin on the proliferation on cultured primate arterial smooth muscle cells. Circ Res 36: 219–237

Swislocki A L, Hoffman B B, Sheu W H, Chen Y D, Reaven G M 1989 Effect of prazosin treatment on carbohydrate and lipoprotein metabolism in patient with hypertension. Am J Med 86: 14–18

Wu C H, Chi J C, Jerng J S et al 1990 Transendothelial macromolecular transport in aorta of spontaneously hypertensive rats. Hypertension 16: 154–161

Zimlichman R, Matas Z, Gass S et al 1995a Hyperinsulinaemia increases blood pressure in genetically predisposed spontaneously hypertensive rats but not in normotensive Wistar-Kyoto rats. J Hypertens 13: 1009–1013

Zimlichman R, Zeidel L, Gefel D et al 1995b Insulin induces medial hypertrophy of myocardial arterioles in rats. Am J Hypertens 8: 915–920

Zimlichman R, Zaidel L, Nofech-Mozes S et al 1997 Hyperinsulinemia induces myocardial infarctions and arteriolar medial hypertrophy in SHR but not in WKY rats. Am J Hypertens In press

H. Daly F. Moscuzza

Anaesthesia for the child with congenital heart disease undergoing non-cardiac surgery

Congenital heart disease (CHD) has a world-wide incidence of 8 per 1000 live births. Approximately 3500 children per year undergo cardiac surgery in the UK. These patients present for corrective or palliative cardiac surgery and for associated or unrelated conditions. Although cardiac surgery for CHD is performed in specialty centres, the improved lifespan of these patients results in more presenting for common, non-cardiac surgical procedures. Anaesthesia for these patients requires a knowledge of the pathophysiology of CHD.

In this review we will initially discuss the pathophysiology of CHD. We will then elucidate treatments of the more common types of CHD and follow this by a review of specific problems that relate to these children and their appropriate management. Finally, we will discuss the anaesthetic management of these children for non-cardiac surgery.

PHYSIOLOGY AND PATHOPHYSIOLOGY

The neonatal circulation must convert from a fetal circulation to an adult type and goes through a transitional phase. In order to discuss this transition it is important to understand the fetal circulation.

NORMAL PHYSIOLOGY

FETAL CIRCULATION

The fetal circulation is a parallel circulation. Oxygenated blood from the placenta flows through the umbilical vein to the fetus. Approximately 50% of

Dr Helen Daly MB BCh BaO LRCS/PI FRCA, Senior Registrar, Anaesthetic Department, Guy's Hospital, St Thomas Street, London SE1 9RT, UK

Dr Franco Moscuzza MB BS FRCA, Senior Registrar, Anaesthetic Department, Guy's Hospital, St Thomas Street, London SE1 9RT, UK

the umbilical venous blood (with an oxygen saturation of 75–80%) bypasses the liver by means of a channel called the ductus venosus which lies on the inferior surface of the liver. This channel allows the oxygenated blood from the umbilical vein to bypass the portal circulation (saturation ~26%) and flow directly to the inferior vena cava (saturation ~70%).

Blood from the inferior vena cava enters the right atrium and is shunted across the foramen ovale into the left atrium and then ejected by the left ventricle into the ascending aorta. Therefore, the coronary and cerebral arteries are perfused with blood having a relatively high oxygen tension (saturation ~65%).

Superior vena caval blood, which is less oxygenated (saturation ~40%), flows into the right ventricle and is ejected into the pulmonary artery where 90% of the flow is shunted across the ductus arteriosus into the descending aorta (saturation ~55–60%).

The right ventricle is dominant during fetal life, its output being approximately twice that of the left ventricle.

At birth the lungs, not the placenta, become the organs of gas exchange and the fetal circulation must convert to an adult (series) type circulation; however, the change to the adult circulation is not immediate and the neonatal circulation passes through an intermediate phase called the transitional circulation.

TRANSITIONAL CIRCULATION (SERIES OR PARALLEL)

Until the foramen ovale and the ductus arteriosus are anatomically closed and while pulmonary vascular resistance remains high, right-to-left shunting of blood may occur. In healthy neonates the instability of the cardiovascular system is well tolerated and self-correcting as normal development progresses. However, in the first weeks of life, many of the normal changes occurring in the circulation may be delayed or reversed by congenital heart disease and also by any of the following factors: prematurity; pulmonary disease; sepsis; acidosis; hypothermia; stress; hypoxia; or hypercarbia. It is important to note that in certain types of congenital heart disease the persistence of transitional circulation is necessary to sustain life until surgery can be undertaken.

MAINTAINING FETAL CIRCULATION

The mechanisms for maintaining fetal circulatory pathways are dependent on the foramen ovale, ductus arteriosus and pulmonary vascular resistance.

Foramen ovale

Functional closure of the foramen ovale occurs in the first few hours after birth, when the mean left atrial pressure exceeds the mean right atrial pressure due to an increase in pulmonary venous return to the left atrium. Anatomical closure usually occurs within the first year of life; however a probe patent foramen ovale persists in 50% of children up to the age of 5 years and in approximately 25% of adults. The septum primum acts as a one-way flow valve thereby preventing left-to-right shunting through the foramen ovale, but pulmonary hypertension increases right ventricular afterload, right ventricular pressure and right atrial pressure. If this pressure exceeds left atrial pressure there is right-to-left shunting across the foramen ovale. Any of the factors listed above may increase pulmonary arterial pressure. Coughing and the Valsalva manoeuvres have also been demonstrated to increase right atrial pressure resulting in right-to-left shunting through the foramen ovale.

Ductus arteriosus

Closure of the ductus arteriosus occurs in two stages in normal neonates. Within 24–48 h, functional closure occurs followed by anatomical closure in the following 2–3 weeks. Functional closure occurs by contraction of muscle in the medial layer of the vessel and this is thought to be due to a rise in ductal blood oxygen in normal mature infants. The response to oxygen in premature infants may be different.

Prostaglandins (PG) E_1 and E_2 relax the ductus arteriosus at low and high oxygen arterial tensions, respectively, and are thought to maintain ductal patency during fetal life.

Before anatomical closure of the ductus arteriosus occurs, it may re-open in response to hypoxaemia or an administration of PGE_1 infusion. The factors listed above can also prolong the patency and shunting can occur in either direction.

Pulmonary vascular resistance

Pulmonary vascular resistance decreases rapidly at birth after expansion of the lungs with air and exposure of the pulmonary resistance vessels to alveolar oxygen. At 24 h of age, pulmonary arterial pressure falls below systemic pressure in normal infants. However the pulmonary arterial tree has to undergo major changes for the pulmonary vascular resistance to decrease to adult levels and these changes occur over the next few years. The pulmonary vascular resistance and pressure decrease relatively quickly throughout the first 5–6 weeks of life and then at a more gradual rate for 2–3 years.

In neonates, the muscular pulmonary vascular bed is very reactive and the degree of hypoxic pulmonary vasoconstriction is much greater than in adults. Any of the factors listed above may delay the rate of reduction in pulmonary vascular pressure. When a neonate is exposed to noxious stimuli, the pulmonary artery pressure may exceed the systemic arterial pressure, resulting in intermittent or continuous right-to-left shunting through the ductus arteriosus, foramen ovale or other cardiac defects.

CLINICAL DIFFERENCES BETWEEN THE NORMAL CHILD AND ADULT HEART

Approximately 30% of muscle mass is composed of contractile elements in the new born myocardium as compared with 60% in the adult, which may explain the increased sensitivity of the immature heart to inhalational anaesthetic agents.

The parasympathetic nervous system of the heart is fully developed at birth and vagal tone is predominant in children, whereas the sympathetic nervous system is incomplete at birth. The ventricles are non-compliant in infants and are very sensitive to increases in volume and have a poor ability to increase stroke volume. The cardiac output is, therefore, rate dependant. The poor compliance and the similarity in size and wall thickness of the ventricles during the first month of life means that when there is failure of one ventricle this rapidly becomes biventricular.

PATHOPHYSIOLOGY OF CHD

There is a large variety of different congenital heart lesions and only the dedicated paediatric cardiac anaesthetist would have a thorough knowledge of all the different pathologies. However, it is important for all anaesthetists to have some general framework with which to classify the different types of lesions, so that an accurate pre-operative assessment can be made and potential problems during anaesthesia anticipated.

CHD is usually divided into cyanotic and non-cyanotic CHD. Cyanotic heart disease may be due to: (i) obstruction of pulmonary blood flow; (ii) mixing in a common chamber; or (iii) separation of pulmonary and systemic circulations. Non-cyanotic heart disease may be due to: (i) pressure overload of the right or left ventricle; or (ii) volume overload of the atria or ventricles (Table 5.1).

FUNCTIONAL GROUPINGS

There are four main functional groups into which these patients are allocated and each group has different anaesthetic significance.

INCREASED PULMONARY BLOOD FLOW

Examples of this include: persistent ductus arteriosus (PDA), septal defects, aorto-pulmonary (A-P) windows, truncus arteriosus, and total anomalous pulmonary venous drainage (TAPVD). In these examples, left-to-right shunting occurs when the pulmonary vascular resistance decreases in the postnatal period. The increase in pulmonary blood flow and pressure causes progressive intimal thickening and hypertrophy of the medial layer of the pulmonary arteries resulting in increased pulmonary vascular resistance.

Anaesthetic implications

Inhalational induction is normal. Respiratory failure may occur due to decreased pulmonary compliance and increased work of breathing. If left untreated, these infants die in cardiac failure or develop pulmonary vascular disease and eventually Eisenmenger's syndrome (i.e. reversal of shunt and pulmonary hypertension). A decrease in systemic vascular resistance can cause reversal of the shunt with severe cyanosis and death.

DECREASED PULMONARY BLOOD FLOW

Examples of this are Fallot's tetralogy, pulmonary stenosis or pulmonary atresia and tricuspid atresia.

Anaesthetic implications

Inhalational induction is slow. Systemic hypotension can increase right-to-left shunting and infundibular spasm leading to severe hypoxia and subsequent acidosis. Severe lesions of this type are dependant on a patent ductus arteriosus and benefit from pre-operative prostaglandin therapy.

OBSTRUCTIVE LESIONS

Left ventricular outflow obstruction occurs in aortic stenosis and aortic arch abnormalities such as coarctation. Those patients presenting with symptoms early in life often have poor cardiac function and require pre-operative support, such as intermittent positive pressure ventilation, intravenous prostaglandins and inotropes.

TRANSPOSITION OF THE GREAT VESSELS

This is a combination of cyanosis and increased pulmonary blood flow due to the main pulmonary artery arising from the left ventricle and the aorta arising from the right ventricle.

The more common conditions and their approximate incidence are listed in Table 5.1.

Table 5.1 The more common congenital heart conditions and their approximate incidence

Cyanotic congenital heart disease	
Obstruction of pulmonary flow	Tetralogy of Fallot (10%) Pulmonary atresia (3%) Tricuspid atresia (2.5%)
Common mixing chamber	Total anomalous pulmonary venous drainage (3%) Truncus arteriosus (1.5%) Single ventricle (2.5%) Double outlet right ventricle (1.5%)
Separation of pulmonary and systemic circulations	Transposition of the great arteries (10%)
Non-cyanotic	
Pressure overload right or left ventricle	Aortic stenosis (2%) Pulmonary stenosis (3.5%) Coarctation of the aorta (8%) Hypoplastic left heart syndrome (1.5%)
Volume overload ventricle or atria	Ventricular septal defect (16.6%) Patent ductus arteriosus (6.5%) Endocardial cushion defect (5%) Atrial septal defect (3.5%)

Figures in brackets are approximate frequencies in children with congenital heart disease.

SPECIFIC TREATMENT OF THE MORE COMMON TYPES OF CONGENITAL HEART DISEASE

PERSISTENT DUCTUS ARTERIOSUS

Medical

In neonates, a trial of indomethacin may be used (usual dose 0.2 mg/kg 8 hourly for 24 h or 0.2 mg/kg daily for 72 h).

Radiological

Transcatheter closure during cardiac catheterisation. This is the method most often performed for closure in the older asymptomatic child.

Surgical

Open surgical ligation via a thoracotomy.

VENTRICULAR SEPTAL DEFECT

Spontaneous closure normally occurs in 30–40% of all ventricular septal defects (VSD) and, in the majority, this happens during the first year of life. Children with VSDs usually show no signs of congestive heart failure until they are 6–8 weeks old as this is the time when the pulmonary vascular resistance falls to a critical level and allows significant left to right shunting.

Medical

Diuretics are the mainstay of treatment and may be combined with digoxin.

Radiological

Transcatheter closure may be indicated in recurrent or residual defects and pre-operatively in complex CHD (Javorski et al 1995).

Surgical

Correction during cardiopulmonary bypass is usually delayed until the child is 1–2 years old due to the higher mortality in infants and neonates. However, early correction may be indicated if there is failure to respond to medical therapy, if there is a large shunt or evidence of an increase in pulmonary vascular resistance.

ATRIAL SEPTAL DEFECT

Medical

Isolated atrial septal defects are usually asymptomatic in childhood. In rare cases, children may develop symptoms of congestive cardiac failure and may be treated with diuretics and digoxin.

Radiological

Secundum defects are suitable for closure by transcatheter techniques.

Surgical

Large secundum and primum defects require closure during cardiopulmonary bypass.

TETRALOGY OF FALLOT

Medical

Prevention of hypercyanotic spells is with propranolol (0.5–1 mg/kg 8 hourly). Treatment of a hypercyanotic spell is aimed at increasing the systemic vascular resistance, reducing sympathetic stimulation and reducing heart rate in order to decrease right ventricular infundibular narrowing. This can be achieved by: (i) administration of 100% oxygen; (ii) intravenous fluids; (iii) placing in the knee chest position to increase systemic vascular resistance; (iv) morphine (0.1 mg/kg i.v.); (v) phenylephrine (1–2 mcg/kg i.v.); (vi) propranolol (0.05 mg/kg i.v.).

Surgical

These usually undergo surgical correction during cardiopulmonary bypass. In certain cases, either where the pulmonary arteries are small or in low birth weight babies, palliative shunts may be performed initially and followed at a later stage by correction. Although there are different types of shunt, the principle is to increase pulmonary blood flow; for example, a Blalock-Taussig shunt is an anastomosis of the right subclavian artery to the right pulmonary artery. Cardiopulmonary bypass is usually required for these procedures.

TRANSPOSITION OF THE GREAT ARTERIES

Palliative procedures involve atrial septostomy to allow mixing of oxygenated and deoxygenated blood within the heart together with pulmonary artery banding to reduce pulmonary blood flow.

Definitive procedures that may be undertaken involve switching of the right and left structures at the atrial (Senning's or Mustard procedure) or ventricular (Rastelli procedure) level. However, the arterial switch, which involves an anatomical correction, is now the most commonly performed operation.

COARCTATION OF THE AORTA

The procedure of choice is resection of the coarctation with end-to-end anastomosis of the aorta. This is often only possible in neonates and younger children because of the aortic elasticity required. Dacron grafts, patch repairs or angioplasty are required in the older child.

COMMON PROBLEMS

CYANOSIS

Patients with chronic hypoxia develop polycythaemia due to an increase in erythropoeitin level resulting in an increased red cell mass. This leads to an increase in blood viscosity as well as producing an iron deficiency. An haematocrit > 65% is associated with renal and cerebral infarcts in infants and children, especially if they become dehydrated.

Coagulopathy may occur in children with elevated haematocrits and manifests as increases in prothrombin and partial thromboplastin times. The exact mechanism of the bleeding disorder has yet to be elucidated.

INFECTIVE ENDOCARDITIS

The majority of patients with CHD, including most patients who have a corrected lesion, should be considered at risk of developing infective endocarditis. The highest risks are in those patients with prosthetic heart valves, systemic to pulmonary anastomoses or post valvotomy aortic stenosis. The exceptions which do not require prophylaxis are considered to be: (i) uncorrected secundum atrial septal defects; (ii) repaired secundum ASD and VSD; or (iii) PDA which are shown to have no residual defect. Oral endotracheal intubation per se does not require prophylaxis, although passage of catheters through the nose is associated with a transient bacteraemia and intubation via the nasal route should, therefore, be covered by antibiotics (Baum & Perloff 1993) For most procedures, two doses of amoxycillin (50 mg/kg given orally 1 h before and up to 8 h post procedure) are adequate. For 'dirty' cases or high risk cases (those with a history of infective endocarditis or prosthetic valves) this should be given intravenously together with 2mg/kg gentamicin. Erythromycin or vancomycin can be used in the patient with a history of penicillin allergy.

SHUNTING

Intracardiac shunting may be from right-to-left resulting in cyanosis or left-to-right resulting in volume overload of the pulmonary circulation. In addition, shunts may be fixed (obligatory) or variable (dependant). Obligatory shunts are those in which there is a constant defect which is independent of the relationship between pulmonary and systemic vascular resistance and where the pressures between the two structures differ by an order of magnitude, such as in atrioventricular canal defects. Variable shunts occur between two structures with similar pressures and depend on the balance between systemic and pulmonary pressures for the magnitude and direction of the shunt. Factors which can alter the pulmonary vascular resistance (PVR) are summarised in Table 5.2.

PARADOXICAL EMBOLI

Paradoxical emboli occur where there is veno-atrial or right-to-left shunting. Precautions need to be taken against venous emboli and meticulous attention

Table 5.2 Factors which can alter the pulmonary vascular resistance (PVR)

Increased PVR	Positive end expiratory pressure Low FiO_2 Acidosis Hypercarbia
Decrease PVR	High FiO_2 Alkalosis Hypocarbia Vasodilators (e.g. nitrates)

to the avoidance of air in venous lines must be taken. Air and particle filters may be placed in peripheral and central venous lines and other techniques such as the use of self sealing caps on access ports should be used. Nitrous oxide should be avoided as any air emboli that may occur will increase in size. It should also be remembered that most left-to-right shunts can be transiently reversed by a valsalva manoeuvre or a bout of coughing.

DYSRHYTHMIAS

Dysrhythmias may due to:

(i) congenital conduction defects;
(ii) underlying cardiac defects;
(iii) medications that the patient is taking; or
(iv) anaesthetic drugs given perioperatively.

Ventricular arrhythmias and conduction problems occur most commonly after correction of Tetralogy of Fallot, ventricular septal defects and complete atrioventricular canal defects.

Congenital heart block or heart block developing following a surgical procedure is usually treated with a permanent pacemaker; however, if this is not present, a temporary pacing wire may be necessary. Patients may be taking antiarrhythmic medication or on treatment for heart failure which can result in electrolyte abnormalities that predispose to further arrhythmias (Strasburger 1991).

MYOCARDIAL DYSFUNCTION

This may be secondary to the congenital heart problem or be related to previous cardiac surgery. Pressure or volume overload of the ventricle results in a decrease in cardiac reserve and a reduction in ejection fraction. A raised end diastolic pressure may lead to pulmonary oedema and an increase in the work of breathing. In infants this is often manifested as a failure to thrive because of difficulty in feeding combined with the increased metabolic demands.

The mainstay of treatment for patients with congestive cardiac failure is 3-fold: diuretics; digoxin; and vasodilators – most commonly angiotensin converting enzyme (ACE) inhibitors. Clearly, anaesthetic techniques which minimise myocardial depression should be adopted.

EXCESS PULMONARY BLOOD FLOW

Excess pulmonary blood flow has detrimental effects on the heart and lungs. An increase in cardiac output results in pressure overload of the right ventricle which results in right ventricular hypertrophy and the increased pulmonary venous return can lead to left atrial dilatation and pulmonary congestion. The increased pulmonary arterial flow leads to enlargement of the pulmonary vasculature which, together with an enlarged left atrium, can obstruct both large and small airways. If the increased pulmonary flow and pressure remain uncorrected, irreversible pulmonary hypertension will result. Patients with pulmonary hypertension are subject to sudden increases in pulmonary vascular resistance which cause acute right ventricular failure. Excess pulmonary flow leads to decreased lung compliance, increased airway resistance and increased work of breathing.

LEFT AND RIGHT VENTRICULAR OUTFLOW OBSTRUCTION

Left ventricular outflow obstruction results in an hypertrophied left ventricle which impairs left ventricular reserve and predisposes the patient to ventricular fibrillation due to the relative imbalance of oxygen supply and demand. Anaesthetic aims should be to maintain good coronary perfusion pressure and prevent sudden increases in left ventricular work.

Right ventricular outflow obstruction leads to an hypertrophied right ventricle and this is subject to ischaemia. Anaesthetic aims are to maintain coronary perfusion and prevent increases in pulmonary vascular resistance.

ANAESTHETIC MANAGEMENT

Pre-operative assessment will include history, physical examination and investigations. In this review, we will place emphasis on the assessment of the CHD.

Most of these children should have their procedures undertaken in a hospital with full paediatric cardiac support, although each child has to be assessed individually as to whether they require referral to a specialist centre.

Some children, such as those with a successfully treated PDA or ASD, may be managed outside specialist centres by paediatric anaesthetists. At the other end of the spectrum, however, those with severe, complex CHD and those who are symptomatic must be treated in specialist centres, regardless of the surgical procedure being undertaken. They will require full paediatric cardiology back up with availability of paediatric high dependency and intensive care facilities.

The middle spectrum of children, such as those with successful correction of TOF, TGA or valvular surgery, may need to be referred to specialist centres depending on present clinical status and the planned surgical procedure. It is necessary in these cases to liaise with the specialist centre with regard to previous cardiological, surgical and anaesthetic history.

When assessing patients with CHD, it is important to appreciate the underlying cardiac problem and to make some assessment of the degree of limitation this imposes upon them. Generally, patients who have little functional limitation, who are clinically well and taking few or no support drugs, will tolerate surgery well. The stresses of the particular surgery that is to be undertaken must also be borne in mind. Certain authors, however, have suggested that even these patients have a higher incidence of perioperative anaesthetic problems than a similar population without underlying CHD (Stafford & Henderson 1991a,b).

HISTORY

The usual pre-operative anaesthetic assessment is performed with special emphasis on the symptoms relating to the current cardiac state. Of particular importance are the presence of cyanosis, squatting, syncope and wheezing. It is also important to ascertain symptoms of congestive heart failure (CHF), such as exercise intolerance and dyspnoea. Failure to thrive and weight loss can be good indicators of the cardiac status. It is important to place these symptoms in the context of the 'normal' state of the patient.

A history of previous anaesthetics for both cardiac and non-cardiac surgery will provide valuable information regarding the problems that may have occurred. A full drug history must be obtained, as many of these children will be taking medications such as β-blockers, diuretics, digoxin, ACE inhibitors and calcium channel blockers.

The cardiologists should be involved at an early stage and should be able to provide information from recent cardiac catheterisations and echocardiography. It is important to note that whilst these infants may have had cardiac surgery performed it should not be assumed that the CHD has been 'cured'.

EXAMINATION

Although specific diagnosis of CHD is often difficult to ascertain by physical examination alone, it will give an indication as to whether the child is active and looks well or is chronically ill. It is important to assess the respiratory rate and pattern and to look for signs of respiratory distress, such as nasal flaring and grunting.

Pulses should be examined in all extremities and their quality assessed. Of extreme importance is the general well-being and activity of the child. Cyanosis at rest or during exercise should be sought for, as should the presence of an enlarged liver, spleen or fullness of the anterior fontelle. Previous operation sites and vascular access scars should also be noted.

INVESTIGATIONS

The extent of pre-operative investigations performed will depend on the underlying pathology and the nature of the planned surgery. An ECG will provide useful information regarding heart rate, rhythm, ventricular hypertrophy and myocardial ischaemia. This is best reviewed by a paediatric cardiologist. Information from a recent echocardiography (echo) and/or cardiac catheterisation will help to define the extent of the lesion precisely and give information regarding ventricular function and the pulmonary vascular state. Blood tests need to be performed as indicated but a haemoglobin estimation in patients with cyanotic heart disease will help identify severe polycythaemia and clotting studies should also be performed in these patients. Children taking diuretics or digoxin should have urea and electrolytes checked. Other tests such as chest x-ray, pulmonary function tests or arterial blood gas estimations may be indicated. Resting pulse oximetry on air is easily performed and provides a baseline oxygen saturation value.

PREMEDICATION

Premedication is considered safe and desirable for children with CHD. A calm and sedated patient has a reduced oxygen consumption compared with the anxious crying child. Although respiratory depression may occur, its effects are generally offset by the reduction in oxygen demand (DeBock et al 1987). Patients with marked cyanosis (oxygen saturations < 75%), however, may have an unpredictable effect from the premedication and this group should have supplementary oxygen and saturation monitoring following premedication (Stow et al 1988). A variety of premedications have been recommended and no one particular drug or combination of drugs appears to confer an advantage. Morphine 0.1 mg/kg with an antisialogogue such as atropine or glycopyrrolate appears to be well tolerated by patients. Alternatively, a benzodiazepine or chloral hydrate (30 mg/kg) may be given orally. All normal medications should be given on the morning of surgery.

MONITORING

Basic monitoring as described by the Association of Anaesthetists should be undertaken in all cases. It may be necessary to commence oxygen saturation monitoring when the premedication is administered in certain patients with cyanotic heart disease. It should be noted that in patients with cyanotic CHD with resting oxygen saturations of < 80%, different types of pulse oximeters may over- or under-estimate the true oxygen saturation (Severinghaus & Naifeh 1987). In this group of patients, the relationship between end tidal and arterial $PaCO_2$ is widened with the end tidal reading underestimating the arterial $PaCO_2$.

Invasive monitoring of blood pressure and central venous pressure will be required in more complex surgery or more complex heart disease. Attention should be paid to the site of previous monitoring lines, and the fact that the type of surgery performed may influence the siting of monitoring lines; for example, invasive pressure monitoring will be inaccurate on the same side as a Blalock-Taussig shunt or below a residual coarctation.

ANAESTHETIC TECHNIQUE

Although ketamine (1–2 mg/kg i.v.) has been regarded as the agent of choice for induction of anaesthesia in patients with cyanotic congenital heart disease, studies have shown that a wide variety of induction techniques (halothane, fentanyl, thiopentone) may all be employed with little clinical difference (Laishley et al 1986, Greeley et al 1986). If obtaining intravenous access is likely to distress the child, a careful inhalational induction with halothane or sevoflurane in oxygen may be undertaken, although it is important to be alert to rhythm changes when using halothane. If the child is too distressed to tolerate an inhalational induction, then intramuscular ketamine (5–10 mg/kg) may be given with atropine 0.02 mg/kg if an antisialogogue has not been administered as part of the premedication.

If there is airway compromise during inhalational induction and intravenous access has not been obtained, then it is acceptable to administer 100% oxygen and to give intramuscular ketamine (5 mg/kg) and suxamethonium (5 mg/kg) with atropine (0.02 mg/kg) as maintenance of the airway is critical. Once the child is anaesthetised and the airway secured, then intravenous access can be obtained.

Most children with CHD have higher oxygen saturation values when anaesthetised than when awake.

Although children with right-to-left shunts may have slower inhalational inductions and those with left-to-right shunts may have slower intravenous inductions, these observations are not usually clinically relevant and no single technique or agent can be recommended, but a regard to the underlying pathophysiology must be undertaken (Burrows 1992).

MAINTENANCE

Maintenance of anaesthesia is usually with volatile agents and supplementary opiates, such as morphine or fentanyl. In some major procedures or in more complex CHD, a high dose fentanyl technique may be employed, but this will require postoperative ventilation. Children with right-to-left shunts and those with pulmonary hypertension are most safely managed by controlled ventilation with a high inspired oxygen concentration.

Pancuronium has been the muscle relaxant of choice in CHD; it may cause a tachycardia and an increase in cardiac output when given as a bolus for intubation, but this is often beneficial in the child with CHD. Atracurium may be given for shorter procedures and in those patients with significant renal impairment. It is extremely important to avoid hypoxia, hypovolaemia and hypotension.

POSTOPERATIVE CARE

Postoperative management depends upon the pre-operative CHD status and the type of procedure performed. Children who have had minor dental or non-invasive x-ray procedures should be extubated immediately following the procedure. In all children, postoperative hypoventilation must be avoided as it may lead to hypoxic pulmonary vasoconstriction and an increase in pulmonary vascular resistance.

In contrast, abdominal and thoracic procedures are likely to require postoperative ventilation in the paediatric intensive care as will children in whom inotropes are required.

Children with polycythaemia (especially if the haematocrit is > 60%)should be given judicious intravenous fluids until they are tolerating oral fluids. It should be stressed that postoperative transport of patients to high dependency or intensive care units requires the same considerations as in the operating theatre as these children are liable to become unstable during transfer.

Key points for clinical practice

- Paediatric anaesthetists should be involved in the management of the child with CHD undergoing non-cardiac surgery.
- Liaison with paediatric cardiologists pre-operatively is essential.
- A full previous cardiological, surgical and anaesthetic history must be obtained.
- Full clinical assessment of respiratory and cardiovascular systems is essential. Investigations are as required but recent echo and cardiac catheter studies should be available.
- Knowledge of management of changes of pulmonary and systemic vascular resistances.
- Technique of anaesthesia is not of the utmost importance but careful administration with a full knowledge of the pathophysiology of the CHD is vital.

ACKNOWLEDGEMENTS

The authors would like to thank Dr C. Bailey, Consultant Anaesthetist, Guy's Hospital, London, UK for his help in reviewing this manuscript.

References

Association of Anaesthetists of Great Britain and Ireland 1988 Recommendations for standards of monitoring during anaesthesia and recovery

Baum V C, Perloff J K 1993 Anesthetic implications of adults with CHD. Anesth Analg 76: 1342–1358

De Bock T L, Petrilli R L, Davis P J et al 1987 Effect of premedication on preoperative arterial oxygen saturation in children with congenital heart disease (ASA Abstract). Anesthesiology 67: A492

Burrows F A 1992 Anaesthetic management of the child with congenital heart disease undergoing non cardiac surgery. Can J Anaesth 39:5 R60–R65

Greeley W J, Bushman G A, Davis D P et al 1986 Comparative effects of halothane and ketamine on systemic arterial oxygen saturation in children with cyanotic heart disease. Anesthesiology 65: 666–668

Javorski J J, Hansen D D, Lausson P C et al 1995 Paediatric cardiac catheterisation: innovations. Can J Anaesth 42: 310–329

Laishley R S, Burrows F A, Lerman J et al 1986 Effect of anaesthetic induction regimens on oxygen saturation in cyanotic congenital heart disease. Anesthesiology 65: 673–677

Lazzell V A, Burrows F A 1991 Stability of the intraoperative arterial to end-tidal carbon dioxide partial pressure difference in children with congenital heart disease. Can J Anaesth 38: 859–865

Severinghaus J W, Naifeh K H 1987 Accuracy of response of six pulse oximeters to profound hypoxia. Anesthesiology 67: 551–558

Stafford M A, Henderson K H 1991a Anesthetic morbidity in congenital heart disease patients undergoing non-cardiac surgery (abstract). Anesthesiology 75: A1056

Stafford M A, Henderson K H 1991b Anesthetic morbidity in congenital heart disease patients undergoing outpatient surgery (abstract). Anesthesiology 75: A866

Stasburger J F 1991 Cardiac arrhythmias in childhood – diagnostic considerations and treatment. Drugs 42: 974–983

Stow P J, Burrows F A, Lerman J et al 1988 Arterial oxygen saturation following premedication in children with congenital heart disease. Can J Anaesth 35: 63–66

Further reading

Ganong F 1991 Review of Medical Physiology, 15th Edn. Lange Medical Books

Kambam J 1994 Cardiac Anaesthesia for Infants and Children. St Louis: Mosby

Katz J, Steward D J 1993 Anaesthesia and Uncommon Paediatric Diseases, 2nd Edn. Philadelphia: Saunders

Last R J 1984 Anatomy Regional and Applied, 7th Edn. Edinburgh: Churchill Livingstone

Sumner E, Hatch D J 1989 Textbook of Paediatric Anaesthetic Practice. London: Baillière Tindall

Hatch D J, Sumner E, Hellman J 1995 The Surgical Neonate; Anaesthesia and Intensive Care, 3rd Edn. London: Edward Arnold

Thomas S J, Kramer J L 1993 Manual of Cardiac Anaesthesia, 2nd Edn. New York: Churchill Livingstone

6

Simon Finfer Graeme Rocker

Mechanical ventilation in intensive care

For many years, simple volume or pressure-cycled ventilators were used in intensive care units (ICUs) with the primary goal of maintaining normal arterial blood gas tensions. At the same time, the hazards of hypoxaemia, hypercarbia and acidaemia were emphasised in the training of anaesthetic and ICU staff. Whilst these lessons and goals are appropriate to patients undergoing short-term ventilation for surgery, their uncritical application in the ICU is not. In this chapter we review the evidence that injudicious mechanical ventilation causes significant lung damage and increases both morbidity and mortality. We also propose guidelines for the rational use of assisted ventilation in the ICU.

VENTILATOR-ASSOCIATED LUNG INJURY

INCIDENCE AND PATHOLOGY

Mechanical ventilation is one of the commonest reasons for admission to an ICU, but the majority of patients require only short-term ventilation and suffer no complication as a result. Patients with relatively normal lungs ventilated for up to 48 h should suffer minimal complications of ventilation. The majority of patients ventilated for longer will suffer complications, mainly ventilator-associated lung injury and nosocomial pneumonia. In those ventilated for acute lung injury (ALI) and the acute respiratory distress syndrome (ARDS), the incidence of ventilator-associated lung injury is particularly high. Usual consequences of ventilator-associated lung injury are pulmonary air leaks

Simon Finfer, Intensive Therapy Unit, Royal North Shore Hospital of Sydney, St Leonard's, NSW 2065, Australia

Graeme Rocker, Intensive Care Unit, Victoria General Site, Queen Elizabeth II Health Sciences Centre, Halifax, Nova Scotia B3H 3A7, Canada

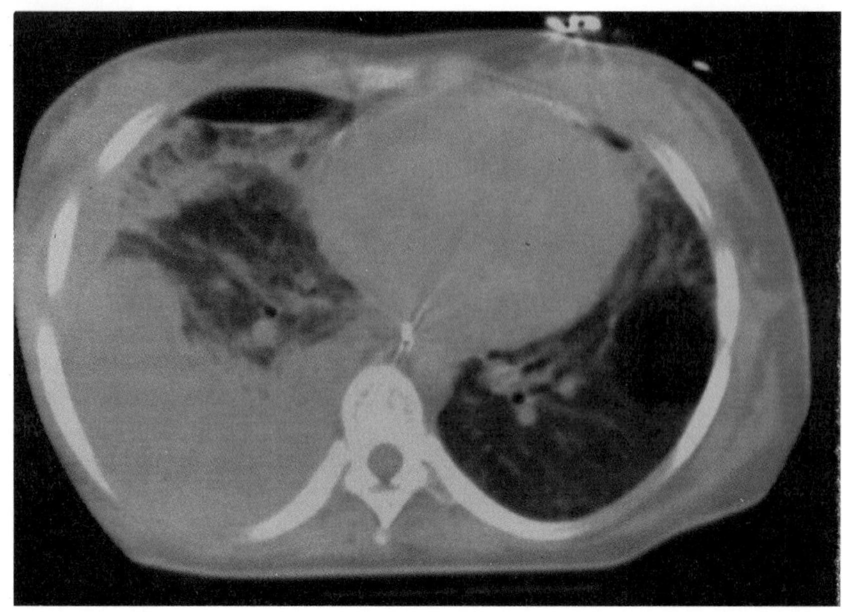

Fig. 6.1 Chest CT scan of previously healthy teenager following 5 weeks' ventilation for ARDS due to non-pulmonary trauma. Scan shows dependent consolidation, right hydropneumothorax, several small aircysts and a large left subpleural cyst. (Reproduced with permission from Finfer & Rocker 1996.)

presenting as pneumothorax, pneumomediastinum, pneumoperitoneum or subcutaneous emphysema. These may present clinically or be detected on routine chest x-rays in 0.5–25% of patients undergoing positive pressure ventilation (Cullen & Caldera 1997, Gammon et al 1992, Petersen & Baier 1983) and in up to 88% of patients with severe acute respiratory failure or ARDS (Gammon et al 1992). More subtle forms of injury such as airspace enlargement, cysts and pulmonary interstitial emphysema are far more common, but much harder to identify. Whilst some airspace enlargement, emphysema and cysts may be detected on chest x-ray, and yet more on chest CT (Fig. 6.1), the true incidence may only be seen by detailed pathological examination. In a recent study, Rouby et al (1993) examined the lungs of 30 young patients who died whilst undergoing mechanical ventilation for acute respiratory failure. The lungs were removed within 20 min of death, inflated to the size of the thoracic cavity, and subjected to detailed histological examination. While only 10 patients (33%) had suffered pneumothoraces, histological examination revealed airspace enlargement in 26 (87%), a similar incidence of pulmonary interstitial emphysema seen in a radiological study (Woodring 1985). These studies suggest that lung damage must be expected in the majority of patients ventilated for acute respiratory failure.

In addition to overt barotrauma and airspace enlargement there is abundant evidence from animal studies that mechanical ventilation can damage the alveolar-capillary membrane producing high permeability pulmonary oedema and a pathological picture indistinguishable from ARDS (Dreyfuss et al 1988, Webb & Tierney 1974). Rats ventilated to a peak inspiratory pressure (PIP) of 14

cmH_2O for 1 h suffered no lung damage, increasing PIP to 30 cmH_2O caused perivascular oedema, and a PIP of 45 cmH_2O resulted in a reduction in respiratory compliance, hypoxaemic respiratory failure, and death. Examination of the lungs revealed marked perivascular and alveolar oedema and haemorrhage (Webb & Tierney 1974). Hernandez and colleagues demonstrated that a mild lung insult plus moderate pressure ventilation produced increased pulmonary capillary permeability when the same insult or ventilation used alone did not (Hernandez et al 1990). These studies suggest that high tidal volume/high pressure ventilation alone produces severe lung damage, and that more moderate airway pressure may be deleterious when applied to already-damaged lungs. These findings, which have been seen in numerous other animal studies, are impossible to validate in clinical practice as there is no indication to ventilate patients with normal lungs using moderate or high airway pressures, and in patients with diseased lungs, it is difficult to separate the effects of ventilation from those of the primary disease process.

MECHANISMS OF LUNG INJURY

Airleaks and pulmonary interstitial emphysema occur more commonly in patients ventilated using high levels of PIP, positive end expiratory pressure (PEEP), respiratory rate (RR), tidal volume (V_T) and minute ventilation (MV) (Gammon et al 1992, Petersen & Baier 1983). As a result the term 'barotrauma' was coined and reinforced the concept that lung damage is due to increased intrathoracic pressure. However, high pressure or volume ventilation is a marker of disease severity and we again face the task of separating the effects of ventilation from those of the underlying disease process. At best, the evidence that high pressure causes lung injury is circumstantial, whereas elegant animal studies and increasing knowledge of lung structure and function during ALI/ARDS provide compelling contrary evidence.

Animal studies

Whereas lung overdistension and high airway pressures will usually coexist in clinical practice, in laboratory studies it is possible to separate them. By binding the chest and abdomen of experimental animals Hernandez et al (1989), Dreyfuss et al (1988) and others have demonstrated that lung damage does not occur, even at very high airway pressures, when lung distension is limited. In addition, Dreyfuss et al demonstrated severe lung damage resulted from using an iron lung to generate high-volume negative pressure ventilation. Thus the evidence from animal studies is consistent and conclusive; it is lung overdistension rather than high pressure that damages the lung.

Evidence from clinical studies

In animals, high pressure ventilation of normally compliant lungs generates V_T several times the physiological norm and lung damage results. If in clinical practice, high pressures are generated ventilating 'stiff lungs' to V_T of 10–15 ml/kg body weight, does lung overdistension occur? At first sight, given that normal vital capacity is 65–75 ml/kg, it would seem unlikely. However,

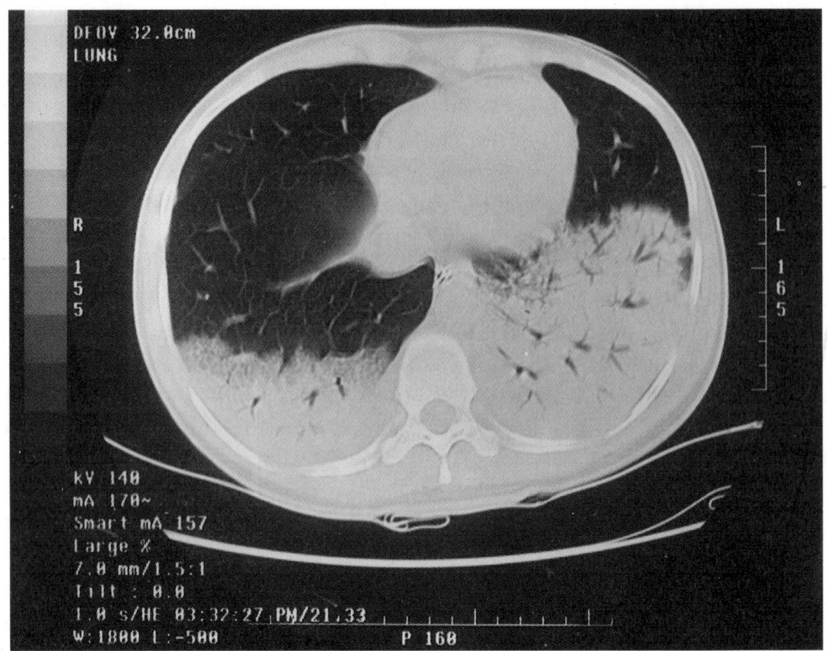

Fig. 6.2 Chest CT of previously healthy 23-year-old with traumatic brain injury and ARDS due to sepsis. CT shows compression atelectasis with dependent consolidation (25% on right, 50% on left) and normally aerated anterior lung.

increasing knowledge of lung structure and pathology during acute respiratory failure suggest otherwise. Although the chest x-ray of a patient with ARDS may suggest a uniform homogenous disease process, chest CT clearly demonstrates marked heterogeneity and that lung structure alters during the evolution and recovery of ARDS (Figs 6.1–6.3 & 6.5,6.6). In a series of elegant CT studies, Gattinoni and colleagues have demonstrated that the lungs of patients with ARDS can be divided into three functional zones: totally collapsed and consolidated lung; collapsed but recruitable lung; and normally aerated lung (Gattinoni et al 1991). To understand these studies some knowledge of the methodology is necessary. CT scan images are produced by reconstructing digitalised measurements of tissue density taken from 360°. As volume and density are known, mass can be calculated and, by analysing the original data, it is possible to calculate the amount of normally aerated and collapsed tissue, and the average weight of lung tissue at any given point in the lung (Gattinoni et al 1988). Using this methodology, Gattinoni and colleagues have demonstrated that the lung weight in ARDS averages twice that of normal, the lung is more dense at all levels, and, like normal lungs, the density increases from non-dependent to dependent zones (i.e. from anterior to posterior in the supine patient). As a consequence, posterior compression atelectasis results with the non-dependent anterior lung remaining normally aerated (Gattinoni et al 1991). These changes differ only in degree from lung CT images of patients undergoing general anaesthesia, where up to 20% of total lung volume may be collapsed or poorly aerated (Reber et al 1996). In patients ventilated for acute respiratory failure, this percentage may be as high as 80% (Fig. 6.2). Significant correlations of lung mechanics and gas exchange with the CT data give further insights into the pathological processes. The degree of hypoxaemia correlates with volume of non-inflated tissue, whilst static lung compliance correlates with volume of normally aerated lung. Compliance corrected for the volume of aerated lung (the specific compliance) is normal (Gattinoni et al 1987). These findings suggest that the lung in ARDS is not truly stiff, rather the amount of lung available for ventilation is reduced (Gattinoni has termed this the 'baby lung'). To avoid overdistending this remaining functional lung, recruitment must be maximised and tidal volume appropriately reduced to match the volume of aerated lung. For example, if we take the extreme case of an 80 kg man with severe ARDS, where 80% of the lung by volume is consolidated, ventilating this patient with a modest tidal volume of 640 ml (8 ml/kg) would be equivalent to a tidal volume of 3.2 l were his lungs normal.

Confirming that overdistension causes ventilator-associated lung injury in patients is difficult, but indirect evidence may come from studying the anatomical distribution of the injury; damage due to overdistension should occur predominantly in the non-dependent lung.

Although Rouby's study did not specifically investigate the anterior-posterior distribution of lung damage, it did report finding pleural aircysts predominantly in the upper lobes and non-dependent lung segments, and that these were consistently associated with underlying alveolar overdistension (Rouby et al 1993). These findings would tend to support our theory. In contrast, Gattinoni and colleagues have addressed this question (Gattinoni et al 1994) and found that bullae were more often found in the **dependent** lung, suggesting that bullae formation occurs due to mechanisms other than alveolar overdistension. Bullae were seen in CTs performed in late ARDS and the authors speculate that infectious or liquifactive necrosis occurs during persistent consolidation; later, when the lung is aerated and again exposed to positive pressure, it breaks down and bullae form. Slutsky has suggested another explanation. Lung at the junction of collapsed and aerated lung may be aerated (recruited) during inspiration and then collapse again (derecruited) during expiration. This constant opening and closing of lung units exerts enormous sheer stresses that may also result in lung damage (Slutsky, 1993).

In our own studies, we have found persistent lung damage in survivors of severe protracted ARDS ventilated with high airway pressures is located predominantly in the non-dependent lung (Finfer & Rocker 1996; Fig. 6.3). In patients with ARDS ventilated using a pressure-limited strategy, we found the dependent lung to be more dense. Fewer bullae were seen than in Gattinoni's patients and, overall, they were distributed in the anterior lung. However, in basal lung slices, bullae were found mainly posteriorly in areas of previously densely consolidated lung (Finfer et al 1997). Owens and colleagues have also reported follow-up CT findings in a population of patients surviving ARDS. They found a persistent reticular pattern that was most marked in lung areas that had been densely consolidated (Owens et al 1994). Although further studies in this area are required, the limited published data suggest that lung damage is caused both by overdistension of aerated non-dependent lung units and by as yet incompletely defined mechanisms occurring in persistently collapsed dependent lung.

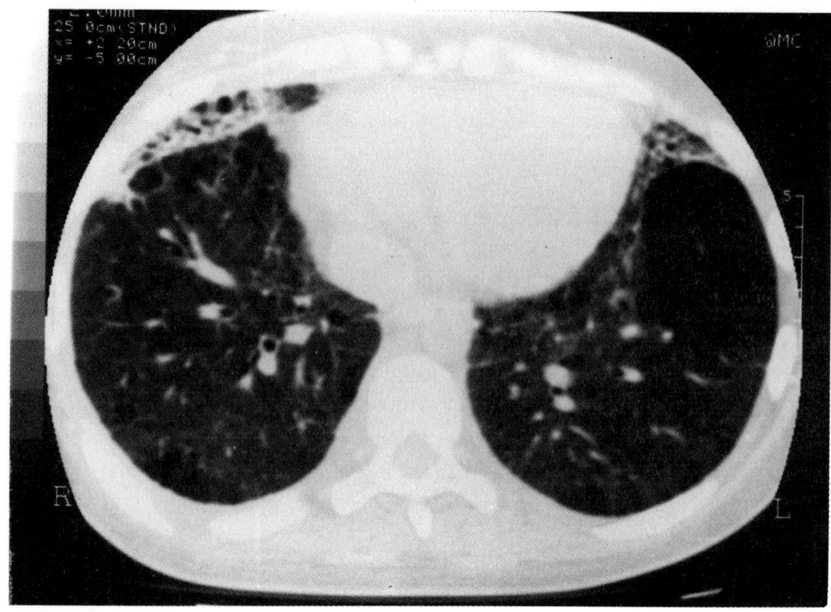

Fig. 6.3 Chest CT 17 months after ICU discharge of same patient as Figure 6.1. CT shows preponderance of damage to anterior lung with peripheral honeycombing, anterior traction bronchiectasis, multiple small subpleural cysts and enlargement of left subpleural cyst. (Reproduced with permission from Finfer & Rocker 1996.)

IMPLICATIONS FOR VENTILATION

PREVENTING COMPRESSION ATELECTASIS

As compression atelectasis results from the superimposed pressure of wet lung, it may be reversed by the application of sufficient PEEP or changing the patient's position.

Positive end expiratory pressure (PEEP)

CT studies demonstrate that PEEP can reverse compression atelectasis. In 22 patients with acute respiratory failure, increasing PEEP from 5 to 15 cmH_2O resulted in progressive clearing of lung densities and improved gas exchange (Gattinoni et al 1988). When PEEP is applied at a level greater than the hydrostatic pressure exerted by overlying lung compression atelectasis can be prevented (Gattinoni et al 1993). It therefore follows that PEEP may need to be applied at a level equal in cmH_2O to the AP diameter of the patients chest, but use of PEEP above this level (8–20 cmH_2O in adults) may be illogical. CT is an excellent research tool but not a practical way to set PEEP in clinical practice. Practical alternatives include examination of the static inspiratory pressure–volume curve of the individual patient, or observed changes in static lung compliance at different levels of PEEP. Early in ARDS, the static pressure–volume has a characteristic shape (Fig. 6.4).The lower inflection point

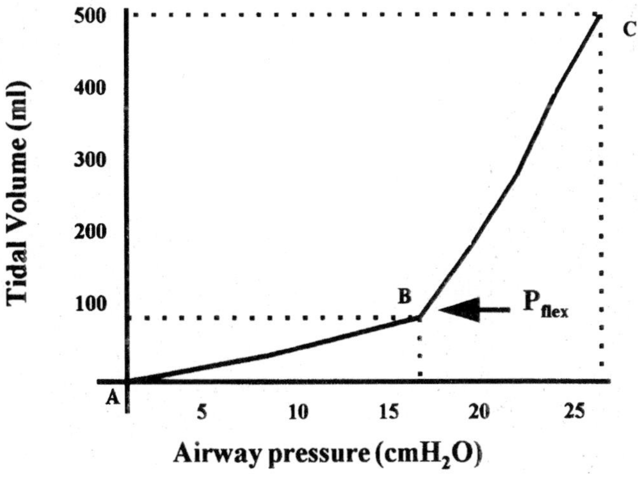

Fig. 6.4 Static inspiratory pressure-volume loop of patient with early ARDS. generated by measuring P_{plat} during randomly ordered breaths of tidal volume 50, 100, 200, 300, 400, and 500 ml from zero end-expiratory pressure. Curve shows lower inflection point (P_{flex}) at 17 cm H_2O.

(P_{flex}) at which compliance appears to improve suddenly is hypothesised to be the pressure at which lung recruitment occurs. Setting PEEP above this level should maintain lung expansion. Amato and colleagues have reported a randomised controlled trial of 'an open lung approach' in severe ARDS (Amato et al 1995). The open lung approach had two aims: first, to recruit collapsed lung and maintain recruitment; and, second, to avoid overdistension and minimise cyclic lung stretch. In the study group PEEP was set at 2 cmH_2O above P_{flex} whilst the control group had PEEP set at 5 cmH_2O or the minimum level required to maintain adequate oxygenation and maintain global oxygen delivery. The mean level of PEEP in the study group on day 1 was 18 cmH_2O, compared with 7 cmH_2O in the control group. The study group achieved significantly better oxygenation, better evolution of pulmonary compliance and had fewer deaths from respiratory failure. The PEEP levels in the two groups converged during the period of the study, with less PEEP being required in the study group and more in the control group. By day 7, there was no significant difference in the level of PEEP between the two groups, but lung function remained significantly better in the study group. Whilst the ventilation strategy varied in other important ways between the two groups, the differences in lung function during the first day or so were most likely due to the different levels of PEEP used.

Another way of setting PEEP is to increase it stepwise whilst observing total thoracic compliance (C_{TH}). PEEP is set at the level above which no further increase in compliance is seen.

As with any medical intervention, PEEP should be used if the potential benefit outweighs the perceived risk. The main drawbacks of the use of PEEP are its effects on the cardiovascular system, and concerns that PEEP itself may be injurious to the lungs.

The adverse cardiovascular effects are a direct result of increased intrathoracic pressure which reduces venous return and lowers cardiac output. These effects, which are most pronounced in fluid depleted patients, can be overcome by temporarily reducing the level of PEEP, ensuring adequate volume resuscitation, and then reapplying the PEEP. The adverse cardiovascular effects are also markedly reduced if PEEP is combined with low tidal volume (5–8 ml/kg) ventilation (Ranieri et al 1995). Although cardiac output may be decreased by PEEP the improvement in oxygenation that occurs usually results in maintenance of global oxygen delivery (Gattinoni et al 1988).

The other main concern that PEEP may damage the lung, and in particular cause airleaks, is also overstated. Miller reported that PEEP of up to 50 cmH_2O in patients with trauma-related ARDS did not cause pneumothoraces (Miller et al 1992) and Gattinoni has found that higher levels of PEEP are associated with a lower incidence of pneumothoraces (Gattinoni et al 1994).

By preventing or reversing lung collapse, PEEP also changes the distribution of ventilation within the lung. In 8 patients with severe ARDS increasing PEEP from zero to 20 cmH_2O increased the proportion of tidal volume distending posterior lung (Gattinoni et al 1995) and this improves ventilation:perfusion relationships. Lung recruitment also decreases the amount of lung collapsing and being recruited during tidal ventilation and so may reduce or prevent the accompanying sheer forces. Two animal studies support this contention. In Webb's study, rats ventilated to a peak pressure of 45 cmH_2O without PEEP developed alveolar oedema and died, the application of 10 cmH_2O of PEEP (a considerable amount in a small animal model) prevented oedema formation and all rats survived (Webb & Tierney, 1974). PEEP was also protective in Dreyfuss' study (1988). In Gattinoni's patients, pneumothoraces occurred not in those ventilated with higher levels of PEEP, but in patients ventilated with increased inflating pressure (the peak pressure to PEEP gradient). Whilst no human study has examined the effect of prophylactic PEEP on outcome in ARDS, current evidence favours the early use of high level PEEP.

Prone positioning

As PEEP acts to prevent compression atelectasis by overcoming the gravitational force exerted by overlying lung, prone positioning may achieve the same end by reversing the direction of those forces. As early as 1976, it was evident that turning patients prone improved gas exchange and that the benefit could be sustained for days (Douglas et al 1977, Phiel & Brown 1976). Interest in this technique since then has been sporadic but, early in 1997, Chatte and colleagues (Chatte et al 1997) reported the largest patient series to date. The effect of prone positioning on short term oxygenation was impressive (PaO_2:FiO_2 ratio improved by 50% at 1 and 4 h) and most patients maintained their improved oxygenation when returned supine. CT studies have suggested that this effect is due to recruitment of collapsed dependent lung (Langer et al 1988; Figs 6.5 & 6.6) and oxygenation improves due to a direct beneficial effect on regional pleural pressure gradient. Factors contributing to the pleural pressure gradient include chest wall and lung shape, weight and mechanics. The lung is effectively triangular with its base along the dorsal plane and this

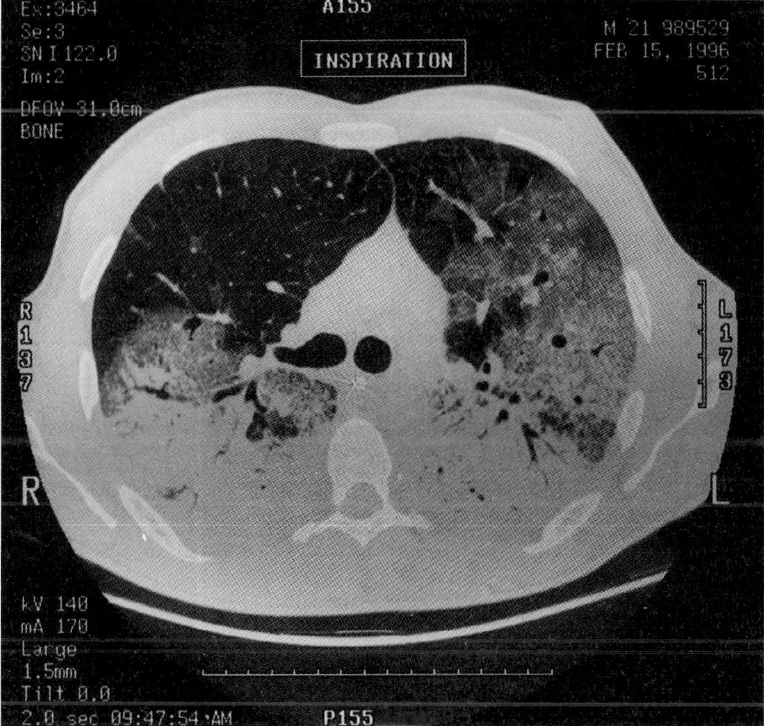

Fig. 6.5 Chest CT of previously healthy young man with ARDS due to near-drowning. Scan taken prone with 15 cmH_2O PEEP and shows widespread consolidation and dependent atelectasis.

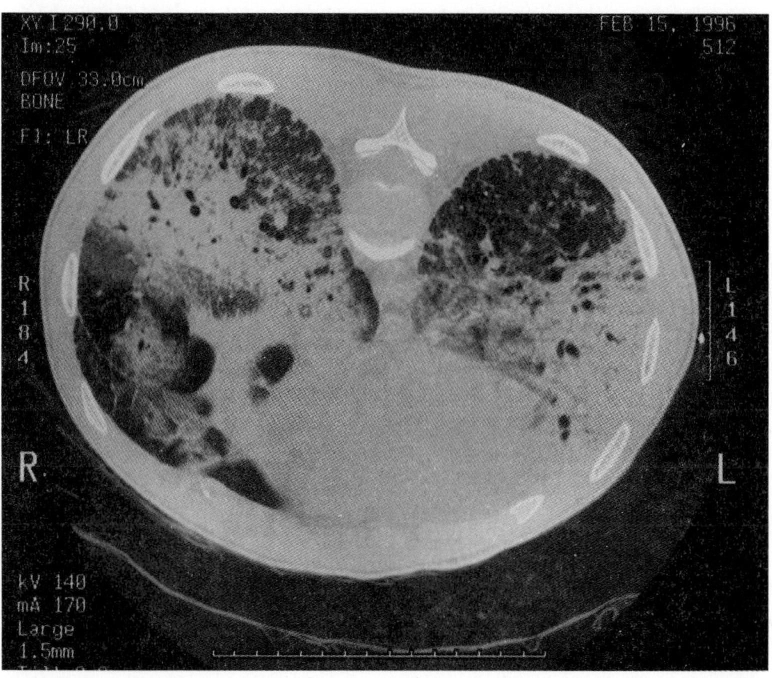

Fig. 6.6 CT scan of same patient after 3 h in prone position. Shows improved aeration of dorsal lung.

results in a greater volume of lung below the prevailing closing airway pressure when supine. In the supine position the weight of the heart, mediastinum, diaphragm, ribs and wet lungs increase the volume of lung in which transalveolar pressure is insufficient to prevent atelectasis. Changes in the pleural pressure gradient also affect regional ventilation, perfusion and their regional ratios. Prone positioning dogs with oleic acid-induced lung injury improves oxygenation and ventilation perfusion ratios, decreases ventilation and perfusion heterogeneity and maintains more uniform and efficient alveolar ventilation over a larger lung volume with a relative increase in ventilation of dorsal lung regions (Lamm et al 1994).

Despite these advantages, turning a patient prone should not be undertaken lightly. It makes intuitive sense for individual ICUs that decide they are going to use this manoeuvre to use it early and plan accordingly. If used only occasionally as a last ditch manoeuvre in the very sickest patients the risk may outweigh the benefit. The manoeuvre requires at least 3 or 4 people to be performed safely. One person should be responsible for the ET tube and ventilator tubing, one for lines, and two others make the turn. Problems are usually relatively minor but may include skin abrasions, facial oedema, extubation, loss of lines and cardiovascular instability. Tubes and lines require careful management, connections must be secure and long enough to reach new positions, hip and shoulder supports should allow the abdomen to protrude. Reasonable contraindications to prone positioning would include haemodynamic instability, a sternal incision, unstable fractures and recent (last day or so) tracheostomy. Once the patient has been turned problems are uncommon. Fridrich et al (1996) reported the effects of 148 cycles of a 20 h prone position, 6 patients were turned back earlier than planned for haemodynamic instability, 3 for nursing needs, and 1 each for loss of ET tube and loss of central venous access. Two patients developed contractures which recovered with physiotherapy (Fridrich et al 1996).

Whether we can protect the lungs of patients with ALI/ARDS by prone positioning remains to be seen. Similarly, the relative effects of prone positioning versus, or combined with, high-level PEEP and/or nitric oxide are only now being investigated. One possible advantage of the prone position over other treatments is that it seems to encourage the drainage of secretions (Langer et al 1988, Phiel & Brown 1976). Although the gas exchange effects of prone positioning are impressive and responders may enjoy a lower ICU mortality rate than non-responders (Chatte et al 1997, Fridrich et al 1996), outcome data from randomised controlled studies currently underway will ultimately determine its role in ICU patients.

AVOIDING ALVEOLAR OVERDISTENSION

Having recruited as much lung as possible, ventilation must be adjusted to avoid overdistension by matching the tidal volume delivered by the ventilator to the volume of functional lung. This poses the question of how do we determine the constantly changing volume of functional lung in a patient with ALI? Lung volumes can only be measured in the ICU with difficulty and a surrogate marker for overdistension must be used. As the lungs in ARDS are not stiff but small and the specific compliance of aerated lung is normal, and knowing that normal lung is fully expanded at a transpleural pressure of 30 cmH_2O, we can design ventilation strategies that aim to prevent transpleural pressure exceeding this level. Pleural pressure can be estimated by an oesophageal balloon, but this technique is not 'user friendly' and has remained a research tool. Consequently it is appropriate to concentrate on the other component of transpleural pressure, the alveolar pressure. Although many studies report peak inspiratory pressure as a marker of the alveolar pressure, measurement of the pause or plateau pressure (P_{plat}) is much more appropriate. The peak pressure is the measured pressure in the ventilator tubing and proximal airway; it reflects the resistance of the ventilator tubing, the endotracheal tube, the airway resistance as well as total respiratory system compliance and it is highly variable depending on inspiratory flow rate. In contrast, a true plateau pressure is measured during a prolonged inspiratory pause when airflow has ceased and pressures have equalised. In this circumstance, P_{plat} is equal to alveolar pressure and if maintained below 35 cmH_2O significant overdistension will be avoided. The advent of pressure/time/volume displays on modern ICU ventilators allows these curves to be observed in patients and permits accurate assessment of alveolar pressure by monitoring the true plateau pressure.

PRESSURE LIMITATION AND PERMISSIVE HYPERCAPNOEA

A ventilator strategy that includes early use of high level PEEP and plateau pressure limitation results in severe limitation of inflating pressure ($P_{infl} = P_{plat} -$ PEEP). If static respiratory system compliance (C_{TH}) is also reduced (and here we are referring to total respiratory system compliance uncorrected for aerated lung volume) then tidal volume will be severely limited. For example, a 70 kg patient with moderate to severe ARDS may have C_{TH} of 20 ml/cmH_2O, if P_{plat} is limited to 35 cmH_2O and 18 cmH_2O PEEP is used, then tidal volume will be 340 ml or 4.9 ml/kg. Unless very high respiratory rate is used this will be inadequate to maintain $PaCO_2$ in the normal range and hypercarbia will result. Is this safe?

There has been concern that acute hypercarbia and respiratory acidosis may impair myocardial performance, and that in patients with head injuries intracranial hypertension may result. Although acidosis impairs myocardial contractility in laboratory experiments, a number of studies have shown that hypercarbia increases cardiac output in ICU patients (Thorens et al 1996), and it may be used cautiously in patients with head injuries if ICP is being monitored.

Despite these concerns, the strategy of allowing $PaCO_2$ to increase above the normal range, referred to as permissive hypercapnia, has become accepted practice in ICUs around the world. Hickling and colleagues reported improved survival in a retrospective series of patients ventilated using this technique and have now reported similar results in a prospective series (Hickling et al 1994). $PaCO_2$ increased up to 19 kPa (140 mmHg) without apparent adverse effects and many others have now reported similar uncontrolled findings. In addition to high-level PEEP, pressure-limitation with permissive hypercapnia formed the other main strand of Amato's 'new approach' ventilation protocol (Amato et al 1995). Patients in the control group were ventilated with an initial tidal volume of 12 ml/kg adjusted up to a maximum of 15 ml/kg to maintain $PaCO_2$ 25–38 mmHg (3.3–5.1 kPa). No attempt was made to control airway pressure. In contrast, pressure limitation was a primary goal in the study group. In these patients, pressure controlled ventilation was used starting with an inspiratory pressure 12 cmH_2O above PEEP. Tidal volume was maintained at less than 6 ml/kg, and PIP less than 40 cmH_2O, respiratory rate was controlled to less than 30 per min with sedation, and an initial $PaCO_2$ of up to 80 mmHg (10.6 kPa) was tolerated. Although full publication of the final results is pending, the study has now been stopped because mortality was significantly reduced in the study group. The study may be criticised on the grounds that the control group underwent more aggressive ventilation than would be normal in many units, but the results can not be ignored. It provides the most compelling evidence to date that a strategy of lung recruitment by high level PEEP, and pressure-limitation with permissive hypercapnia may improve survival in patients with severe acute respiratory failure. However, it remains to be seen if others can duplicate this result particularly as a French-led international study of pressure-limited ventilation has been stopped because no benefit appeared possible from the treatment (Brochard et al 1997). This study is published only in abstract form and so its significance is difficult to judge. Nevertheless the results are at odds with Amato's study and the reasons for this must await the final reports of both studies. Of note is that Brochard's study used the same level of PEEP in both the study and treatment groups.

Mode of ventilation

Lung recruitment and permissive hypercapnia can be achieved using either pressure or volume-cycled ventilation. If pressure-cycled ventilation is used the patient cannot be subjected to an airway pressure above that set. This provides great safety but careful observation of tidal volume is necessary as this may change dramatically as resistance and compliance vary or patient-ventilator asynchrony occurs. Equivalent safety can be achieved with volume-cycled ventilation if the upper pressure alarms are set appropriately. Most modern ventilators will cycle to expiration if airway pressure reaches the upper alarm limit, as a result the set tidal volume will not be delivered and similar vigilance is needed as for pressure-cycled ventilation. The advantage of using volume controlled ventilation is that the set volume may be delivered at a lower pressure if compliance is improving. Ultimately either mode may be used as long as the medical and nursing staff managing ventilation are familiar with the mode employed and the underlying principles to be followed.

NON-ALI/ARDS PATIENTS

Most of the evidence in favour for a high PEEP, volume/pressure-limited ventilation strategy comes from patients with, or animal models of, ALI/ARDS. It is reasonable to ask whether the findings should be generalised to all ICU patients. The occurrence of increased airway pressure in any ICU patient should ring warning bells and prompt a search for the cause. Possibilities include equipment problems such as a blocked or kinked endotracheal tube, or patient problems such as bronchospasm or pneumothorax. With the exception of equipment problems which should be rectified, and patients at risk from increased ICP, adjusting ventilation to limit P_{plat} offers benefit without risk in the majority of ICU patients. In particular, pressure limited ventilation with permissive hypercapnia has been used with great success in patients with asthma (Darioli & Perret 1984). The use of high level PEEP should be reserved for those with early ALI/ARDS in which lung weight is increased. PEEP remains controversial in patients with expiratory airflow limitation (Tuxen 1989) as most have significant intrinsic PEEP and compression atelectasis does not occur. However, increasing CPAP in those breathing spontaneously will reduce work of breathing when intrinsic PEEP is elevated.

THE PRESENT AND THE FUTURE

There is a fair international consensus on the conduct of ventilation in patients with acute lung injury (Slutsky 1994). Pressure and tidal volume limitation with resultant hypercapnia are widely accepted, but there is less consensus on the use of high-level PEEP. Several exciting innovations are currently undergoing clinical evaluation, and these may radically alter the way we ventilate patients in the future. Some of these are discussed briefly below.

Inhaled nitric oxide

Inhaled nitric oxide has received enormous attention (Rossaint et al 1995), and its easy availability led to its introduction into clinical use without rigorous scientific evaluation. There is no doubt that it can improve oxygenation in many patients and prospective randomised controlled trials of its effect on mortality are underway. The largest study to date using well-matched historical controls does not suggest it will have major impact on outcome (Rossaint et al 1993).

Partial liquid ventilation

In partial liquid ventilation the lungs are filled to FRC with perfluorocarbon and the patient is ventilated in a conventional fashion. Partial liquid ventilation is possible because of the unique physico-chemical properties of perfluorocarbons which are simple organic compounds in which the hydrogen atoms are replaced by halogens. Liquid ventilation has been reported in neonates, infants, children and adults (Hirschl et al 1995). It causes dramatic improvements in gas exchange and lung mechanics, appears safe, and randomised controlled trials are underway. Whilst liquid ventilation is an exciting development, we must await the results of properly constructed trials and it may prove most useful in the neonatal and paediatric ICU.

Tracheal gas insufflation

Tracheal gas insufflation refers to the insufflation of fresh gas (usually pure oxygen) into the airway as close as possible to the main carina in combination with conventional ventilation. This results in improved carbon dioxide removal by eliminating anatomical dead space. The technique is simple and non-

Key points for clinical practice

- A minority of patients admitted to ICU will require long term ventilation but in these patients injudicious conduct of mechanical ventilation may increase morbidity and mortality.
- In ALI/ARDS, compression atelectasis results in ventilation of a much reduced lung volume (the 'baby lung').
- The baby lung has normal specific compliance but tidal volume must be reduced to avoid lung overdistension.
- Plateau airway pressure is the best bedside marker of overdistension and should be kept below 35 cmH_2O.
- Early use of high-level PEEP prevents and reverses compression atelectasis improves gas exchange and makes lung damage less likely.
- Hypercarbia is well-tolerated and Pa_{CO_2} should be allowed to increase above normal rather than expose the lung to higher plateau airway pressure.
- A ventilation strategy based on opening the lung with high level PEEP, with strict pressure, tidal volume and respiratory rate limitation has been reported to improve survival in patients with ARDS.
- Tracheal gas insufflation, partial liquid ventilation and non-invasive ventilation are promising new developments.

invasive, can be used without expensive or complex equipment, requires no alteration in the conduct of mechanical ventilation, and may result in improved gas exchange (Belghith et al 1995). Its role in the management of severe respiratory failure remains to be clarified, but its simplicity and inherent safety may justify its use in individual patients without awaiting rigorous outcome data.

Non-invasive ventilation

Recently, renewed interest has been shown in the provision of non-invasive pressure support ventilation (NIPSV) by face mask for acute respiratory failure. Interest is based on its success in avoiding intubation in 70% of patients with exacerbations of chronic obstructive pulmonary disease. Mortality from ARDS has long been associated with multiple organ failure rather than death from hypoxaemic respiratory failure *per se*, and when intubation is avoided the risk from nosocomial pneumonia/sepsis may be substantially reduced. Data on the efficacy of NIPSV in patients with acute lung injury and ARDS are very limited. Rocker has reported its use on 12 occasions in 10 severely hypoxaemic patients with early ARDS (Rocker et al 1997). When NIPSV was used as the primary assisted ventilation strategy intubation was avoided in 6 of 9 episodes. In 3 patients it was used for acute respiratory distress followed self or planned extubations but all 3 required reintubation. Duration of successful NIPSV was approximately 60 h followed by ICU discharge in the next 24–48 h. Survival to hospital discharge was 70%. These promising results suggest the possibility of using NIPSV as an initial ventilation strategy for haemodynamically stable patients with ALI/ARDS.

DEDICATION

This chapter is dedicated to the memory of our co-author Dr John Neville Shephard MB BS FRCA MD who died during its preparation.

References

Amato M B, Barbas C S, Medeiros D M et al 1995 Beneficial effects of the 'open lung approach' with low distending pressures in acute respiratory distress syndrome. A prospective randomized study on mechanical ventilation. Am J Respir Crit Care Med 152: 1835–1846

Belghith M, Fierobe L, Brunet F, Monchi M, Mira J 1995 Is tracheal gas insufflation an alternative to extrapulmonary gas exchangers in severe ARDS? Chest 107: 1416–1419

Brochard L, Roudot-Thoraval F and the Collaborative Group on Vt Reduction 1997 Tidal volume (Vt) reduction in acute respiratory distress syndrome (ARDS): a multicenter randomized study [Abstract]. Am J Respir Crit Care Med 155: A505

Chatte G, Sab J, Dubois J, Sirodot M, Gaussorgues P, Robert D 1997 Prone position in mechanically ventilated patients with severe acute respiratory failure. Am J Respir Crit Care Med 155: 473–478

Cullen D J, Caldera D L 1997 The incidence of ventilator-induced pulmonary barotrauma critically ill patients. Anesthesiology 50: 185–190

Darioli R, Perret C 1984 Mechanical controlled hypoventilation in status asthmaticus. Am Rev Respir Dis 129: 385–387

Douglas W W, Rehder K, Beynen F M, Sessler A D, Marsh H M 1977 Improved oxygenation in patients with acute respiratory failure: the prone position. Am Rev Respir Dis 115: 559–566

Dreyfuss D, Soler P, Basset G, Saumon G 1988 High inflation pressure pulmonary oedema. Respective effects of high airway pressure, high tidal volume, and positive end-expiratory pressure. Am Rev Respir Dis 137: 1159–1164

Finfer S, Rocker G 1996 Alveolar overdistension is an important mechanism of persistent lung damage following severe protracted ARDS. Anaesth Intensive Care 24: 569–573

Finfer S, Wilcox T, Brigs G 1997 Lung injury in ARDS: a computerised tomography study [Abstract]. Anaesth Intensive Care 25: In press

Fridrich P, Krafft P, Hochleuthner H, Mauritz W 1996 The effects of long-term prone positioning in patients with trauma-induced adult respiratory distress syndrome. Anesth Analg 83: 1206–1211

Gammon R B, Shin M S, Buchalter S E 1992 Pulmonary barotrauma in mechanical ventilation. Patterns and risk factors. Chest 102: 568–572

Gattinoni L, Bombino M, Pelosi P et al 1994 Lung structure and function in different stages of severe adult respiratory distress syndrome. JAMA 271: 1772–1779

Gattinoni L, D'Andrea L, Pelosi P, Vitale G, Pesenti A, Fumagalli R 1993 Regional effects and mechanism of positive end-expiratory pressure in early adult respiratory distress syndrome. JAMA 269: 2122–2127

Gattinoni L, Pelosi P, Crotti S, Valenza F 1995 Effects of positive end-expiratory pressure on regional distribution of tidal volume and recruitment in adult respiratory distress syndrome. Am J Respir Crit Care Med 151: 1807–1814

Gattinoni L, Pelosi P, Pesenti A et al 1991 CT scan in ARDS: clinical and physiopathological insights. Acta Anaesthesiol Scand Suppl 95: 87–94

Gattinoni L, Pesenti A, Avalli L, Rossi F, Bombino M 1987 Pressure-volume curve of total respiratory system in acute respiratory failure. Computed tomographic scan study. Am Rev Respir Dis 136: 730–736

Gattinoni L, Pesenti A, Bombino M et al 1988 Relationships between lung computed tomographic density, gas exchange, and PEEP in acute respiratory failure. Anesthesiology 69: 824–832

Hernandez L A, Coker P J, May S, Thompson A L, Parker J C 1990 Mechanical ventilation increases microvascular permeability in oleic acid-injured lungs. J Appl Physiol 69: 2057–2061

Hernandez L A, Peevy K J, Moise A A, Parker J C 1989 Chest wall restriction limits high airway pressure-induced lung injury in young rabbits. J Appl Physiol 66: 2364–2368

Hickling K G, Walsh J, Henderson S, Jackson R 1994 Low mortality rate in adult respiratory distress syndrome using low-volume, pressure-limited ventilation with permissive hypercapnia: a prospective study. Crit Care Med 22: 1568–1578

Hirschl R B, Pranikoff T, Gauger P, Schreiner R J, Dechert R, Bartlett R H 1995 Liquid ventilation in adults, children, and full-term neonates. Lancet 346: 1201–1202

Lamm W J E, Graham M M, Albert R K 1994 Mechanism by which the prone position improves oxygenation in acute lung injury. Am J Respir Crit Care Med 150: 184–193

Langer M, Mascheroni D, Marcolin R, Gattinoni L 1988 The prone position in ARDS patients. A clinical study. Chest 94: 103–107

Miller R S, Nelson L D, DiRusso S M, Rutherford E J, Safcsak K, Morris Jr J A 1992 High-level positive end-expiratory pressure management in trauma-associated adult respiratory distress syndrome. J Trauma 33: 284–290

Owens C M, Evans T W, Keogh B F, Hansell D M 1994 Computed tomography in established adult respiratory distress syndrome. Correlation with lung injury score. Chest 106: 1815–1821

Petersen G W, Baier H 1983 Incidence of pulmonary barotrauma in a medical ICU. Crit Care Med 11: 67–69

Phiel M A, Brown R S 1976 Use of extreme position changes in respiratory failure. Crit Care Med 4: 13–14

Ranieri V M, Mascia L, Fiore T, Bruno F, Brienza A, Giuliani R 1995 Cardiorespiratory effects of positive end expiratory pressure during progressive tidal volume reduction (permissive hypercapnia) in patients with acute respiratory distress syndrome. Anesthesiology 83: 710–720

Reber A, Engberg G, Sporre B et al 1996 Volumetric analysis of aeration in the lungs during general anaesthesia. Br J Anaesth 76: 760–766

Rocker G M, Mackenzie M-G, Williams B, Shields K, Logan P M 1997 Non-invasive pressure support ventilation: successful outcome in acute lung injury/ARDS [Abstract]. Am J Respir Crit Care Med 155: A410

Rossaint R, Falke K J, Lopez F, Slama K, Pison U, Zapol W M 1993 Inhaled nitric oxide for the adult respiratory distress syndrome. N Engl J Med 328: 399–405

Rossaint R, Gerlach H, Schmidt Ruhnke H et al 1995 Efficacy of inhaled nitric oxide in patients with severe ARDS. Chest 107: 1107–1115

Rouby J J, Lherm T, Martin de Lassale E et al 1993 Histologic aspects of pulmonary barotrauma in critically ill patients with acute respiratory failure. Intensive Care Med 19: 383–389

Slutsky A S 1993 Barotrauma and alveolar recruitment. Intensive Care Med 19: 369–371

Slutsky A S 1994 Consensus conference on mechanical ventilation – January 28–30, 1993 at Northbrook, Illinois, USA. Intensive Care Med 20: 64–79

Thorens J, Jolliet P, Ritz M, Chevrolet J 1996 Effects of rapid permissive hypercapnia on hemodynamics, gas exchange, and oxygen transport and consumption during mechanical ventilation for the acute respiratory distress syndrome. Intensive Care Med 22: 182–191

Tuxen D V 1989 Detrimental effects of positive end-expiratory pressure during controlled mechanical ventilation of patients with severe airflow obstruction. Am Rev Respir Dis 140: 5–9

Webb H H, Tierney D F 1974 Experimental pulmonary edema due to intermittent positive pressure ventilation with high inflation pressures. Protection by positive end expiratory pressure. Am Rev Respir Dis 110: 556–565

Woodring J H 1985 Pulmonary interstitial emphysema in the adult respiratory distress syndrome. Crit Care Med 13: 786–791

S. Clare Stanford

Imidazol(in)es and α_2-adrenoceptors

α_2-ADRENOCEPTOR LIGANDS IN ANAESTHESIA: PROBLEMS AND DEVELOPMENTS

The physiological changes induced by α_2-adrenoceptor agonists include: promotion of platelet aggregation; mydriasis; reduced spillover of plasma catecholamines; inhibition of lipolysis and increased growth hormone secretion. Of particular relevance in the anaesthetic context are their centrally mediated effects. Some of these, such as a reduction in blood pressure (coupled with bradycardia and possible sinus arrest) and hypothermia, can be problematic. Others, such as muscle relaxation, sedation, anxiolysis, analgesia, decreased salivary secretion and haemodynamic stabilising effects are advantageous.

From a pharmacological point of view, one limitation of most α_2-adrenoceptor agonists is their lack of selectivity. Many of these agents show appreciable binding to receptor systems for other neurotransmitters and they all bind to α_1-adrenoceptors to some extent. Poor efficacy can also be a problem: clonidine has only partial agonist activity at α_2-receptors, for example. Consequently, development of novel agents has aimed to improve their α_2-adrenoceptor selectivity and efficacy.

Many α-adrenoceptor ligands are substituted imidazoles or imidazolines (Table 7.1). Although some of these compounds (e.g. cirazoline) are regarded as selective α_1-adrenoceptor ligands, most (e.g. clonidine) bind preferentially to α_2-adrenoceptors. The imidazole, medetomidine, has been added to the portfolio comparatively recently and the development of this compound has been documented thoroughly. Briefly, it has been found to share actions typical of α_2-agonists, albeit with greater potency and selectivity.

Medetomidine is a racemic mixture but only the *d*-stereoisomer (dexmedetomidine) reduces blood pressure in anaesthetised rats. Dexmedetomidine is

Dr S. Clare Stanford, Department of Pharmacology, University College London, Gower Street, London WC1E 6BT, UK

Table 7.1 Classification of common a-adrenoceptor ligands

Imidazoles	Imidazolines	Oxazolines	Guanidines	Alkaloids
Atipamezole	Clonidine	Rilmenidine	Amiloride	Rauwolscine
Cimetidine	Cirazoline		Guanabenz	Yohimbine
Dexmedetomidine	Efaroxan		Guanfacine	
Imidazole-4-acetic acid	Idazoxan			
Histamine	Lofexidine			
Medetomidine	Monoxidine			
Mivazerol	Naphazoline		**Phenylethylamines**	
	Oxymetazoline		Adrenaline	
	p-Aminoclonidine		α-Methylnoradrenaline	
	Phentolamine		Methoxamine	
	Tolazoline		Noradrenaline	
			Phenylephrine	

also a more potent analgesic than the *l*-stereoisomer (Savola & Virtanen 1991). In fact, dexmedetomidine is the most selective α_2-agonist to have been developed so far and has an α_2-/α_1-adrenceptor selectivity ratio of approximately 1600-fold. This compound is already used routinely as an adjunct in veterinary anaesthesia and has proved beneficial in tests as a preanaesthetic agent in humans (see Hyashi & Maze 1993).

At the cellular level, dexmedetomidine reduces noradrenaline release in the periphery and CNS. This latter effect is likely to be due, at least in part, to activation of α_2-adrenoceptors in the locus coeruleus (Jorm & Stamford 1993) which will reduce neuronal firing rate. Activation of α_2-adrenoceptors on noradrenergic nerve terminals will also cause feedback inhibition of transmitter release in the terminal field. Since the locus coeruleus is the major source of central noradrenergic neurones in the brain, and is thought to have a pivotal role in arousal, both these actions of dexmedetomidine are entirely consistent with its prominent sedative/hypnotic effects.

Of particular note is the reduction in anaesthetic requirement associated with the use of dexmedetomidine. This has been reported for volatile and other anaesthetics from several generic groups (Bloor et al 1992a). For instance, dexmedetomidine has maximal anaesthetic sparing effect of approximately 90% when used in conjunction with isoflurane. This action can be reversed by an α_2-antagonist (Segal et al 1988) and is not modified by neurotoxin- or reserpine-induced depletion of noradrenaline stores. This suggests that it arises through activation of postsynaptic α_2-adrenoceptors. The greater α_2-adrenoceptor selectivity and efficacy of dexmedetomidine compared with that of the partial agonist, clonidine, would explain why the anaesthetic sparing action of the former compound is considerably greater than that of the latter. However, competitive inhibition of microsomal cytochrome P450 enzymes in the liver by dexmedetomidine and, consequently, the metabolism of anaesthetic could also contribute to the reduced anaesthetic requirement when these agents are co-administered. This action, common to both stereoisomers of medetomidine, is likely to be shared by other substituted imidazoles (Kharasch et al 1992), although clonidine does not seem to have this effect. Notwithstanding evidence that this inhibition occurs in vitro, there is cause to question whether the concentration of dexmedetomidine attained in the anaesthetic context is sufficient to exert such a pharmacokinetic interaction (Pelkonen et al 1991). Inhibition of mitochondrial P450 enzymes by imidazoles also has a marked effect on steroidogenesis and it is thought that this inhibition can adversely affect surgical outcome. Whereas this is a prominent effect of the imidazole, etomidate, this too is thought not to occur at clinically relevant doses of dexmedetomidine (Maze et al 1991).

In healthy human volunteers, intravenous infusion of relatively high doses of α_2-agonists causes a transient increase in blood pressure. This is due to activation of α_2-adrenoceptors in the peripheral vasculature which causes vasoconstriction (Bloor et al 1992b). Such an increase in systemic vascular resistance would be a problem in patients with impaired cardiac function but can be avoided by using slow infusion rates. Later, a hypotensive response is manifest because centrally mediated actions of these drugs predominate: there is a dose-dependent fall in mean arterial and diastolic pressure (see *Imidazolines and the cardiovascular system*).

Despite this biphasic change in mean arterial pressure, heart rate is reduced throughout. In the hypertensive phase, this is presumably due to activation of the baroreceptor reflex. The bradycardia which parallels hypotension is the result of a reduction in sympathetic outflow (indexed by a reduction in plasma catecholamines) and increased vagal tone. Cardiac output is also reduced during both phases of the response, possibly because of the net increase in systemic vascular resistance combined with a reduced sympathetic outflow in the heart. Yet, in anaesthetised dogs, dexmedetomidine does not reduce blood pressure. This is thought to be because the hypotensive effects of this agent are offset by the reduction in the requirement for isoflurane which itself causes vasodilatation (Bloor et al 1992a). Such a net increase in vascular tone with isoflurane anaesthesia can be expected to apply to all species to some extent. A dose-dependent respiratory depression, which is paralleled by hypoxia and hypercapnia, has also been reported with dexmedetomidine (Zornow 1991).

Attention has also been devoted to the development of more selective α_2-antagonists. One such compound, the imidazole atipamezole, has a higher affinity (< 1 nM) for α_2-receptors than its predecessors and an α_2/α_1 selectivity of 8500 (Scheinin et al 1988). Its use in reversal of medetomidine-induced sedation is already established practice in veterinary anaesthesia.

α_2-ADRENOCEPTORS: DISTINCTIVE INTERACTIONS WITH IMIDAZOL(IN)ES AND PHENYLETHYLAMINES?

Despite the evident efficacy of imidazoles and imidazolines as α_2-adrenoceptor agonists and antagonists, the endogenous ligands for α_2-adrenoceptors, adrenaline and noradrenaline, come from a generically unrelated group of compounds. These catecholamines have a phenylethylamine molecular nucleus (Fig. 7.1). The receptor (and clinical) efficacy of synthetic phenylethylamines is evident from their use in treatment of acute hypotension (e.g. methoxamine and phenylephrine) or hypertension (e.g. methyldopa). In so far as the effects of

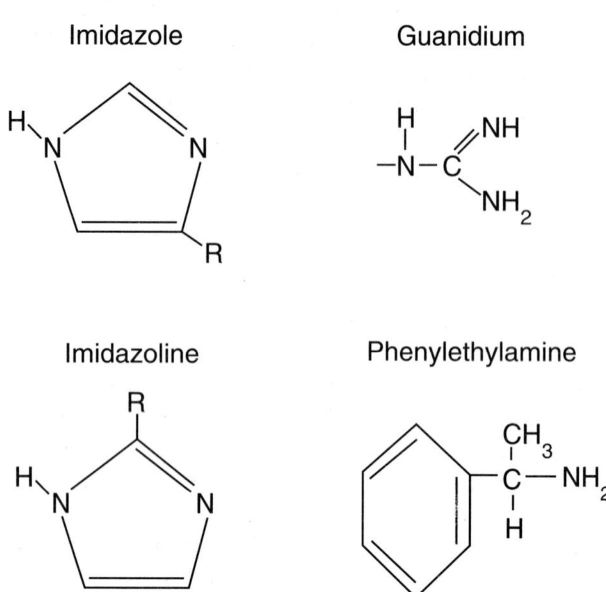

Fig. 7.1 Molecular structure of α_2-adrenoceptor ligands

imidazol(in)es are effected by α_2-adrenoceptors, the molecular derivations of these two groups of compounds should make little difference to their physiological effects. However, it is now clear that they have a distinctive pharmacology which could have a profound impact on their use in anaesthesia.

HISTORY

Over recent years, evidence has accumulated to indicate that not all α_2-adrenoceptor ligands bind to the same site on the α_2-adrenoceptor. One of the first suggestions for this came from comparisons of the centrally-mediated effects of imidazol(in)es and phenylethylamines on blood pressure. This is discussed in detail below (see *Imidazol(in)es) and the cardiovascular system*).

Other early indications that imidazolines and phenylethylamines do not have the same pharmacological profile came from studies of the neurochemical modulation of noradrenergic transmission. Normally, activation of (presynaptic) α_2-adrenoceptors on noradrenergic nerve terminals causes feedback inhibition of transmitter release. When uptake of noradrenaline was inhibited, thereby increasing its concentration in the synapse, the inhibition of noradrenaline release by the imidazoline α_2-agonist, clonidine, was diminished as anticipated. Presumably, this reflected the increased activation of α_2-adrenoceptors resulting from the increased concentration of noradrenaline in the synapse. However, the inhibition of release by the phenylethylamine, α-methylnoradrenaline (the active metabolite of α-methyldopa), was unaffected. This led to the tentative suggestion that the pharmacological inhibition of noradrenaline uptake had somehow disrupted the receptor binding or efficacy of imidazolines, but not that of phenylethylamines (see Starke 1987). Further evidence indicating that these two groups of drugs bind to distinct sites emerged from studies of functional desensitization of tissue responses to α_2-adrenoceptor agonists. For instance, in the rat vas deferens, under conditions where there was overt desensitisation of the response to imidazolines, this desensitisation did not generalize to phenylethylamines (Ruffolo et al 1977).

RADIOLIGAND BINDING

More recently, radioligand binding studies have provided definitive evidence for the existence of binding sites for imidazolines which are not only different from those for phenylethylamines but which are unrelated to the α_2-adrenoceptor. The first convincing support for this came from quantitative analysis of the binding of the radiolabelled imidazoline and α_2-adrenoceptor ligand, [^{3}H]-*p*-aminoclonidine, to tissues derived from the bovine ventrolateral medulla. The binding of [^{3}H]-*p*-aminoclonidine could be displaced completely by α_2-adrenoceptor ligands which had an imidazol(in)e molecular structure, but only about 70–75% could be displaced by phenylethylamines. This suggested that there were two binding sites for [^{3}H]-*p*-aminoclonidine but only one of these was accessible to phenylethylamines. The residual binding after maximal displacement by phenylethylamines could be displaced by imidazoles such as cimetidine; about 30% of the [^{3}H]-*p*-aminoclonidine binding sites had a high affinity for these compounds (Ernsberger et al 1987). These sites appear to have a high affinity and selectivity for imidazoles, therefore.

Even more striking support came from studies of radioligand binding to tissue from the human nucleus reticularis lateralis (NRL) (Bricca et al 1989). Here, phenylethylamines had no effect at all on [^{3}H]-clonidine binding. Yet, imidazolines such as cirazoline, oxymetazoline and idazoxan competed strongly for nearly all the bound radioligand. Similar findings are reported for [^{3}H]-idazoxan binding in the liver. This suggests that, in these tissues, all the imidazoline binding sites are of a non-adrenoceptor type. These findings were complemented by results from autoradiographic studies: the number of binding sites for the α_2-adrenoceptor antagonist, [^{3}H]-idazoxan, was consistently greater, and more widely distributed throughout the brain, than those for the alkaloid α_2-adrenoceptor antagonists, rauwolscine and yohimbine, which lack an imidazol(in)e nucleus (Boyajian & Leslie 1987).

Collectively, this evidence suggested that the alkaloid antagonists, yohimbine and rauwolscine, bind selectively to α_2-adrenoceptors but that idazoxan binds to an additional, non-adrenoceptor site. That this is unrelated to the α_2-adrenoceptor was confirmed by studies of radioligand binding to membranes derived from a transfected COS-7 cell line expressing the cloned human α_2-adrenoceptor (Michel at al 1990). Here, there was no indication of any binding to a non-adrenoceptor site, i.e. the two sites are not co-expressed.

It is now acknowledged that not all ligands for these non-adrenoceptor binding sites are imidazol(in)es: guanidium compounds, such as guanabenz and amiloride, are notable examples (Table 7.1). Conversely, some imidazol(in)es (e.g. the experimental compound, RX 810002) bind preferentially to α_2-adrenoceptors. Nevertheless, these non-adrenoceptor binding sites are now known as imidazoline (I-) receptors and are characterised by their low affinity for phenylethylamines and the alkaloid α_2-antagonists, yohimbine and rauwolscine, but a high affinity for cirazoline. This imidazoline does bind appreciably to α_1-adrenoceptors but has negligible interactions with α_2-adrenoceptors. Using these criteria, I-receptors have been now identified in tissues from a wide range of species. In humans, they are found, *inter alia,* in the kidney, liver, platelets, adrenal medulla, adipocytes, myometrium and brain tissue.

IMIDAZOLINE RECEPTOR SUBTYPES

More recent and detailed characterization of the pharmacological profiles of imidazol(in)e binding led to the conclusion that there are subtypes of the I-receptor. For example, clonidine is a weak displacer of [^{3}H]-idazoxan binding yet guanabenz, which potently competes with [^{3}H]-idazoxan binding, does not displace [^{3}H]-clonidine. Conversely, the imidazoles, histamine and cimetidine, will displace [^{3}H]-clonidine but not [^{3}H]-idazoxan binding. As as result of such evidence, two imidazoline receptor subtypes, designated I_1- and I_2-receptors, are now acknowledged. Both bind cirazoline and idazoxan, but I_1-receptors are characterised by their high affinity for clonidine.

Several other imidazol(in)es are now known to bind preferentially to I_1-receptors. The antihypertensive agents, rilmenidine and monoxidine are examples and the generally accepted affinity profile for I_1-receptors is: monoxidine > clonidine > cirazoline > idazoxan > amiloride. These receptors also have a high affinity for the imidazoles cimetidine, histamine and the histamine metabolite, imidazole-4-acetic acid. However, the marked species differences means that details of the pharmacological profile of I_1-receptors is not assured and the possibility that there are further subtypes should be left open.

In contrast, I_2-receptors have a low affinity for clonidine but a high affinity for benzazepines and guanidium compounds. The accepted affinity profile is: cirazoline > idazoxan > amiloride > monoxidine > clonidine. However, in some tissues, the affinity of the guanidium compound, amiloride, for this receptor is especially high. This has led to the proposal, now generally accepted, that there are subtypes of the I_2-receptor (Michel & Insel 1989, Renouard et al 1993). These have been tentatively ascribed the status of I_{2A} (amiloride sensitive, found in human placenta) and I_{2B} (amiloride insensitive, found in human kidney, liver and adipocytes) receptors (Parini et al 1996).

Further evidence for I_2-receptor subtypes came from studies of displacement of [^{3}H]-clonidine binding by the *d*- and *l*-enantiomers of medetomidine in the guinea-pig. The displacement profile for these stereoisomers was quite different in the brain from that in the ileum (Wikberg et al 1991). Moreover, the binding of the imidazoline, naphazoline, to I_2-receptors is also best described by a two-site fit. Whether these subtypes correspond with those distinguished by amiloride is uncertain.

Finally, evidence is accumulating for a third type of imidazoline receptor in pancreatic islets of Langerhans. It is thought that activation of this receptor closes ATP-sensitive K^+ channels which, by causing membrane depolarisation, augments insulin secretion. Many imidazol(in)es stimulate insulin secretion as does the putative endogenous ligand for I-receptors, 'clonidine displacing substance' (see *Endogenous ligands;* Chan et al 1997). However, the pharmacological profile of this action does not seem to conform to that of either I_1- or I_2-receptors. Since the response is evoked by the selective I_1-ligand, efaroxan, which binds to I_1-receptors but shows negligible binding to I_2-receptors, an I_1-receptor mediated effect is most likely, However, reports of the effects of the I_1-receptor ligand, monoxidine, on insulin secretion are inconsistent; whether such discrepancies can be resolved by the characterisation of an I_3-receptor remains to be seen.

SUBCELLULAR LOCALIZATION OF I_2-RECEPTORS

Liver cells are ideal for studying I_2-receptors because there are few (or no) α_2-adrenoceptors in this tissue. After differential centrifugation of homogenates of human or rabbit liver, the subcellular distribution of I_2 binding sites correlated positively with that of cytochrome oxidase, a marker for mitochondria. Further separation of the inner and outer membranes of mitochondria confirmed that this I_2-receptor co-localised with the enzyme monoamine oxidase (MAO) on the mitochondrial outer membrane (Tesson et al 1991). It was thought originally that the density of the I_2-receptor in different tissues correlated with that of MAO_B, only. However, the link between I_2-receptors and MAO seems to apply to both the MAO isoenzymes (MAO_A and MAO_B). This is inferred from studies showing that I_2-binding sites are evident after transfection of yeast cells and expression of recombinant cDNA for either human MAO_A or MAO_B (Tesson et al 1995). Nevertheless, there seem to be differences in the pharmacological profile of I_2-binding sites on the two MAO isoenzymes. It has even been suggested that the I_2-receptor on MAO_A corresponds to the amiloride-sensitive I_{2A}-receptor while binding to MAO_B corresponds to the amiloride-insensitive I_{2B} subtype (Raddatz et al 1995).

The question arises as to whether the I_2 receptor site is the same as the catalytic site on MAO which is responsible for metabolising endogenous monoamines. This is supported by evidence that the rank order of potency for inhibition of MAO enzymic activity by I_2-ligands parallels their affinity for the I_2-receptor, albeit with much lower affinity. However, there are many reasons to rule out the possibility that the I_2-receptor is the same as the enzyme catalytic site. Amongst these is the more restricted tissue distribution of I_2-receptors when compared with that of MAO. This is best illustrated by the presence of I_2-binding sites on MAO_B derived from human liver, but not on MAO_B isolated from human platelets. So far, reasons for this disparity are unresolved but one obvious possibility is that only a subpopulation of MAO incorporates an I_2-binding site. Another is that the I_2 site in platelets is masked in a way which prevents the binding of radioligands.

Definitive evidence that the I_2 receptor and MAO catalytic site are not one and the same, comes from radioligand binding studies of rat liver tissue. First, there is a great deal of variation in the extent to which MAO inhibitors bind to the I_2 receptor: whereas the MAO inhibitors, pargyline and clorgyline, are weak displacers of $[^3H]$-idazoxan binding, tranylcypromine has a comparatively high affinity for this receptor site. Importantly, the affinity for binding of MAO inhibitors to the I_2-receptor does not correspond with their enzyme inhibiting potency (Carpene et al 1995). It is less certain that this is also the case in the brain, however. Secondly, some I_2-receptor ligands reversibly inhibit MAO enzymic activity but, with most of these agents (e.g. naphazoline and idazoxan), this occurs only at high concentrations or not at all. Thirdly, the inhibition of MAO activity by imidazolines has non-competitive kinetics. This is borne out by the fact that binding of I_2-receptor ligands does not compete with that of MAO inhibitors (Tesson et al 1995, Raddatz et al 1995). In view of all this evidence, it seems extremely unlikely that the I_2-receptor is the same as the catalytic site of MAO. One suggestion is that the I_2 receptor has a regulatory role such that binding to this receptor has an allosteric effect on the catalytic site of the enzyme. This is controversial, however (Alemany et al 1995).

Interestingly, chronic, but not acute, administration of clorgyline or pargyline and phenelzine (see Alemany et al 1995) reduces the density of I_2 sites in the rat cerebral cortex. This has raised considerable interest in the possible role of imidazolines in the therapeutic effects of MAO inhibitors in depression, especially since the density of I_2-receptors in human platelets is increased in this disorder. It is noteworthy that reversible inhibitors do not seem to have this effect (Alemany et al 1995). This could suggest that the apparent downregulation of I_2-receptors in vivo is, in fact, an artefact arising from accumulation of an irreversible inhibitor. However, this has been ruled out. Instead, it is thought that an indirect mechanism, as yet unidentified, is responsible for this downregulation.

It has also been discovered that chronic administration of the imidazol(in)es, cirazoline or idazoxan, increases the density of I_2-receptors in the brain (Olmos et al 1994). Recent studies suggest that this change might be confined to I_2-receptors on glial cells and, specifically, regulate the expression of glial fibrillary acidic protein (GFAP). This raises the interesting possibility that I_2-receptors are involved in neurochemical changes arising from neurodegenerative conditions in which there is marked astrocytic hypertrophy (see Olmos et al 1994). This would be consistent with the burgeoning evidence that glial cells have a key role in modulating neuronal transmission in the brain. It also strengthens links between I_2-receptors and inhibition of MAO since MAO inhibitors are thought to have neuroprotective effects in some neurodegenerative conditions.

ENDOGENOUS LIGANDS FOR THE I-RECEPTOR?

The discovery of an imidazoline receptor provoked the question of whether there is an endogenous ligand for this receptor? As early as 1984, experiments had shown that extracts of calf brain, and later from human plasma, contained a substance which displaced [^{3}H]-clonidine binding from sites that were presumed to be α_2-adrenoceptors (see Atlas 1991). The active agent, known as 'clonidine displacing substance' (CDS) mimics the physiological effects of clonidine in a range of peripheral tissues, including the promotion of insulin secretion (Chan et al 1997). In the cat, infusion of CDS into the rostro ventrolateral medulla triggers hypertension. However, in the rat such local infusions cause hypotension (Meeley et al 1986). Reasons for this disparity are unclear at present. Like the actions of clonidine itself, the hypotensive effect of CDS was blocked by idazoxan but not by alkaloid α_2-adrenoceptor antagonists. Consequently, it was clear that the effects of CDS could not be explained by an interaction with α_2-adrenoceptors (Atlas 1991). Since CDS displaces [^{3}H]-clonidine binding to non-adrenoceptors, research has progressed on the assumption that this extract was (or contained), by definition, an endogenous ligand for I_1-receptors.

Recently, it has been proposed that CDS is in fact agmatine, an endogenous metabolite of *l*-arginine (Li et al 1994). Although agmatine is an endogenous compound, there are several reasons to rule out the possibility that it is the same as CDS: (i) agmatine has a relative molecular mass considerably less than that of CDS; (ii) unlike CDS, binding of agmatine to α_2-adrenoceptors does not evoke a physiological response in a range of peripheral tissues (Pinthong et al 1995); (iii) the binding profiles of agmatine and CDS to a range of different tissues are not the same (Piletz et al 1995); and (iv) unlike CDS, there is little agmatine in plasma. Consequently, either CDS is not the same as agmatine or there is more than one active agent in the extract containing CDS.

IMIDAZOL(IN)ES AND THE CARDIOVASCULAR SYSTEM

One important action of α_2-adrenoceptor ligands concerns their antidysrhythmic effects. In dogs, adrenaline-induced dysrhythmia under halothane anaesthesia is prevented by dexmedetomidine. This action (manifest as a rise in the plasma concentration of adrenaline at which dysrhythmias occur) was abolished by vagotomy. It was also blocked by imidazoline α_2-adrenoceptor antagonists, idazoxan and atipamezole, but not rauwolscine (Kamibayashi et al 1995). This suggests that the cardiac stabilising effect of dexmedetomidine is mediated by I-receptors rather than α_2-adrenoceptors. Clearly, there is scope for investigating this potentially important action of I-receptor ligands in anaesthesia.

A role for I-receptors in haemodynamic regulation is not restricted to cardiac excitabilty. It has been generally believed that the hypotensive effect of all α_2-adrenoceptor agonists is attributed to activation of α_2-adrenoceptors in the CNS. Thus, activation of postsynaptic α_2-adrenoceptors is thought to result in reduced sympathetic, and increased parasympathetic tone. However, it has become increasingly apparent that the hypotensive effects of imidazol(in)es and phenylethylamines are not mediated by the same mechanisms.

The first indication that this was the case came from an early report that, when injected into the nucleus reticularis lateralis (NRL) in the rostral ventrolateral medulla, the hypotension and bradycardia induced by I-receptor ligands correlated more closely with their binding to I-receptors than to α_2-adrenoceptors (see Ernsberger et al 1990). In fact, imidazoles with no appreciable activity at α_2-adrenoceptors reliably reduced blood pressure. In contrast, α-methylnoradrenaline infusion in this brain region has no effect on blood pressure. The hypotensive effects of clonidine are inhibited by local infusion of idazoxan into the NRL whereas equivalent local infusion of yohimbine is without effect. From such evidence it was inferred that the hypotensive effects of clonidine are mediated by I-receptors rather than α_2-

adrenoceptors. Since I-receptors in the NRL have a high affinity for [^{3}H]-*p*-aminoclonidine, they are, by definition, of the I_1-subtype. As a result of such findings, the antihypertensive effects of monoxidine and rilmenidine have been attributed to their actions at I_1-receptors rather than their α_2-adrenoceptor agonist activity. This is supported by their minimal sedative activity, an α_2-adrenoceptor mediated response, by comparison with that of clonidine.

It is interesting that concentrations of idazoxan which prevent the hypotensive effects of clonidine have no effect on the clonidine-induced inhibition of neuronal firing in the locus coeruleus. Conversely, concentrations of yohimbine which prevent the effects of clonidine on locus firing rate have no effect on the hypotension. This raises the exciting possibility that it might be feasible to separate the sedative and hypotensive effects of the α_2-agonists (Tibirica et al 1991). Such compounds would have obvious applications in anaesthesia and one such agent, mivazerol, is at an advanced stage of development.

Despite this re-appraisal of central mechanisms underlying the effects of the imidazol(in)es on the cardiovascular system, recent evidence indicates that these actions are not due entirely to activation of I-receptors. This is because idazoxan infusion into the NRL does not prevent clonidine-induced bradycardia. Also, the hypotensive effects of systemic administration of clonidine in the pithed rat and in the spontaneously hypertensive rat were prevented by administration of SKF 86466, a selective α_2-antagonist. Similarly, the hypotension induced by peripheral administration of rilmenidine (Szabo et al 1993) and monoxidine (Urban et al 1995) is prevented by yohimbine. Such findings raise the possibility that these agents could well have haemodynamic effects mediated by α_2-adrenoceptors in regions beyond the NRL. Possible areas in which α_2-adrenoceptors might regulate blood pressure could include the nucleus tractus solitarius, the dorsal vagal nucleus or even spinal regions. A recent report suggests yet more mechanisms for the effects of clonidine on heart rate since neither I-receptor nor α_2-adrenoceptor antagonists prevented the effects of intrathecal administration of clonidine (Kroin et al 1996). Evidently, more research is need to resolve this question.

α_2–ADRENOCEPTOR ACTIVATION WITHOUT HYPOTENSION

The fact that not all α_2-adrenoceptors inevitably reduce blood pressure is underlined by the actions of mivazerol. This compound shows negligible binding to I-receptors and, although showing preferential binding to α_2-adrenoceptors (Noyer et al 1994), does not induce hypotension. As yet, few studies with this compound have been published but the potential wider applications in anaesthesia for a selective α_2-agonist which does not cause hypotension are clear.

Despite its lack of effect on mean arterial blood pressure, mivazerol does reduce heart rate and cardiac output in experimental coronary artery stenosis in anaesthetised dogs. It is likely that this effect is due, at least in part, to inhibition of noradrenaline release as a result of activation of presynaptic α_2-adrenoceptors on noradrenergic nerve terminals (Zhang et al 1995). A recent study also suggests that, with the exception of the epicardium, mivazerol preserves myocardial blood flow during ischaemia and increases coronary vascular resistance only in the subepicardial layer. Therefore, coupled with a reduced myocardial oxygen demand (Rockaerts et al 1996), this compound could have beneficial applications in prevention of damage ensuing from myocardial ischaemia during surgery. Clinical trials to test for this application are underway. There is also considerable interest in its possible use in cerebral ischaemia. In vitro, at least, the inhibition of stress-evoked release of noradrenaline by mivazerol is prevented by α_2-antagonists. This compound also prevents release of the excitatory amino acid transmitter, glutamate, in some brain regions. Since noradrenergic neurones in the locus coeruleus are activated by glutamate, either of these actions could contribute to the prevention by mivazerol of hyperadrenergic activity in perioperative patients. Also, because the neurotoxic effects of glutamate are thought to account for much ischaemic damage, the effects of mivazerol on glutamate secretion could help to explain its anti-ischaemic effects.

IMIDAZOL(IN)ES AND ANALGESIA

In experimental models, the analgesic effects of α_2-adrenoceptor agonists depend to some extent on the type of pain experienced: such agents are generally more effective in tests involving mechanical stimulation than thermal stimulation. One problem is that sedative effects of α_2-agonists can interfere with measurements of pain threshold which depend on a motor response. Another is that both the hypothermic and sedative effects of these drugs can effect measures of thermal and, possibly, inflammatory pain. The analgesic effects of these drugs are thought to involve α_2-adrenoceptor activation in the locus coeruleus and the dorsal horn of the spinal cord. This is supported by evidence that in humans, with the possible exception of ischaemic pain, analgesia induced by dexmedetomidine is evident only at sedative doses. Also, the analgesic effects of clonidine are prevented by yohimbine as well as idazoxan (Monroe et al 1995) so a role for I-receptors in analgesia is extremely unlikely. This is consistent with the lack of any analgesia on administration of the I-receptor ligand, cirazoline. Nevertheless, in the light of accumulating evidence for multiple I-receptors, and the now well established multiple subtypes of α_2-adrenoceptors, it might be possible to develop compounds with minimal adverse haemodynamic effects but which retain their sedative and/or analgesic actions.

References

Alemany R, Olmos G, Garcia-Sevilla J A 1995 The effects of phenelzine and other monoamine oxidase inhibitor antidepressants on brain and liver I_2-imidazoline preferring receptors. Br J Pharmacol 114: 837–845

Atlas D 1991 Clonidine-displacing substance (CDS) and its putative imidazoline receptor Biochem Pharmacol 41: 1541–1549

Bloor B C, Frankland M, Alper G, Raybould D, Weitz J, Shurtliff M 1992a Hemodynamic and sedative effects of dexmedetomidine in dog. J Pharmacol Exp Ther 263: 690–697

Bloor B C, Ward D S, Belleville J P, Maze M 1992b Effects of intravenous dexmedetomidine in humans. Anesthesiology 77: 1134–1142

Boyajian C L, Leslie F M 1987 Pharmacological evidence for α_2-adrenoceptor heterogeneity: differential binding properties of [^{3}H]-rauwolscine and [^{3}H]-idazoxan. J Pharmacol Exp Ther 241: 1092–1098

Bricca G, Dontenwill M, Molines A, Feldman J, Belcourt A, Bousquet P 1989 The imidazoline preferring receptor: binding studies in bovine, rat and human brainstem. Eur J Pharmacol 162: 1–9

Carpene C, Collon P, Remaury A et al 1995 Inhibition of amine oxidase activity by derivatives that recognise imidazoline I_2 sites. J Pharmacol Exp Ther 272: 681–688

Chan S L F, Atlas D, James R F L, Morgan N G 1997 The effect of the putative endogenous imidazoline receptor ligand, clonidine-displacing substance, on insulin secretion from rat and human islets of Langerhans. Br J Pharmacol 120: 926–932

Ernsberger P, Meeley M P, Mann J J, Reis D J 1987 Clonidine binds to imidazole binding sites as well as α_2-adrenoceptors in the ventrolateral medulla. Eur J Pharmacol 134: 1–13

Ernsberger P, Giuliano R, Willette R N, Reis D J 1990 Role of imidazole receptors in the vasodepressor response to clonidine analogs in the rostral ventrolateral medulla. J Pharmacol Exp Ther 253: 408–418

Hayashi Y, Maze M 1993 Alpha$_2$ adrenoceptor agonists and anaesthesia. Br J Anaesth 71: 108–118

Jorm C M, Stamford J A 1993 Actions of the hypnotic anaesthetic, dexmedetomidine, on noradrenaline release and cell firing in rat locus coeruleus slices. Br J Anaesth 71: 447–449

Kamibayashi T, Mammoto T, Hayashi Y et al 1995 Further characterization of the receptor mechanism involved in the antidysrhythmic effect of dexmedetomidine on halothane/epinephrine dysrhythmias in dogs. Anesthesiology 83: 1082–1089

Kharasch E D, Herrmann S, Labroo R 1992 Ketamine as a probe for medetomidine stereoisomer inhibition of human liver microsomal drug metabolism. Anesthesiology 77: 1208–1214

Kroin J S, McCarthy R J, Penn R D, Lubenow T R, Ivankowich A D 1996 Intrathecal clonidine and tizanidine in conscious dogs: comparison of analgesic and hemodynamic effects. Anesth Analg 82: 627–635

Li G, Regunathan S, Barrow C J, Eshraghi J, Cooper R, Reis D J 1994 Agmatine: an endogenous clonidine-displacing substance in the brain. Science 263: 966–969

Maze M, Virtanen R, Daunt D, Banks S J M, Stover E P, Feldman D 1991 Effects of dexmedetomidine, a novel imidazole sedative-anesthetic agent, on adrenal steroidogenesis in vivo and in vitro studies. Anesth Analg 73: 204–208

Meeley M P, Ernsberger P R, Granata A R, Reis D J 1986 An endogenous clonidine-displacing substance from bovine brain: receptor binding and hypotensive actions in the ventrolateral medulla. Life Sci 38: 1119–1126

Michel M C, Insel P A 1989 Are there multiple imidazoline binding sites? Trends Pharmacol Sci 10: 342–344

Michel M C, Regan J W, Gerhardt M A, Neubig R R, Insel P A, Motulsky H J 1990 Nonadrenergic [^{3}H]-idazoxan binding sites are physically distinct from α_2-adrenergic receptors. Mol Pharmacol 37: 65–68

Monroe P J, Smith D L, Kirk H R, Smith D J 1995 Spinal nonadrenergic imidazoline receptors do not mediate the antinociceptive action of intrathecal clonidine in the rat. J Pharmacol Exp Ther 273: 1057–1062

Noyer M, de Laveleye F, Vauquelin G, Gobert J, Wulfert E 1994 Mivazerol, a novel compound with high specificity for α_2 adrenergic receptors: binding studies on different human and rat membrane preparations. Neurochem Int 24: 221–229

Olmos G, Alemany R, Escriba P V, Garcia-Sevilla J A 1994 The effects of chronic imidazoline drug treatment on glial fibrillary acidic protein concentrations in rat brain. Br J Pharmacol 111: 997–1002

Parini A, Moudanos C G, Pizzinat N, Lanier S M 1996 The elusive family of imidazoline binding sites. Trends Pharmacol Sci 17: 13–16

Pelkonen O, Puurunen J, Arvela P, Lammintausta R 1991 Comparative effects of medetomidine enantiomers on in vitro and in vivo microsomal drug metabolism. Pharmacol Toxicol 69: 189–194

Piletz J E, Chikkala D N, Ernsberger P 1995 Comparison of the properties of agmatine and endogenous clonidine-displacing substance at imidazoline and alpha-2 adrenergic receptors. J Pharmacol Exp Ther 272: 581–587

Pinthong D, Wright I K, Hanmer C et al 1995 Agmatine recognizes α_2-adrenoceptor binding sites but neither activates nor inhibits α_2-adrenoceptors. Naunyn-Schmiedeberg's Arch Pharmacol 351: 10–16

Raddatz R, Parini A, Lanier S M 1995 Imidazoline/guanidinium binding domains on monoamine oxidases. J Biol Chem 270: 27961–27968

Renouard A, Widdowson P S, Cordi A 1993 [^{3}H]-idazoxan binding to rabbit cerebral cortex recognises multiple imidazoline I_2-type receptors: pharmacological characterization and relationship to monoamine oxidase. Br J Pharmacol 109: 625–631

Rockaerts P M H J, Prinzen F W, Willigers H M M, de Lange S 1996 The effects of α_2-adrenergic stimulation with mivazerol on myocardial blood flow and function during coronary artery stenosis in anesthetized dogs. Anesth Analg 82: 702–711

Ruffolo R R, Turowski B S, Patil P N 1977 Lack of cross desensitization between structurally dissimilar α-adrenoceptor agonists. J Pharm Pharmacol 29: 378–380

Savola J-M, Virtanen R 1991 Central α_2-adrenoceptors are highly stereoselective for dexmedetomidine, the dextro enantiomer of medetomidine. Eur J Pharmacol 195: 193–199

Scheinin H, MacDonald E, Scheinin M 1988 Behavioural and neurochemical effects of atipamezole, a novel α_2-adrenoceptor antagonist. Eur J Pharmacol 151: 35–42

Segal I S, Vickery R G, Walton J K, Doze V A, Maze M 1988 Dexmedetomidine diminishes halothane anesthetic requirements in rats through a postsynaptic alpha$_2$ adrenergic receptor. Anesthesiology 69: 818–823

Starke K 1987 Presynaptic α-autoreceptors. Rev Physiol Biochem Pharmacol 107: 73–146

Szabo B, Urban R, Starke K 1993 Sympathoinhibition by rilmenidine in conscious rabbits: involvement of α_2-adrenoceptors. Naunyn-Schmiedeberg's Arch Pharmacol 348: 593–600

Tesson F, Prip-Buus C, Lemoine A, Pegorier J-P, Parini A 1991 Subcellular distribution of imidazoline-guanidium-receptive sites in human and rabbit liver. J Biol Chem 266: 155–160

Tesson F, Limon-Boulez I, Urban P et al 1995 Localisation of I_2-imidazoline binding sites on monoamine oxidases. J Biol Chem 270: 9856–9861

Tibirica E, Feldman J, Mermet C, Gonon F, Bousquet P 1991 An imidazoline-specific mechanism for the hypotensive effect of clonidine: a study with yohimbine and idazoxan. J Pharmacol Exp Ther 256: 606–613

Urban R, Szabo B, Starke K 1995 Involvement of α_2-adrenoceptors in the cardiovascular effects of monoxidine. Eur J Pharmacol 282: 19–28

Wikberg J E S, Uhlen S, Chajlani V 1991 Medetomidine stereoisomers delineate two closely related subtypes of idazoxan (imidazoline) I-receptors in the guinea-pig. Eur J Pharmacol 193: 335–340

Zhang X, Kindel G H, Wulfert E, Hanin I 1995 Effects of immobilization stress on hippocampal monoamine release: modification by mivazerol, a new α_2-adrenoceptor agonist. Neuropharmacology 34: 1661–1672

Zornow M H 1991 Ventilatory, hemodynamic and sedative effects of the α_2 adrenergic agonist, dexmedetomidine. Neuropharmacology 30: 1065–1070

Jennifer M. Hunter

New neuromuscular blocking drugs

HISTORY

In 1942, Griffith and Johnson of Montreal administered 'Intocostrin', a mixture of alkaloids with neuromuscular blocking properties, derived from the South American plant *Chondrodendron tomentosum*, to a patient undergoing an appendicectomy; this event heralded a new era in anaesthetic practice. But it was not fully appreciated at that time that respiration had to be supported if neuromuscular blocking drugs were administered; otherwise, complications sufficient to cause death could ensue. In 1946, Gray and Halton in Liverpool described a series of patients given the purified extract of 'Intocostrin', *d*-tubocurarine, in whom respiration was fully assisted and an anticholinesterase used at the end of the procedure. The new technique gained popularity only slowly; initially small, sub-paralysing doses of tubocurarine were often given, an anticholinesterase was not used, and respiration not always supported. But, by the end of the 1950s, and mainly as a result of the development of artificial ventilators, many anaesthetists were appreciating the benefits of complete paralysis and support of respiration during major surgery.

Tubocurarine has disadvantages: it can cause histamine release with flushing of the skin, vasodilatation and a fall in blood pressure. It is also a long-acting drug, which is mainly eliminated unchanged in the urine. It can, therefore, have a prolonged effect if renal function is either temporarily or permanently impaired. The search began for an ideal neuromuscular blocking agent and, 50 years later, still continues.

Jennifer M. Hunter MB ChB PhD FRCA, Reader in Anaesthesia and Honorary Consultant Anaesthetist, Department of Anaesthesia, University Clinical Department, The Duncan Building, Royal Liverpool University Hospital, Liverpool L69 3GA, UK

CHEMICAL STRUCTURE

New developments in the pharmacology of neuromuscular blocking drugs have, in Europe and the US, centred around aminosteroid and benzyliso-quinolinium compounds.

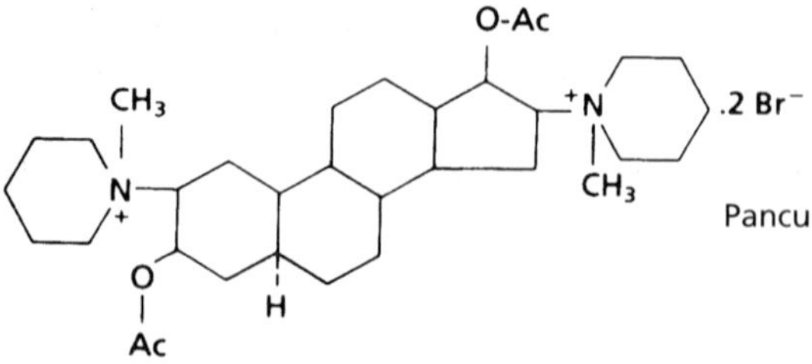

Pancuronium bromide

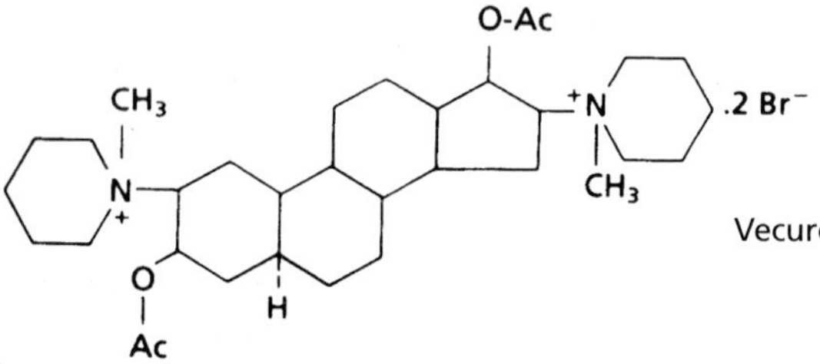

Vecuronium bromide

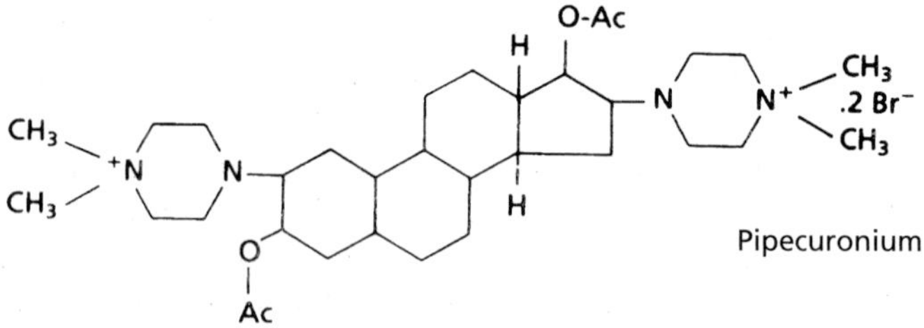

Pipecuronium bromide

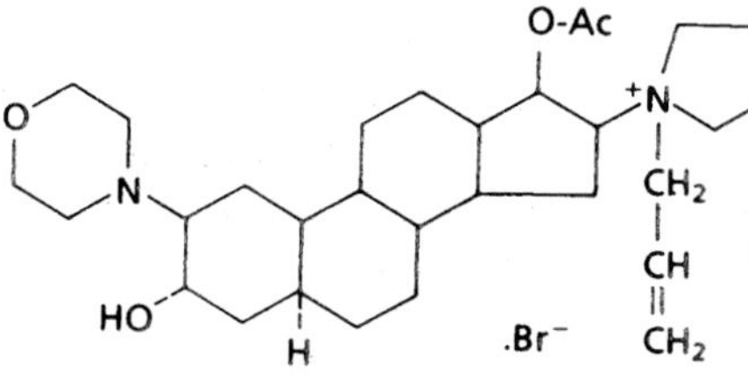

Rocuronium

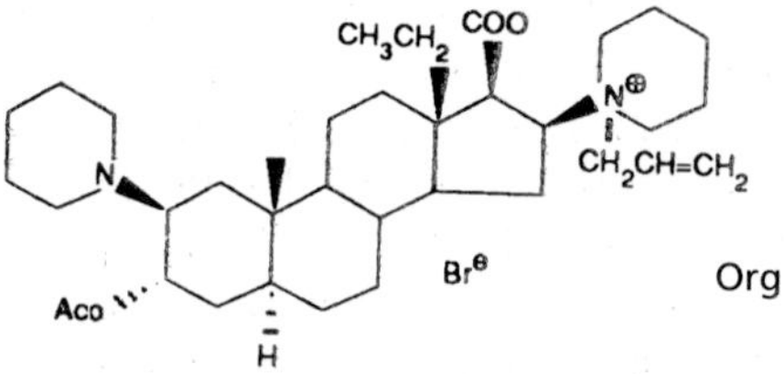

Org 9487

Fig. 8.1 The chemical structure of the aminosteroid neuromuscular blocking drugs, pancuronium, vecuronium, pipecuronium, rocuronium and Org 9487. Acetyl (Ac-O) groups are present in some of these structures at the 3C, and 17C positions (bottom left and top right corners, respectively, of the molecular structures). These acetyl groups are removed during the first step in the metabolism of aminosteroid drugs. The deacetylated 3 carbon metabolites have neuromuscular blocking properties.

AMINOSTEROIDS

The first aminosteroid to be developed was pancuronium in 1964 (Fig. 8.1). This drug was produced in an attempt to overcome the disadvantageous cardiovascular effects of tubocurarine, but pancuronium has vagolytic and sympathomimetic effects. It is also as long acting as tubocurarine, and undergoes significant renal excretion as well as hepatic metabolism. Vecuronium was developed to produce an agent free of cardiovascular effects, and with a shorter duration of action than pancuronium. In 1992, pipecuronium became available in many parts of Europe and the US (Stanley et al 1991). It has a similar onset and duration of action to pancuronium, but is free of cardiovascular effects. In 1995, rocuronium was introduced. This aminosteroid has a rapid onset of action, but a similar duration of effect to vecuronium. It may have a slight vagolytic action (Booth et al 1992). Another aminosteroid, Org 9487, is at present undergoing Phase III clinical trials. It is thought to have a similar onset of action to rocuronium, but a shorter duration of effect (Weirda et al 1993).

BENZYLISOQUINOLINIUMS

These drugs have a slim carbon chain linking the quaternary ammonium radicals ($N^+(CH_3)_3$) present in all neuromuscular blocking agents, which attach to the α subunits of the post-synaptic nicotinic receptor (Fig. 8.2). This carbon chain is vulnerable to breakdown in the plasma. Atracurium undergoes Hofmann degradation and ester hydrolysis; mivacurium is broken down by plasma cholinesterase. Doxacurium undergoes only a small amount of breakdown in the plasma (6%), but was the first benzylisoquinolinium not to have a propensity to release histamine (Basta 1992). It undergoes significant organ dependent elimination; it is mainly excreted unchanged in the urine (Cashman et al 1990). This drug has a long onset of action and a very variable and prolonged duration of effect. It is not expected that it will become available in the UK, although it is available in the US.

Atracurium is a mixture of 10 isomers. The 1R *cis*–1′R *cis* isomer, cisatracurium, is now available. It is a more potent agent than atracurium; a lower dose is required to produce neuromuscular block. It is also thought to be free of histamine releasing effects (Lien et al 1995).

Isomerism

Many anaesthetic agents, including neuromuscular blocking drugs, exhibit chirality; the same chemical structure exists in more than one form. Atracurium has four chiral centres; at each site the drug can exist in two forms (Fig. 8.2). Because of molecular symmetry, the 16 theoretical isomers of atracurium are reduced to 10 (Wastila et al 1996). The optical and geometric configurations of these 10 isomers exist in the *cis* or *trans*, and R or S forms respectively. The *cis* isomers are known to be longer acting and to stimulate less histamine release than the *trans* isomers. The 1R *cis*–1′R *cis* isomer was selected for clinical investigation and is now available as cisatracurium.

Mivacurium (Fig. 8.2) is a mixture of three stereoisomers. The two short-acting isomers, the *cis–trans* and *trans–trans*, have very short half-lives of about 2 min; the much less potent *cis–cis* isomer has only one-tenth of the neuromuscular blocking potency of the other two isomers and undergoes some renal excretion as well as being broken down by plasma cholinesterase. The shorter acting isomers are broken down almost entirely by plasma cholinesterase (Head-Rapson et al 1994).

AN IDEAL NEUROMUSCULAR BLOCKING DRUG

Such a drug would possess the properties listed in Table 8.1. It would be a non-depolarising agent, free of the side-effects of suxamethonium, such as muscle pains, hyperkalaemia, and malignant hyperthermia, and yet have as rapid an onset of action, with a slightly longer duration of effect.

Mivacurium

Doxacurium

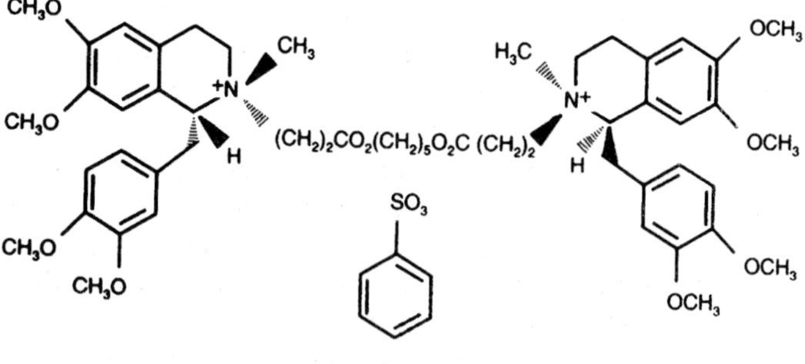

Cisatracurium

R, *cis*-R', *cis* isomer

Fig. 8.2 The structure of the benzylisoquinoliniums, mivacurium, doxacurium and cisatracurium. The isomeric sites of cisatracurium are highlighted by the solid and broken arrows, which signify the forward (solid) or backward (broken) direction of the adjacent carbon or hydrogen atom to the chiral centre.

Table 8.1 The ideal properties of a new neuromuscular blocking drug

- Non-depolarising
- Rapid onset: within one minute
- Short duration
- Predictable effect
- Breakdown independent of organ function
- Non-cumulative
- No adverse cardiovascular effects
- No histamine release
- Easily antagonised

RATE OF ONSET

A rapid onset is desirable if a patient with a full stomach is being anaesthetised; it is also preferable if tracheal intubation is about to be attempted in a patient with a difficult airway. A rapid onset of action has been one of the most difficult challenges in the development of an ideal neuromuscular blocking drug; some believe that it will prove impossible to develop a non-depolarising agent which has as rapid an onset as suxamethonium. It is thought that a drug of low potency within a chemical series of agents, is more likely to have a rapid onset of action than a very potent drug. A less potent drug is given in a larger dose; a larger number of molecules reach the post-synaptic nicotinic receptor at the neuromuscular junction, causing a more rapid onset of effect (Bowman et al 1988).

Rocuronium is the only non-depolarising agent with an onset of action similar to suxamethonium (Table 8.2). It has a low potency, with an ED_{95} (see below) of 0.3 mg/kg (Booth et al 1992). In comparison, pancuronium and vecuronium have an ED_{95} of 0.05 mg/kg. The onset of action of rocuronium 0.6 mg/kg ($2 \times ED_{95}$) is about 75 s; this is 15 s longer than suxamethonium 1.0 mg/kg, which has an onset of 1 min. In addition, the onset of rocuronium is more variable than suxamethonium, a disadvantageous property with any neuromuscular blocking drug. If $4 \times ED_{95}$ of rocuronium (1.2 mg/kg) is given, it has an onset very similar to suxamethonium but a duration of effect comparable with pancuronium. Org 9487 has an even lower potency than rocuronium; it has an ED_{95} of 1.0 mg/kg. It has a similar onset of action to rocuronium (Table 8.2).

Cisatracurium is more potent than atracurium, and its onset of action, in equipotent doses, is longer than its parent compound (Boyd et al 1995; Table 8.2). Mivacurium, if given in equipotent doses, has a similar onset of action to atracurium, but the intubating dose initially recommended ($2 \times ED_{95}$ = 0.15 mg/kg) was too low. This was advised in an attempt to prevent the adverse cardiovascular effects produced by mivacurium from histamine release, but resulted in an impression that neuromuscular block was difficult to obtain with this drug. Three times the ED_{95} (0.2 mg/kg), is a preferable dose for tracheal intubation. Doxacurium and pipecuronium have a long onset of action, at least as slow as pancuronium and tubocurarine (Table 8.2). This is a marked disadvantage of these two new agents.

Table 8.2 Two of the pharmacodynamic properties of 2 × ED_{95} of the new neuromuscular blocking drugs compared to equipotent doses of pancuronium, vecuronium and atracurium (Hunter 1995, van den Broek et al 1994)

	Time to maximum block (min)	20% recovery (T_1/T_0) (min)
Aminosteroids		
Pancuronium	2.9	86
Vecuronium	2.4	44
Pipecuronium	2.5	95
Rocuronium	1.25	43
Org 9487	1.9	2.7
Benzylisoquinoliniums		
Atracurium	2.4	38
Doxacurium	5.9	83
Mivacurium	1.8	16
Cisatracurium	4.8	46

CARDIOVASCULAR EFFECTS

In addition to developing a neuromuscular blocking drug which is free from histamine releasing properties, it is also preferable that the agent be free from the vagal effects of suxamethonium, and has no vagolytic or sympathomimetic properties, as seen with pancuronium or gallamine. Attempts have been made to produce a benzylisoquinolinium compound which was broken down in the plasma, but did not release histamine. Atracurium and mivacurium release about one-third of the amount of histamine released by tubocurarine in equipotent doses (Naguib et al 1995). Mivacurium probably releases slightly more histamine than atracurium (Loan et al 1995). Neither atracurium, mivacurium, doxacurium or cisatracurium have any direct effects on the cardiovascular system. Doxacurium only very rarely stimulate histamine release and cisatracurium, at this early stage of its development, also seems to be free from histamine releasing effects (Lien et al 1995). The aminosteroids, pipecuronium and rocuronium, do not release histamine. Rocuronium may have a slight vagolytic effect, as may Org 9487, but it is not as marked as with pancuronium.

DURATION OF EFFECT

A fixed dose of an ideal neuromuscular blocking agent would have a similar duration of action in a large group of individuals, with little variability of effect. This was a particular disadvantage of the older agents, tubocurarine and pancuronium. Doxacurium and pipecuronium are no improvement in this respect. Atracurium was a major development; it was the first non-depolarising neuromuscular blocking agent with a predictable duration of action.

A non-depolarising agent with a duration of action of 10–15 min is preferred by many anaesthetists. If the agent is required for a prolonged procedure it can be given by continuous infusion; if the surgical procedure is short, it can be reversed promptly. Mivacurium has these characteristics, in the presence of normal plasma cholinesterase (see below).

CUMULATIVE EFFECTS

If a neuromuscular blocking drug is given in repeated bolus doses without neuromuscular monitoring, a prolonged effect may occur. This is a particular risk with drugs which are metabolised in the liver or excreted unchanged in the urine; repeated bolus doses elevate the plasma concentration of the agent causing a prolonged effect. As the aminosteroid agents undergo organ-dependent elimination, cumulation of these agents is more likely to occur than with the benzylisoquinoliniums, which are broken down in the plasma.

ANTAGONISM

Ideally, a non-depolarising neuromuscular blocking drug would have the potential to be antagonised at any time after its administration. This is difficult to achieve. Recovery from neuromuscular block depends primarily on the diffusion of neuromuscular blocking agent away from the neuromuscular junction, down a concentration gradient, as the plasma concentration of the drug falls. The initial decline in plasma concentration after a single bolus dose of such a drug depends on redistribution; it is not related to metabolism of the drug in the liver or excretion through the kidney. No breakdown of a neuromuscular blocking drug occurs at the neuromuscular junction.

Successful antagonism of block with an anticholinesterase requires recovery to have commenced, regardless of which neuromuscular blocking agent or anticholinesterase is being used. Rapid recovery from neuromuscular block can only be assured if at least two twitches of the train-of-four twitch response are palpable or visible before the anticholinesterase is given. Clinical detection of the first twitch of the train occurs at about 10% recovery T_1/T_0; the second twitch is usually visible by 20% recovery T_1/T_0. The times to 20% recovery T_1/T_0 after $2 \times ED_{95}$ dose of the new neuromuscular blocking drugs are given in Table 8.2. Spontaneous recovery from mivacurium is so rapid in the presence of normal plasma cholinesterase that the use of an anticholinesterase such as neostigmine, given when $T_1/T_0 = 20\%$, only hastens recovery by a few minutes (Phillips & Hunter 1992).

Neostigmine inhibits plasma as well as acetylcholinesterase; the shorter acting anticholinesterase, edrophonium, has no such effect (Mirakhur et al 1982, Mirakhur 1986). Edrophonium has been shown to be more effective in reversing residual block produce by mivacurium than neostigmine (Bevan et al 1996).

PHARMACODYNAMICS

It is essential when comparing the onset and recovery of neuromuscular blocking drugs that equipotent doses are used. Neuromuscular blocking drugs are compared in multiples of their effective doses – the effective dose being the dose in mg/kg which, for instance, causes 95% depression of the twitch response. This would be designated the ED_{95}. Alternatively, the ED_{50} or ED_{90} is sometimes quoted. As there is a variation within the general population in the response to a neuromuscular blocking drug, it is recommended that two to three times the ED_{95} of a non-depolarising agent is given to assure adequate conditions for tracheal intubation.

To determine accurately the onset and recovery characteristics of any neuromuscular blocking drug, it is essential to record the electrical (electromyographic) or mechanical (mechanomyographic) response of a peripheral muscle to stimulation of its motor nerve. The train-of-four (TOF) response is useful in clinical practice and research; it is more sensitive that the twitch response, and yet does not produce residual pain postoperatively, as can be experienced with fast, tetanic rates of stimulation. The ratio of the fourth twitch of the train to the first (T_4/T_1) is known as the train-of-four ratio. The degree of decrement of this ratio varies with neuromuscular blocking drugs; the greater the degree of fade, the greater the degree of presynaptic effect. It is thought to be desirable that a new agent has purely a postsynaptic effect. It was recommended that 70% recovery T_4/T_1 was necessary before extubation could be effected safely. Recent work has suggested that, if electromyographic monitoring is being used, such as a Datex Relaxograph, then 80% recovery T_4/T_1 is preferable (Engbaek et al 1989).

PHARMACOKINETICS

Redistribution of a bolus dose of any neuromuscular blocking drug, all of which are highly ionised and water soluble compounds, only occurs to a small extent outside the intravascular compartment; the volumes of distribution of these agents are relatively small (Table 8.3). During redistribution, recovery from block commences, and thus the elimination of a single dose of such a drug through the liver or kidney plays little part in its clinical effect. The value of the elimination half-life for such drugs has little relevance in these clinical circumstances (Fisher 1996). If, however, the drug is given in repeated bolus doses, or by continuous infusion, then elimination will contribute to recovery from block.

METABOLISM

The breakdown products of neuromuscular blocking drugs can also have pharmacological activity. The active metabolites of neuromuscular blocking drugs are of two main types: those with the same effects as the parent compound; and those with different properties from the parent compound.

METABOLITES WITH NEUROMUSCULAR BLOCKING ACTIVITY

The metabolism in the liver of the aminosteroid compounds occurs in two stages; initially the drug is deacetylated, and then glucuronidation to a more

Table 8.3 The clearance (Cl ml/min/kg) and volume of distribution at steady state (Vd_{ss} ml/kg) for the newer non-depolarising neuromuscular blocking drugs compared with pancuronium, atracurium and vecuronium (Hunter 1995, van den Broek 1994)

	Cl (ml/min/kg)	Vd_{ss} (ml/kg)
Aminosteroids		
Pancuronium	1.8	241
Vecuronium	5.3	199
Pipecuronium	3.0	350
Rocuronium	2.9	207
Org 9487	8.5	293
Benzylisoquinoliniums		
Atracurium	6.6	87
Doxacurium	2.7	220
Mivacurium		
cis–trans	95.0	210
trans–trans	70.0	200
cis–cis	5.2	266
Cisatracurium	5.1	153

water soluble form takes place. Deacetylation occurs at the 3C and 17C positions, if an acetyl group is linked to that carbon (Fig. 8.1). The 3-desacetyl metabolites have up to 50% of the neuromuscular blocking properties of the parent compound and are more water soluble. As the metabolites are excreted almost entirely through the kidney, they may contribute to neuromuscular block if these drugs are given for prolonged periods, or in high doses. In critically ill patients with acute renal failure who have received a continuous infusion of vecuronium in an intensive care unit, the 3-desacetyl metabolite has been shown to be detectable in the plasma for longer than the parent compound. This metabolite is thought to contribute to prolonged neuromuscular block in such circumstances (Segredo et al 1992). Rocuronium does not possess an acetyl group at the 3C position (Fig. 8.1) and should not, therefore, possess a metabolite with neuromuscular blocking activity; this may be an advantage of the agent over vecuronium in patients with renal dysfunction. Org 9487 has an acetyl group attached to 3C (Fig. 8.1), and is known to have a deacetylated metabolite with neuromuscular blocking activity – Org 9488. It is, as yet, uncertain whether this metabolite will, in any clinical circumstances, contribute to neuromuscular block.

The 17-desacetyl metabolites of pancuronium, vecuronium, pipecuronium and rocuronium have only minimal neuromuscular blocking properties, which are unlikely to contribute to neuromuscular block, even in patients with organ dysfunction.

ACTIVE METABOLITES WITH OTHER PROPERTIES

Hofmann degradation of atracurium produces laudanosine, which is known in pharmacological doses in animals to produce epileptiform fits (Chapple et al

1987). Ester hydrolysis of atracurium produces monoquaternary alcohol, which also undergoes Hofmann degradation to laudanosine. Thus two molecules of laudanosine are produced from the breakdown of each molecule of atracurium.

Laudanosine

Laudanosine is more lipid soluble than atracurium; it is metabolised in the liver, and also excreted unchanged in the urine. In dogs, cerebral irritation has been demonstrated at plasma laudanosine levels of 14.0 μg/ml and at 17.0 μg/ml, convulsive activity occurs (Chapple et al 1987). In small animal species, the plasma threshold is lower; in rabbits, abnormal cerebral activity occurs at 5 μg/ml.

In humans, plasma laudanosine levels peak at around 0.3 μg/ml after a bolus dose of atracurium 0.5 mg/kg. The plasma level is slightly higher in patients with chronic renal failure (Fahey et al 1985). There have been no adverse effects reported from laudanosine in man, but plasma levels are significantly higher in patients with multiple organ failure, receiving continuous infusions of atracurium for many days in an intensive therapy unit (see below).

As cisatracurium is much more potent than atracurium (ED_{95} = 0.05 and 0.23 mg/kg, respectively) it may be expected that lower levels of laudanosine would be generated when cisatracurium is used. In healthy and renal failure patients given cisatracurium 0.1 mg/kg, peak laudanosine levels were around 0.025 μg/ml; 10 times lower than after an equipotent dose of atracurium (Eastwood et al 1995).

Mivacurium and doxacurium do not possess any active metabolites.

NEUROMUSCULAR BLOCKING DRUGS : EXTREMES OF AGE

CHILDREN

The neuromuscular junction at birth is not mature; it takes about three months for the subunits of the postsynaptic nicotinic receptor to convert from the fetal to the adult form. Fetal receptors are the same as those that develop extra-junctionally in, for instance, burned patients and patients with neuromuscular disorders. They are slightly resistant to the action of non-depolarising neuromuscular blocking drugs.

Neonates have a higher extracellular fluid volume as a proportion of body weight than adults. Neuromuscular blocking drugs will, therefore, initially be distributed in a larger volume in respect of body weight than in adults. All these factors can lead to relative resistance to non-depolarising neuromuscular blocking drugs in the healthy neonate. If the neonate is immature or born at a premature date, however, then organ function, in particular liver and renal function, may not be fully developed. In such sickly infants, sensitivity to neuromuscular blocking drugs may be encountered.

Plasma cholinesterase activity is not fully developed until 6 months of age. Neonates may, therefore, be sensitive to suxamethonium. The use of mivacurium is this age group has not yet been detailed.

In children up to adolescence, extracellular fluid volume remains a higher proportion of body weight than in adults and thus the relative resistance to non-depolarising neuromuscular blocking drugs continues.

ELDERLY PATIENTS

Even in healthy patients, renal and hepatic function deteriorate with increasing age. Glomerular filtration rate and renal plasma flow gradually fall and plasma creatinine rises. The rate of hepatic metabolism decreases. These changes only become marked in healthy adults by the age of 80 years, but in less fit patients they will be detectable at an earlier age. These organ changes will have pharmacokinetic effects; all neuromuscular blocking drugs excreted in the urine or metabolised in the liver could have an altered action. This was demonstrated with pancuronium (McLeod et al 1979) and can occur with vecuronium (Lien et al 1991). Rocuronium may also have a prolonged effect in the elderly (Matteo et al 1993).

The newer benzylisoquinolinium agents, which are less dependent on organ disposition, are less likely to have altered effects with increasing age. The pharmacokinetics of atracurium were shown to be unaltered by increasing age (Kent et al 1989), although the plasma laudanosine levels were slightly higher in the elderly. There is only a marginal difference in the pharmacokinetics of cisatracurium in the elderly compared with the young: onset of block may be delayed because of slower biophase equilibration (Sorooshian et al 1996).

There is evidence that plasma cholinesterase activity may decrease with increasing age. This is though to explain the slightly longer effect of mivacurium in the elderly (Basta et al 1989).

NEUROMUSCULAR BLOCKING DRUGS IN DISEASE STATES

RENAL DISEASE

Many of the older non-depolarising neuromuscular blocking drugs, both aminosteroids and benzylisoquinoliniums, were excreted to a significant degree in the urine. If these drugs were given in excess, then persistent neuromuscular block could ensue. Gallamine, a trisquaternary amine, is almost entirely excreted by the kidney; persistent block was reported repeatedly in patients with renal dysfunction given this agent. It would now be negligent to use gallamine in this group of patients.

The development of atracurium and vecuronium was significant in this respect; for the first time, non-depolarising neuromuscular blocking drugs became available which did not depend primarily on the kidney for their disposition. Early pharmacodynamic work suggested no statistically significant difference between the recovery characteristics in healthy or chronic renal failure patients given atracurium or vecuronium (Hunter et al 1984). But pharmacokinetic studies subsequently demonstrated a greater clearance of atracurium in chronic renal failure patients (Fahey et al 1984). In contrast, the clearance of vecuronium is reduced in patients with renal disease (Lynam et al 1988). The increased clearance of atracurium is probably due to the increased volume of distribution in the oedematous diseased state. Atracurium can break down wherever it exists in the body if the pH is the same as that of plasma.

Cisatracurium has been shown to undergo more Hofmann degradation and less ester hydrolysis than atracurium (Wastila et al 1996). It probably also undergoes slightly more renal excretion (Table 8.4). Pharmacodynamic studies of

Table 8.4 The 24 h urine excretion (%) of a bolus dose of the new neuromuscular blocking drugs compared with pancuronium, vecuronium and atracurium (Hunter 1995, van den Broek et al 1994)

		%
Aminosteroids		
	Pancuronium	40
	Vecuronium	15
	Pipecuronium	38
	Rocuronium	9
	Org 9487	15
Benzylisoquinoliniums		
	Atracurium	10
	Doxacurium	20–30
	Mivacurium	< 10
	Cisatracurium	15

cisatracurium 0.1 mg/kg have shown a slightly longer onset time in renal patients which may be due to a slower circulation time (Boyd et al 1995). There was no significant difference in the recovery variables between the two groups, but pharmacokinetic data obtained from the same patients showed a slightly lower clearance and increased elimination half-life of cisatracurium in the renal patients (Eastwood et al 1995). The safety net of Hofmann elimination is still present however; there is no evidence of a prolonged effect after cisatracurium in chronic renal failure patients

Plasma cholinesterase activity may be reduced in chronic renal failure, and this is thought to explain the 50% increase in the duration of block found in renal failure patients given mivacurium compared with healthy controls (Phillips & Hunter 1992). The clearances of the *cis–trans* and *trans–trans* isomers of mivacurium in healthy and renal failure patients have been shown to be highly correlated with plasma cholinesterase activity (Head-Rapson et al 1995).

Studies on rocuronium in chronic renal failure patients have produced conflicting results. In renal transplant patients, no difference was found between onset or recovery characteristics in the renal failure and healthy patients (Szenohradzky et al 1992). An increased volume of distribution was thought to explain the increased elimination half-life of rocuronium in the disease state. But in anephric patients undergoing vascular access surgery, longer recovery times were found compared with healthy controls (Cooper et al 1993). There was also more variability in the recovery characteristics in the disease state. Rocuronium is unlikely to replace atracurium or cisatracurium in this group of patients. Doxacurium (Cashman et al 1990), and pipecuronium (Cameron et al 1994) may also have a prolonged effect in the presence of renal disease.

HEPATIC CIRRHOSIS

These patients are often oedematous with significant ascites, and thus will also have an increased volume of distribution of water-soluble non-depolarising muscle relaxants. The effect may produce resistance to onset of block. But then any non-depolarising agent metabolised in the liver may have a prolonged effect. This has been demonstrated for pancuronium, vecuronium and pipecuronium (Duvaldestin et al 1978, Lebrault et al 1985, D'Honneur et al 1992). The pharmacodynamics and pharmacokinetics of atracurium are little changed in cirrhosis; resistance to onset of block may occur but, if anything, recovery will be faster than in health (Bell et al 1985), due to an increased rate of clearance in the disease state (Parker & Hunter 1989). Cisatracurium has also been shown to have similar onset and recovery characteristics in liver transplant patients to healthy controls; an increased clearance of cisatracurium was found in the liver patients (de Wolf et al 1996). Plasma laudanosine levels were estimated in this study; the mean peak concentration in the transplant patients was 21 μg/ml. These levels are 10 times lower than those reported after atracurium in cirrhotic patients (Parker & Hunter 1989). As laudanosine is in part metabolised in the liver, it is preferable to use cisatracurium in this group of patients. The effect of doxacurium is also unaltered by liver disease (Cook et al 1991).

Plasma cholinesterase is synthesised in the liver. Mivacurium has a prolonged effect in hepatic cirrhosis, which is inversely related to cholinesterase activity (Devlin et al 1993). There is little indication for its use in cirrhosis.

The first study of rocuronium in patients with liver disease suggested a decreased clearance which did not reach statistical significance (Khalil et al 1994). A subsequent study, using old controls, failed to substantiate these findings (Magorian et al 1995), but more recently, in a larger study, a decreased clearance and prolonged recovery has been found in cirrhotic patients given rocuronium 0.6 mg/kg (van Miert et al 1997). There is no benefit of rocuronium over atracurium or cisatracurium in liver disease.

MYASTHENIA GRAVIS

These patients were recognised to be very sensitive to the older non-depolarising neuromuscular blocking drugs; doses as small as tubocurarine 3 mg could produce complete neuromuscular block (Foldes & McNall 1962). It was, therefore, common to avoid the use of non-depolarising neuromuscular blocking drugs in patients with myasthenia gravis. Usually this did not limit anaesthetic management, except perhaps when such a patient presented for upper abdominal or thoracic surgery. Often anticholinesterase or corticosteroid therapy was stopped pre-operatively and the patient could easily be ventilated using potent inhalational agents only. The advent of the intermediate-acting agents, atracurium and vecuronium, allowed for the first time the more predictable management of neuromuscular block in myasthenic patients. It was demonstrated that, if about one- to two-fifths of the normal dose of these agents was given, and neuromuscular block was monitored throughout surgery, good recovery could be obtained with normal doses of neostigmine (Bell et al 1984, Hunter et al 1985). In addition, it was not necessary to stop routine therapy pre-operatively, which the patient preferred. Mivacurium has also been used successfully in small doses in myasthenic patients (Seigne & Scott 1994).

MULTI-SYSTEM ORGAN FAILURE

In critically ill patients undergoing intensive therapy, artificial ventilation can usually be managed using sedatives and analgesics alone; it is not necessary also to administer neuromuscular blocking drugs. But, occasionally, these drugs are a useful adjunct to patient management, for instance if the patient has adult respiratory distress syndrome or severe burns. In the presence of hepatic or renal dysfunction, however, the older agents such as pancuronium or alcuronium could have a prolonged effect (Vandenbrom & Wierda 1988, Smith et al 1987). This is in part due to decreased renal elimination, and with pancuronium, because of the additional effect of its active metabolite, 3-desacetyl pancuronium.

Atracurium became the first neuromuscular blocking drug to have a similar effect in the critically ill and healthy patient. Recovery of T_1/T_0 to 70%, without the use of an anticholinesterase, was similar in both groups of patients – about 60 min – even if the drug had been given for several days by continuous infusion (Griffiths et al 1986). The only concern was laudanosine; the plasma levels were higher in critically ill patients, especially in the presence of renal or hepatic dysfunction, when values of around 5.0 μg/ml were commonplace (Parker et al 1988). The highest reported laudanosine level of 8.6 μg/ml, in a neurosurgical patient with normal renal and hepatic function, produced no adverse effect (Gwinnutt et al 1990). More recent studies of atracurium and cisatracurium in the critically ill have reported similar laudanosine levels in the atracurium group, around 5 μg/ml, but the highest laudanosine level in the cisatracurium patients was 1.2 μg/ml (Boyd et al 1996). For those clinicians worried about the potential effects of laudanosine in the critically ill, cisatracurium will have a marked advantage.

Doxacurium has been compared with pancuronium in the critically ill patient; both drugs were given in incremental doses with routine neuromuscular monitoring (Murray et al 1995). Cardiovascular stability was more marked and recovery of T_1/T_0 to 70% was slightly quicker in the doxacurium group. It, nevertheless, took 180 min compared with 268 min after pancuronium; these are different orders of recovery compared with atracurium and cisatracurium.

Pipecuronium has also been demonstrated to be useful, if given in bolus doses and with regular neuromuscular monitoring, in the management of the critically ill patient (Khuenl-Brady et al 1994). There is little indication for the use of mivacurium in the critically ill; its effect would be too unpredictable in patients with many potential causes for decreased cholinesterase activity.

The most important, yet often most neglected aspect of the use of these drugs in the critically ill patient, is the necessity for regular and simple neuromuscular monitoring if prolonged block is to be avoided.

ATYPICAL CHOLINESTERASE

One in 200 of the Caucasian population possess one abnormal gene for plasma cholinesterase. As the inheritance of this gene is autosomal recessive, one in 40 000 of the population are potentially homozygote carriers of two abnormal cholinesterase genes. In addition to causing a prolonged neuromuscular block after suxamethonium, an even more pronounced effect can occur if mivacurium is given in standard doses to such patients. In heterozygote patients, 25% recovery T_1/T_0 after mivacurium 0.15 mg/kg will take 35 min, compared with 17 min in patients with normal plasma cholinesterase (Ostergaard et al 1993). In such circumstances, mivacurium, therefore, has a similar length of action to atracurium. But, if a similar dose of mivacurium is given to a homozygous patient, several anecdotal reports suggest that neuromuscular block can persist for several hours (Fox & Hunt 1995, Sockalingham & Green 1995). In such circumstances, the clinical management is as with a suxamethonium (scoline) apnoea; keep the patient asleep and monitor neuromuscular block until recovery is complete. The use of fresh frozen plasma is questionable as its content of plasma cholinesterase cannot be quantified. However, genetically engineered plasma cholinesterase has now been developed and is undergoing clinical trials (Naguib et al 1995); such a preparation would be useful when unexpectedly prolonged block after mivacurium is demonstrated using neuromuscular monitoring.

NEW AGENTS UNDERGOING CLINICAL TRIALS

ORG 9487

This aminosteroid has a similar onset to rocuronium, but 25% recovery T_1/T_0 only takes about 8 min (Wierda et al 1993). This is longer than at first predicted; it was expected that it may be possible to antagonise this agent within a few minutes of administration (Van den Broek et al 1994; Table 8.2). Org 9487 may, like rocuronium, have a slight vagolytic effect. There is some evidence of bronchospasm occurring after its administration; this may be due to histamine release, although this is unusual with an aminosteroid compound. It is not necessarily accompanied by cutaneous flushing. As this aminosteroid has such a high plasma clearance (Table 8.3), it is possible that it undergoes spontaneous degradation in the plasma as well as deacetylation in the liver.

SUMMARY

Three new neuromuscular blocking drugs are available in clinical practice in the UK. Mivacurium, in equipotent doses, has a similar onset of action to atracurium but, in the presence of normal plasma cholinesterase activity, the shortest duration of action of any non-depolarising drug. Cisatracurium is more potent than atracurium; it has a slightly longer onset and duration of action than the parent drug. It is free of histamine releasing properties and produces less laudanosine than atracurium.

Rocuronium has the most rapid onset of any available non-depolarising drug, but a duration of effect similar to vecuronium. It has a slight vagolytic action. Org 9487 is not yet available for clinical use. This aminosteroid has a similar onset of action to rocuronium, but a duration of effect comparable with mivacurium.

Doxacurium and pipecuronium are not available in the UK. Both drugs have a long and variable onset and duration of effect, but are free from adverse cardiovascular side-effects.

References

Basta S J, Dresner D L, Shaff L P et al 1989 Neuromuscular effects and pharmacokinetics of mivacurium in elderly patients under isoflurane anesthesia. Anesth Analg 68: S18

Basta S J 1992 Modulation of histamine release by neuromuscular blocking drugs. Curr Opin Anaesth 5: 572–576

Bell C F, Florence A M, Hunter J M et al 1984 Atracurium in the myasthenic patient. Anaesthesia 39: 961–968

Bell C F, Hunter J M, Jones R S et al 1985 Use of atracurium and vecuronium in patients with oesophageal varices. Br J Anaesth 57: 160–168

Bevan J C, Tousigant C, Stephenson C et al 1996 Dose responses for neostigmine and edrophonium as antagonists of mivacurium in adults and children. Anesthesiology 84: 354–361

Booth M G, Marsh B, Bryden F M M et al 1992 A comparison of the pharmacodynamics of rocuronium and vecuronium during halothane anaesthesia. Anaesthesia 47: 832–834

Bowman W C, Rodger I W, Houston J et al 1988 Structure: action relationships among some desacetoxy analogues of pancuronium and vecuronium in the anesthetized cat. Anesthesiology 69: 57–62

Boyd A H, Eastwood N B, Parker C J R et al 1995 Pharmacodynamics of the 1R *cis*- 1'R *cis* isomer of atracurium (51W89) in health and chronic renal failure. Br J Anaesth 74: 400–404

Boyd A H, Eastwood N B, Parker C J R et al 1996 Comparison of the pharmacodynamics and pharmacokinetics of an infusion of *cis*-atracurium (51W89) or atracurium in critically ill patients undergoing mechanical ventilation in an intensive therapy unit. Br J Anaesth 76: 382–388

Cameron EM, Lisbon A, Moorman R et al 1994 Prolonged neuromuscular blockade with pipecuronium in a patient with renal insufficiency. Eur J Anaesthesiol 11: 237–239

Cashman J N, Luke J J, Jones R M 1990 Neuromuscular block with doxacurium (BWA938U) in patients with normal or absent renal function. Br J Anaesth 64: 186–192

Chapple D J, Miller A A, Ward J B et al 1987 Cardiovascular and neurological effects of laudanosine: studies in mice and rats and in conscious and anaesthetized dogs. Br J Anaesth 59: 218–225

Cook D R, Freeman J A, Lai A A et al 1991 Pharmacokinetics and pharmacodynamics of doxacurium in normal patients and in those with hepatic or renal failure. Anesth Analg 72: 145–150

Cooper R A, Maddineni V R, Mirakhur R K et al 1993 Time course of neuromuscular effects and pharmacokinetics of rocuronium bromide (Org 9426) during isoflurane anaesthesia in patients with and without renal failure. Br J Anaesth 71: 222–226

De Wolf A M, Freeman J A, Scott V L et al 1996 Pharmacokinetics and pharmacodynamics of cisatracurium in patients with end-stage liver disease undergoing liver transplantation. Br J Anaesth 76: 624–628

Devlin J C, Head-Rapson A G, Parker C J R et al 1993 Pharmacodynamics of mivacurium chloride in patients with hepatic cirrhosis. Br J Anaesth 71: 227–231

D'Honneur G, Khalil M, Dominique C et al 1993 Pharmacokinetics and pharmacodynamics of pipecuronium in patients with cirrhosis. Anesth Analg 77: 1203–1206

Duvaldestin P, Agoston S, Henzel D et al 1978 Pancuronium pharmacokinetics in patients with liver cirrhosis. Br J Anaesth 50: 1131–1136

Eastwood N B, Boyd A H, Parker C J R et al 1995 Pharmacokinetics of 1R-*cis* 1'R-*cis* atracurium besylate (51W89) and plasma laudanosine concentrations in health and in chronic renal failure. Br J Anaesth 75: 431–435

Engbaek J, Ostergaard D, Viby-Mogensen J et al 1989 Clinical recovery and train-of-four ratio measured mechanically and electromyographically following atracurium. Anesthesiology 71: 391–395

Fahey M R, Rupp S M, Fisher D M et al 1984 The pharmacokinetics and pharmacodynamics of atracurium in patients with and without renal failure. Anesthesiology 61: 699–702

Fahey M R, Rupp S M, Canfell C et al 1985 Effect of renal failure on laudanosine excretion in man. Br J Anaesth 57: 1049–1051

Fisher D M 1996 (Almost) everything you learned about pharmacokinetics was (somewhat) wrong! Anesth Analg 83: 901–903

Foldes F F, McNall P G 1962 Myasthenia gravis: a guide for anesthesiologists. Anesthesiology 23: 837–872

Fox M H, Hunt P C W 1995 Prolonged neuromuscular block associated with mivacurium. Br J Anaesth 74: 237–238
Griffiths R B, Hunter J M, Jones R S 1986 Atracurium infusions in patients with renal failure on an ITU. Anaesthesia 41: 375–381
Gwinnutt C L, Eddleston J M, Edwards D et al 1990 Concentrations of atracurium and laudanosine in cerebrospinal fluid and plasma in three intensive care patients. Br J Anaesth 65: 829–832
Head-Rapson A G, Devlin J C, Parker C J R et al 1994 Pharmacokinetics of the three isomers of mivacurium and pharmacodynamics of the chiral mixture in hepatic cirrhosis. Br J Anaesth 73: 613–618
Head-Rapson A G, Devlin J C, Parker C J R et al 1995 Pharmacokinetics and pharmacodynamics of the three isomers of mivacurium in health, in end-stage renal failure and in patients with impaired renal function. Br J Anaesth 75: 31–36
Hunter J M 1995 New neuromuscular blocking drugs. N Engl J Med 332: 1691–1699
Hunter J M, Jones R S, Utting J E 1984 Comparison of vecuronium, atracurium and tubocurarine in normal patients and in patients with no renal function. Br J Anaesth 56: 941–951
Hunter J M, Bell C F, Florence A M et al 1985 Vecuronium in the myasthenic patient. Anaesthesia 40: 848–853
Kent A P, Parker C J R, Hunter J M 1989 Pharmacokinetics of atracurium and laudanosine in the elderly. Br J Anaesth 63: 661–666
Khalil M, D'Honneur G, Duvaldestin P et al 1994 Pharmacokinetics and pharmacodynamics of rocuronium in patients with cirrhosis. Anesthesiology 80: 1241–1247
Khuenl-Brady K S, Reitstatter B, Schlager A et al 1994 Long term administration of pancuronium and pipecuronium in the intensive care unit. Anesth Analg 78: 1082–1086
Lebrault C, Berger J L, D'Hollander A A et al 1985 Pharmacokinetics and pharmacodynamics of vecuronium (ORG NC45) in patients with cirrhosis. Anesthesiology 62: 601–605
Lien C A, Matteo R S, Ornstein E et al 1991 Distribution, elimination, and action of vecuronium in the elderly. Anesth Analg 73: 39–42
Lien C A, Belmont M R, Abalos A et al 1995 The cardiovascular effects and histamine-releasing properties of 51W89 in patients receiving nitrous oxide/opioid/barbiturate anesthesia. Anesthesiology 82: 1131–1138
Loan P B, Elliot P, Mirakhur R K et al 1995 Comparison of the haemodynamic effects of mivacurium and atracurium during fentanyl anaesthesia. Br J Anaesth 74: 330–332
Lynam D P, Cronnelly R, Castagnoli K P et al 1988 The pharmacodynamics and pharmacokinetics of vecuronium in patients anesthetized with isoflurane with normal renal function or with renal failure. Anesthesiology 69: 227–231
McLeod K, Hull C J, Watson M J 1979 Effects of ageing on pharmacokinetics of pancuronium. Br J Anaesth 51: 435–438
Magorian T, Wood P, Caldwell J et al 1995 The pharmacokinetics and neuromuscular effects of rocuronium bromide in patients with liver disease. Anesth Analg 80: 754–759
Matteo R S, Ornstein E, Schwartz A E et al 1993 Pharmacokinetics and pharmacodyamics of rocuronium (Org 9426) in elderly surgical patients. Anesth Analg 77: 1193–1197
Mirakhur R K, Lavery T D, Briggs L P et al 1982 Effects of neostigmine and pyridostigmine on serum cholinesterase activity. Can J Anaesth 29: 55–58
Mirakhur R K 1986 Edrophonium and plasma cholinesterase activity. Can J Anaesth 33: 588-590
Murray M J, Coursin D B, Scuderi P E et al 1995 Double blind randomised, multicenter study of doxacurium vs. pancuronium in intensive care unit patients who require neuromuscular blocking agents. Crit Care Med 23: 450–458
Naguib M, Daoud W, El-Gammal M et al 1995 Enzymatic antagonism of mivacurium-induced neuromuscular blockade by human plasma cholinesterase. Anesthesiology 83: 694–701
Naguib M, Samarkandi A H, Bakhamees H S et al 1995 Histamine release haemodynamic changes produced by rocuronium, vecuronium, mivacurium, atracurium and tubocurarine. Br J Anaesth 75: 588–592
Ostergaard D, Jensen F S, Jensen E et al 1993 Mivacurium-induced neuromuscular blockade in patients with atypical plasma cholinesterase. Acta Anaesthesiol Scand 37: 314–318

Parker C J R, Jones J E, Hunter J M 1988 Disposition of infusions of atracurium and its metabolite, laudanosine, in patients in renal and respiratory failure in an ITU. Br J Anaesth 61: 531–540

Parker C J R, Hunter J M 1989 Pharmacokinetics of atracurium and laudanosine in patients with hepatic cirrhosis. Br J Anaesth 62: 177–183

Phillips B J, Hunter J M 1992 Use of mivacurium chloride by constant infusion in the anephric patient. Br J Anaesth 68: 492–498

Segredo V, Caldwell J E, Matthay M A et al 1992 Persistent paralysis in critically ill patients after long-term administration of vecuronium. N Engl J Med 327: 524–528

Seigne R D, Scott R P F 1994 Mivacurium chloride and myasthenia gravis. Br J Anaesth 72: 468–469

Smith C L, Hunter J M, Jones R S 1987 Prolonged paralysis following an infusion of alcuronium in a patient with renal dysfunction. Anaesthesia 42: 522–525

Sockalingam I, Green D W 1995 Mivacurium-induced prolonged neuromuscular block. Br J Anaesth 74: 234–236

Sorooshian S S, Stafford M A, Eastwood N B et al 1996 Pharmacokinetics and pharmacodynamics of cisatracurium in young and elderly adult patients. Anesthesiology 84: 1083-1091

Stanley J C, Mirakhur R K, Bell P F et al 1991 Neuromuscular effects of pipecuronium bromide. Eur J Anaesthesiol 8: 151–156

Szenohradszky J, Fisher D M, Segredo V et al 1992 Pharmacokinetics of rocuronium bromide (ORG 9426) in patients with normal renal function or patients undergoing cadaver renal transplantation. Anesthesiology 77: 899–904

Van den Broek L, Wierda J M K H, Smeulers N J et al 1994 Pharmacodynamics and pharmacokinetics of an infusion of Org 9487, a new short-acting steroidal neuromuscular blocking agent. Br J Anaesth 73: 331–335

Vandenbrom R H G, Wierda J M K H 1988 Pancuronium bromide in the intensive care unit: a case of overdose. Anesthesiology 69: 996-997

van Miert M M, Eastwood N B, Boyd A H et al 1997 The pharmacokinetics and pharmacodynamics of rocuronium in patients with hepatic cirrhosis. Br J Clin Pharmacol 44: 139–144

Wastila W B, Maehr R B, Turner G L et al 1996 Comparative pharmacology of cisatracurium (51W89), atracurium, and five isomers in cats. Anesthesiology 85: 169–177

Wierda J M K H, van den Broek L, Proost J H et al 1993 Time course of action and endotracheal intubating conditions of Org 9487, a new short-acting steroidal muscle relaxant: a comparison with succinylcholine. Anesth Analg 77: 579–584

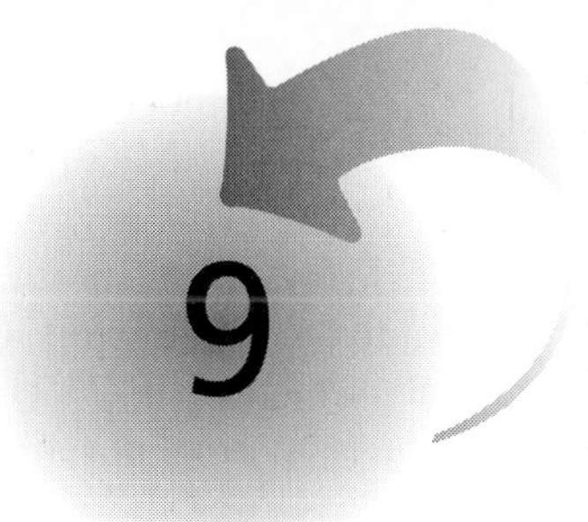

Geraldine O'Sullivan

Regional analgesia/ anaesthesia in obstetrics

A question of efficacy, safety and the provision of information to the mother?

The pain of labour is rarely surpassed (Melzack 1984) and frequently exceeds the mother's pre-partum expectation (Capogna et al 1996). Thus a mother who during pregnancy had decided that epidural analgesia would be unnecessary for her or who had adopted a 'wait and see' policy can demand regional analgesia at a time when her ability to comprehend a verbal explanation of the advantages and disadvantages of the impending technique is impaired. Since 1985 the Committee on Professional Liability of the American Society of Anesthesiologists (ASA) has been conducting an ongoing study of insurance company liability files involving anaesthetists (Chadwick 1996). Files that are no longer active are reviewed by practising anaesthetists, abstracted, double checked by the ASA Closed Claims Committee and then entered into a computer database. An analysis of the obstetric anaesthesia database found that obstetric complaints included a large proportion of relatively minor injuries which was in marked contrast to the non-obstetric files. It was felt by those reviewing the files that, in many instances, mothers were unhappy with the care provided and felt themselves ignored, mistreated or assaulted. Anaesthetists must deal sympathetically with mothers such that she will not be motivated to seek redress for an unexpected or unhappy outcome (MacArthur et al 1993). The importance of establishing and maintaining a good rapport with the mother throughout labour and delivery cannot be over emphasised. The fall in maternal mortality and the increasing knowledge and sophistication of many of the mothers presenting for pain relief in labour means that the issue of 'quality care' is paramount. The aim of those involved in obstetric anaesthesia should be to achieve effective analgesia and anaesthesia, to minimise all risks for both mother and child and to provide

Dr Geraldine O'Sullivan, Anaesthetic Department, St Thomas' Hospital, Lambeth Palace Road, London SE1 7EH, UK

mothers with realistic expectations and knowledge of the potential major and minor risks associated with regional analgesia/anaesthesia (Fig. 9.1).

Dissatisfaction with childbirth experience has been related to inadequate analgesia, long labour and instrumental delivery (Paech 1991), unfriendly midwives or doctors and with lack of sympathy and reassurance during labour (Lindt & Hoel 1989). Maternal satisfaction is high when effective analgesia is achieved but is low when pain persists after the provision of analgesia (Capogna et al 1996).

Changing Childbirth (HMSO 1993) is committed to increasing maternal freedom of choice and aims to ensure that the mother is well informed on the choices available to her. This means that those anaesthetists involved in the provision of obstetric analgesia and anaesthesia must strive to ensure that the maternal population in their care fully comprehend the advantages and disadvantages of obstetric regional analgesia. A survey of 320 American mothers, 57% of whom were Caucasian and 28% of whom had some postgraduate education showed that although 82% of the mothers attempted to obtain information about anaesthesia before labour, 28% did not feel adequately informed and the majority (59%) would have wanted a pre-labour visit by the anaesthetist (Beilin et al 1996). Obstetric anaesthetists must, therefore, have a formal input into ante-natal education, each ante-natal class should see a trained obstetric anaesthetist and written and visual aids, such as the OAA/Poole Hospital video, should be used to disseminate information. Recall of information has been shown to be significantly better in mothers who attended ante-natal education classes but not all mothers attend such classes, which means, therefore, that leaflets explaining the process of epidural analgesia should be available at all ante-natal clinics (Swan & Borshoff 1994). Nevertheless, when a mother requests epidural analgesia during labour information concerning the risks and benefits of epidural analgesia, inevitably modified by the prevailing clinical conditions, must be provided. The issue of how best to ensure 'informed consent' during labour is controversial and the

Pain Relief?
Headache
Backache
Prolonged labour
Forceps
Caesarean
Bladder
CNS

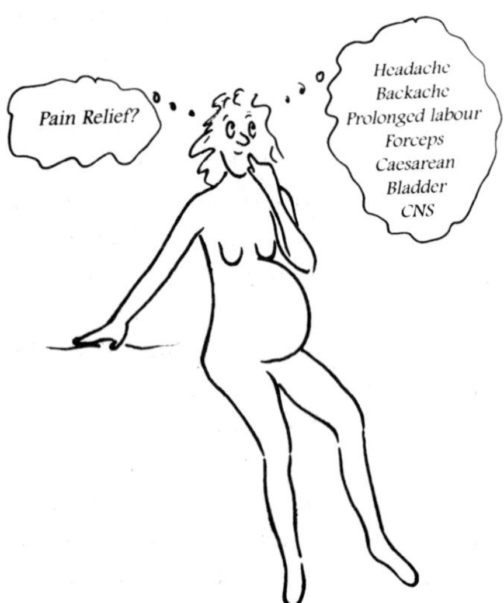

Fig. 9.1 Maternal sequelae of epidural analgesia.

> **Issues to be raised with mothers and explored in a detail dictated by the situation, e.g. ante-natal class or active labour, include:**
>
> The efficacy of regional analgesic techniques during labour and delivery.
>
> The effect of epidural analgesia on uterine activity and the outcome of labour.
>
> Complications and long term sequelae of epidural analgesia in labour.

prudent anaesthetist would be well advised to document briefly in the notes an outline of the issues discussed with the mother. It is important also for the anaesthetist to visit the mother post-partum to discuss any perceived deficiencies in management or more happily to receive praise for a job well done.

Issues to be raised with mothers and explored in a detail dictated by the situation, e.g. ante-natal class or active labour, include: the efficacy of regional analgesic techniques during labour and delivery; the effect of epidural analgesia on uterine activity and the outcome of labour; and complications and long term sequelae of epidural analgesia in labour.

THE EFFICACY OF REGIONAL ANALGESIC TECHNIQUE DURING LABOUR AND DELIVERY

Most women use some form of pain relief in labour. A survey, by the National Birthday Trust, of 10 353 women who delivered in 293 obstetric units in the last week of June 1990 showed that Entonox was available in 99% of maternity units and was used by 60% of mothers, pethidine was available in 98% of units, and was used by 37% whilst epidural analgesia was available in 63.3% and was used by 25% of women in units where the technique was available as a 24 hour service. The survey also showed that a major cause of dissatisfaction in women was when epidural analgesia was promised but not provided (Chamberlain et al 1993). A mother who requests epidural analgesia expects effective pain relief and in view of the media interest in the 'Walking Epidural' might also anticipate to be relatively mobile throughout labour. A spontaneous vaginal delivery will be the aim of most mothers but, if a caesarean section or an instrumental vaginal delivery is required, the mother who has chosen epidural analgesia is entitled to a painless delivery. Mothers must, however, be advised that the analgesia provided by an epidural can on some occasions be inadequate. The anaesthetist should re-assure the mother that every attempt will be made to rectify the situation by providing supplementary top-ups or, if necessary, by resiting the epidural. A mother recently took a successful medico-legal action against an anaesthetist for not providing adequate anaesthesia for an instrumental delivery and manual removal of a retained placenta. The claim, against the anaesthetist was: (i) that an insufficient volume of local anaesthetic had been administered; (ii) insufficient time was allowed for the local anaesthetic (despite the insufficient volume) to work; and (iii) for failing to check that the epidural top-up had achieved the desired level of sensory block before allowing the obstetrician to perform a forceps delivery

The claim, against the anaesthetist was:

(i) that an insufficient volume of local anaesthetic had been administered;

(ii) insufficient time was allowed for the local anaesthetic (despite the insufficient volume) to work; and

(iii) for failing to check that the epidural top-up had achieved the desired level of sensory block before allowing the obstetrician to perform a forceps delivery with subsequent manual evacuation of the retained products of conception.

with subsequent manual evacuation of the retained products of conception. The anaesthetist must, therefore, be as diligent in providing effective anaesthesia for an operative vaginal delivery as he would be for ensuring a pain free caesarean delivery.

Effective epidural analgesia during labour is now most commonly achieved by using low concentration/high volume local anaesthetic and opioid mixtures. Some advocate that analgesia should be achieved initially by the technique of combined spinal-epidural (CSE). This involves puncturing the dura with a long atraumatic spinal needle which is passed through a previously sited epidural needle and following intrathecal drug administration and removal of the spinal needle a catheter is passed into the epidural space (Collis et al 1995). In this situation, initial analgesia can be achieved by injecting 1 ml 0.25% bupivacaine (2.5 mg) and 0.5 ml (25 μg) fentanyl into the cerebrospinal fluid. When analgesia from the initial spinal injection has worn off, a 10–15 ml top-up of a pre-mixed solution of 0.1% bupivacaine with fentanyl 2.0 μg/ml is administered by the anaesthetist, subsequent 10–15 ml top-ups of the same solution are administered as required by the midwife responsible for the mother's care. Alternatively, an epidural infusion (8–12 ml/h) of the same pre-mixed solution can be commenced 30–60 min after the initial intrathecal injection. The main advantage of the CSE technique is the speed of onset of analgesia (less than 5 min to achieve the first painless contraction) and the relative absence of motor block allowing the mother to remain relatively mobile during her labour. Disadvantages of the starter spinal include dural puncture with the potential for post dural puncture headache (PDPH), technical failure and a documented risk of meningitis (Harding et al 1994, Cassio & Heath 1996).

Analgesia of similar quality but of slower onset, 15–20 min to achieve the first painless contraction, can be achieved by inducing analgesia with 15 ml of pre-mixed 0.1% bupivacaine with 2 μg/ml fentanyl and maintaining analgesia with 10–15 ml top-ups or by continuous infusion (10–12 ml/h) of the same pre-mixed solution. 0.0625% bupivacaine with 2.5 μg fentanyl has also been shown to produce excellent analgesia in labour (Russell et al 1995), whilst in the US and Europe sufentanil is frequently used in preference to fentanyl.

The success of low dose local anaesthetic/opioid mixtures depends on attention to detail and ongoing interaction between mother, midwife and anaesthetist. Standard practice should be to record details of the epidural analgesia on a specifically designed chart. The efficacy of the initial epidural or spinal injection and the subsequent top-ups or continuous infusion must be regularly checked: this should include direct questioning of the mother in respect of the analgesia achieved and clinical testing of the block. The upper and lower level of sensory block, the motor power of the lower limbs and the temperature of the feet (warm or cold) should be assessed at hourly intervals. Attending the woman only when called by the midwife is not sufficient. If the mother complains of inadequate analgesia, e.g. unilateral block, perineal, low back or supra pubic pain, the anaesthetist must, without delay, attempt to rectify the situation. In the first instance, it is appropriate to administer a 10 ml bolus of the pre-mixed solution or less frequently a stronger solution, such as bupivacaine 0.25%, may be required. If satisfactory analgesia is not achieved within 30–45 min, the anaesthetist should consider re-siting the epidural.

In the majority of cases, the **analgesia** achieved with local anaesthetic/opioid mixtures is excellent but cannot be guaranteed to provide effective **anaesthesia** for an operative vaginal delivery. If an operative vaginal delivery is required, the level of sensory block should be checked and 10–15 ml of 0.25 % or 0.5% bupivacaine could be required to render the mother pain free. The efficacy of the epidural block must be ensured before the obstetrician is allowed to deliver the baby by either forceps or vacuum extraction. A similar situation pertains with respect to delivery by caesarean section. **Anaesthesia** must be extended to a T4 level and again it is essential that the efficacy of the regional block is established before the surgical procedure is allowed to commence. Both the technique employed (cold, touch, pin prick to test the block) and the final level of anaesthesia achieved must be checked and recorded before allowing surgery to commence. It should be remembered that loss of temperature sensation is cephalad to pin prick and is cephalad to light touch. In a prospective study, Russell (1995) recorded levels of analgesia (loss of sharp pin prick sensation) and anaesthesia (loss of touch sensation) in 220 women during caesarean section under regional anaesthesia (70 epidurals, 150 spinals). The results suggested that assessing the adequacy of block by sharp pin prick could be misleading and that in the absence of spinal or epidural narcotics a level of anaesthesia (loss of touch) up to and including T5 is required to prevent pain during caesarean section. However, a recent survey (Bourne et al 1997) on how British anaesthetists test their regional blocks showed that 64% of those surveyed employed loss of temperature sensation to check the adequacy of the block and T4 was the most frequent upper level the surveyed anaesthetists sought to achieve. There is, therefore, a discrepancy between the theoretical ideal of Russell's study and actual clinical practice. On the basis of Russell's paper, a temperature block to T4 could potentially be inadequate in some women and he speculates that this may be due to a diverse range of extra-spinal afferent routes for visceral pain to the upper thoracic cord. This paints a confusing picture for the anaesthetist but, in clinical practice, these potential problems of an adequate block can be overcome by the addition of opioids and/or adrenaline to the epidural solutions. The difficulty in Russell's study of obtaining an adequate level of epidural block with plain 0.5% bupivacaine was obvious from the large volumes used and means that there is little or no place in current practice for attempting to perform a caesarean section under **epidural** anaesthesia using plain solutions of bupivacaine.

In a study (Noble et al 1991) in which (i) adrenaline (ii) fentanyl and (iii) adrenaline and fentanyl were used as adjuncts to bupivacaine 0.5% for epidural anaesthesia for caesarean section, the combination of bupivacaine with fentanyl and adrenaline provided the best analgesia with the least requirements for analgesic supplements, the best observer rating and the best visual analogue scores. The fentanyl only group ranked second for the same assessments. Epidural anaesthesia for caesarean section should be achieved using 0.5% plain bupivacaine supplemented with fentanyl (100 μg) and adrenaline (1 :200 000) or fentanyl only if there is a contra-indication to the use of adrenaline. If unsupplemented bupivacaine 0.5% is used for caesarean section, a proportion of mothers may experience unacceptable discomfort which is most probably visceral pain. When a caesarean section is being carried out under epidural anaesthesia, the anaesthetist should establish the cephalad and caudal distribution of the block as some sparing of the sacral roots is occasionally seen with epidural anaesthesia. It is clinically well recognised that spinal anaesthesia guarantees a complete sensory block below the most cephalad level of sensory loss and there is no requirement to check the caudal extent of a spinal block.

Mothers, no matter how well informed and prepared, are usually somewhat apprehensive when undergoing caesarean section under regional anaesthesia and will require enormous moral support and sympathy from her anaesthetist. The mother should be aware of the option of general anaesthesia in the event of severe pain and, in such circumstances, the anaesthetist must not hesitate in requesting that surgery cease and general anaesthesia should be induced before surgery is allowed to proceed further. Otherwise the anaesthetist risks medico-legal action which he/she will almost certainly lose.

THE EFFECTS OF EPIDURAL ANALGESIA ON UTERINE ACTIVITY AND THE OUTCOME OF LABOUR

The effect of maternal pain relief on the course and outcome of labour has recently been the subject of intense debate in both the obstetric and anaesthetic literature (Miller 1997). The marked difference in study design, retrospective or prospective, blinded or open, the stage in labour when epidural analgesia is administered, the volume and concentration of the local anaesthetic used and the individual labour and its obstetric management makes evaluation of the available data very difficult. In addition, few studies have attempted to compare epidural analgesia with the other less effective techniques which are offered to mothers during labour.

There would appear to be some relationship between the use of epidural analgesia and delay in both the first (Carli et al 1993) and second stages of labour and the need for instrumental delivery (Chestnut et al 1987). It has also been suggested that epidural analgesia has contributed to the rise in the caesarean section rate (Thorp et al 1993) but are these associations always that of cause and effect?

There is clear evidence from the National Birthday Trust Survey that the longer the duration of labour the more likely is the mother to choose epidural analgesia (Fig. 9.2). Therefore, it is reasonable to argue that a labour which is prolonged, painful or complicated will indeed prompt the women to seek epidural analgesia. Studies can be used to selectively support or refute the arguments pertaining to the effect of epidural analgesia on labour but the problem is that few, if any, studies are similar in design and many of the earlier

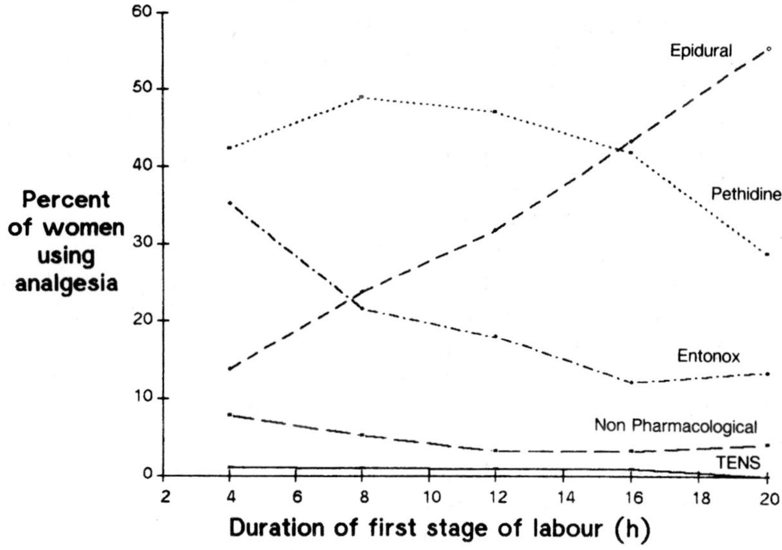

Fig. 9.2 The percentage of nulliparae using a dominant method of analgesia by the duration of labour (reproduced from Pain and its Relief in Childbirth).

studies will have employed stronger solutions of local anaesthetic than are currently utilised and thus are irrelevant in the context of modern obstetric analgesic techniques which utilise low dose local anaesthetic/opioid solutions. Cheek et al (1996) have shown that women who received a 1000 ml intravenous fluid bolus exhibited a decrease in uterine activity for 20 min after the fluid bolus, yet those who had received a 500 ml bolus did not exhibit any change in activity. The use of low concentration local anaesthetic/opioid mixtures should now obviate the need for fluid pre-loading of greater than 500 ml.

Two recent (Thorp et al 1993, Ramin et al 1995) randomised, prospective but unblinded studies of epidural versus narcotic analgesia in labour have provoked much controversy. In both studies, epidural analgesia was established with 0.25% bupivacaine and maintained with a continuous infusion of 0.125% bupivacaine and fentanyl 2 µg/ml and was compared to an intravenous meperidine (pethidine)/promethazine mixture. Thorp et al (1993), who studied 93 nulliparae, found that the epidural group had a significant prolongation of the first and second stages of labour, an increased use of oxytocin and the caesarean section rate for dystocia was 16.7% in the epidural group as opposed to 2.2% for the non-epidural group. Ramin et al (1995) studied 1330 mothers of mixed parity in spontaneous uncomplicated labour; the route of delivery and complications in relation to the type of labour analgesia are illustrated in Table 9.1. Although these two randomised studies are superior to many of the previous studies, it is almost impossible to blind patient and obstetrician to the method used. Most importantly, it is the obstetric management that will influence the progress of labour and the need for instrumental or caesarean delivery, indeed it is noteworthy that one of the factors contributing to the lower incidence of caesarean section in Ramin's study was the more aggressive use of oxytocin than in Thorp's study.

Table 9.1 Route of delivery and complications in relation to type of labour analgesia (reproduced from Ramin et al 1995)

Delivery complications	Epidural (*n* = 432)	Meperidine (*n* = 437)	*P*
Vaginal delivery			
Spontaneous	352 (81%)	407 (93%)	< 0.001
Outlet forceps*	8 (2%)	8 (2%)	NS
Low forceps**	33 (8%)	5 (1%)	< 0.001
Shoulder dystocia	2	2	NS
Caesarean delivery	39 (9%)	17 (4%)	0.002
Dystocia	21 (5%)	7 (1.6%)	0.007
Fetal distress	18 (4%)	10 (2.3%)	NS

NS = significant
Data are presented as *n* (%)
*Outlet forceps: fetal head at the perineum
**Low forceps: +2 cm to +4 cm below the ischial spines.

Obstetric management, which will inevitably vary between units, is probably one of the most significant factors affecting labour outcome. At the National Maternity Hospital, Dublin, Eire, where the active management of labour originated, the increase in the epidural rate from 10% to 45% occurred with minimal effect on the instrumental or caesarean delivery rate (Robson et al 1993a). More cynically, Neuhoff et al (1989) have shown that caesarean section for dystocia was much more common for private patients than clinic patients even though the two groups received epidural analgesia with the same frequency. By adopting an aggressive approach towards the management of labour and adhering to strict criteria for the definition of dystocia, it should be possible to administer epidural analgesia to spontaneously labouring women without increasing the incidence of caesarean section for dystocia.

The weight of evidence suggests that epidural analgesia does influence the course and outcome of labour, the effect on the first stage is complex while the second stage is prolonged but without detriment to the baby. The need for instrumental deliveries is increased whilst the effect on the rate of caesarean section requires further careful evaluation. Mothers who request epidural analgesia should be advised to expect slightly longer labours and that the need for amniotomy and oxytocin augmentation are increased. Most mothers will consider that the benefits of epidural analgesia will outweigh the disadvantages. What must not be forgotten is that epidural analgesia is the only truly effective option available to mothers desiring a pain free delivery. There is no justification for denying this method of analgesia to those mothers who request it.

COMPLICATIONS AND LONG TERM SEQUELAE OF EPIDURAL ANALGESIA

Epidural analgesic is unrivalled in its efficacy in providing pain relief for the parturient. An expertly managed and carefully audited obstetric anaesthetic service should ensure that the maternal sequelae of epidural analgesia are minor and self-limiting. Unfortunately, surveys and case reports testify to the morbidity relating to epidural analgesia and anaesthesia.

SITING THE EPIDURAL

This should be a painless procedure for the mother and the incidence of that most incapacitating complication, post dural puncture headache (PDPH) should be minimised by meticulous attention to teaching and maintaining a careful technique for epidural insertion. This is particularly important in teaching units with a large throughput of trainee anaesthetists. A sterile technique is mandatory, the operator should wear a sterile gown and gloves whilst the use of a face mask is a matter of some debate. The frequency of case reports concerning epidural abscesses and meningitis in the obstetric population means that there is no place for relaxing sterile procedures. The left or right lateral position is probably the most commonly employed for siting an epidural although in very obese patient identification of the midline is facilitated by the sitting position. It has been suggested that the technique of identifying the epidural space using a loss of resistance to air should be abandoned in favour of a loss of resistance to saline (Yentis 1997). Loss of resistance to air has been implicated in several case reports of complications associated with epidural analgesia. These have included an increased incidence of dural tap and patchy block, cauda equina compression, pneumocephalus and air embolism. Whilst obviously the question of air versus saline would be best addressed by a prospective randomised controlled study, the evidence to date suggests that saline rather than air should be used to locate the epidural space.

Igarashi et al (1996) in Japan assessed the cephaled spread in analgesia in 491 patients undergoing lumbar epidural anaesthesia and found that the cephaled spread was greater in those without a history of previous epidural cannulation. In addition, they examined the epidural space using a flexible epiduroscope in a further 32 patients and concluded that epidural anaesthesia may cause aseptic inflammatory changes in the epidural space which may reduce the spread of analgesia. This interesting study raises more questions than it answers and closer scrutiny reveals that although wide variations in the level of analgesia were seen in the patients with repeated epidural blockade, these variations were similar to those encountered in those receiving their first epidural. Similarly, an American study (Blanche et al 1994) has suggested that a previous inadvertent dural puncture does not reduce the success rate of subsequent epidural analgesia in labour, although the chance of another inadvertent dural puncture was considered to be significant. In this study, 47 women with inadvertent dural puncture were evaluated; 19 of these women developed a PDPH and 9 received an epidural blood patch, neither of which were considered to have adversely affected the quality of analgesia during subsequent epidural blockade. These two studies are, therefore, somewhat contradictory suggesting that further studies are required to clarify the situation.

Post-dural puncture headache and extradural blood patch

Most mothers are aware of and many seek information on the relationship between headache and epidural analgesia. Few, however, realise that the headache is a result of a complication of the procedure rather than being intrinsically linked with the technique per se. A carefully managed and audited unit should have available the annual dural puncture rate which should ideally be not greater than 1% and the mother reassured accordingly. Complications associated with dural puncture include persistent headache, cranial nerve abnormalities, coning and subdural haematoma, so it is vital that PDPH is carefully managed.

Management of PDPH

Dural puncture with removal of the Tuohy needle immediately following the puncture

The sudden and unexpected sight of CSF pouring from the end of an epidural needle probably evokes a reflex response in most anaesthetists; they immediately withdraw the offending needle! This action inevitably dictates the subsequent clinical management of the mother. The anaesthetist should site the epidural catheter at an adjacent interspace and should employ a low concentration local anaesthetic opioid mixture to relieve pain in labour. This can be administered by infusion or by fractionated top-up and must be administered by the anaesthetist. In the past it was advised that mothers with a dural puncture should avoid pushing in the second stage and should have an elective forceps delivery. However, current practice is that the management of the second stage need not be altered in mothers with a dural puncture (Robson et al 1993b). If the mother requires a caesarean section, the epidural must not be topped with a stronger concentration of bupivacaine as this practice has been implicated as causing a total spinal block. Anaesthesia for caesarean should be achieved with a single shot spinal or a general anaesthetic.

Catheter dural puncture or anaesthetist deliberately sites the epidural catheter intrathecally following dural puncture

In this context epidural analgesia should be managed by continuous spinal analgesia. Intrathecal bupivacaine 0.25% (1 ml) and fentanyl 25 μg (0.5 ml) are commonly used to achieve initial analgesia in labour as part of a CSE technique before proceeding to subsequent epidural analgesia. If the epidural catheter is sited intrathecally, intermittent injections of the same solutions can be administered, as required, throughout labour. If a caesarean section is required, 0.5% bupivacaine heavy can be administered to achieve an anaesthetic level to T4.

Epidural blood patch

If a mother develops a **significant** PDPH, an epidural blood patch is probably the only treatment which will provide complete pain relief and allow her to return to an active and busy post partum life. The risks and benefits of the procedure should be explained to the mother who should give written consent for the procedure. Ideally, the mother should remain horizontal for 1 h prior to the procedure, in order to minimise the leak and ensure that the epidural space is free of cerebrospinal fluid. The epiduralist and venepuncturist must take full aseptic precautions. The mother should be placed in the left lateral position and a tourniquet should be placed on her left arm. The epiduralist paints the back with an antiseptic solution after which the venepuncturist places a sterile paper under the patient's arm, paints it generously and covers the lower forearm with a sterile drape. After the epiduralist has entered the epidural space, the venepuncturist should take 20 ml of blood aseptically and pass the syringe to the epiduralist. The venepuncturist should then continue to take a further 10 ml of blood for blood culture (this step may be omitted if you are confident there is no bacteraemia). The blood should be injected slowly into the epidural space. It should go in **very** easily. The mother may complain of pain and a tight feeling in the legs. Slow down or pause but you should aim to inject a minimum of 15 ml. Before removing the Tuohy needle, inject 1 ml of saline from the loss of resistance device. This minimises the entry of blood into the needle tract, which causes back pain. Apply an adhesive dressing and turn the mother supine. She should remain lying down for at least 2 h, thereafter she can gradually be raised to the sitting position. The mother should be advised to avoid coughing and straining and, if possible, not to lift heavy objects for 2 weeks.

EPIDURAL ANALGESIA AND NEUROLOGICAL DEFICITS

Scott and Tunstall (1995) carried out a prospective study of the complications (excluding post dural puncture headache) of epidural and spinal block in obstetrics during 1990 and 1991. There were 467 491 deliveries in participating units and 108 133 mothers received epidural block and 14 356 received a spinal block. There were 128 complications and peripheral neuropathies were the commonest complication. The neuropathies were almost all related to a single spinal or peripheral nerve and all recovered completely in 1–12 weeks. Table 9.2 illustrates the most common injuries in the obstetric anaesthesia files of the ASA Closed Claims Committee and, if maternal mortality and post dural puncture headache is excluded, neuropathies account for a large number of the complications. The potential for nerve trauma is pertinent to the practice of the obstetric anaesthesia as the anaesthetist is invariably involved when a mother who has had epidural analgesia develops a post partum neurological defect.

In a one year survey of 48 066 deliveries in the North Thames region, which included 13 636 regional blocks, 19 women were judged to have suffered a neurological complication of whom 7 had a continuing neurological disability for more than one year. Thirteen of the 19 women had received a regional block but of these only one mother was considered to have had the complications attributable to an epidural anaesthetic (Holdcroft et al 1995). This survey and other work has shown that neurological problems are more likely to be related to trauma/obstruction, fetal malposition, cephalopelvic disproportion, difficult vaginal delivery and excessive use of the lithotomy position results in overstretching of the sciatic nerve or compression of the lateral femoral cutaneous nerve or the peroneal nerve at the knee. Epidural and spinal anaesthesia are, therefore, associated with a significant incidence of neurological defects and the causes are likely to be traumatic, vascular, compressive/infective and neurotoxic.

A large variety of noxious substances have been injected into the epidural space without resulting neurological sequelae which is in sharp contrast to the subarachnoid space, where the unprotected cord has been shown to be extremely vulnerable to a large variety of agents. Human error plays a large part in these disasters, so careful checking of drugs and adherence to carefully constructed guidelines play an important part in the safe running of an obstetric anaesthetic service.

Ischaemic damage is relatively unusual in the obstetric population but there have been several recent reports of infective/compressive lesions. Compressive lesions will cause paraplegia or cauda equina syndrome whereas trauma from an epidural catheter or spinal needle should be limited to a single nerve root. Complaints of paraesthesia on inserting the spinal needle or epidural catheter are not uncommon in those women who subsequently develop minor neurological deficits.

It has been suggested in a major American textbook, *Obstetric Anaesthesia* (Bromage 1994), that the anaesthetist should seek a history of neurological symptoms in the lower extremities during pregnancy and labour and perform a brief neurological examination of the lower extremities prior to regional analgesia. The author advises an evaluation of motor function, tendon and Babinski reflexes and sensation of the lateral surfaces of the lower leg and foot.

If a neurological deficit does occur post partum, a careful history and neurological examination are essential. A pyrexia might suggest an infective process (Lindler et al 1996) whilst the development of a clotting defect might cause a deficit secondary to a bleed or haematoma. A MRI is the most useful investigative procedure whilst neurophysiological studies give useful information in isolated nerve lesion.

Whilst most deficits will resolve spontaneously in days to weeks, a neurological opinion should be sought if the mother deteriorates or fails to improve. The mother must not be lost to follow-up until it has been clearly demonstrated that the neurological deficit has resolved or at least is resolving. It is pertinent

Table 9.2 Most common injuries in obstetric anaesthesia files (reproduced from Chadwick 1996)

	Obstetric files *n* = 434	**Regional anaesthesia** *n* = 290*	**General anaesthesia** *n* = 133*
Maternal death	83 (19%)	31 (11%)	52 (39%)*
Newborn brain damage	82 (19%)	51 (18%)	28 (21%)
Headache	64 (15%)	61 (21%)	2 (2%)*
Nerve damage	43 (10%)	38 (13%)	5 (4%)*
Pain during anesthesia	37 (9%)	36 (12%)	0 (0%)*
Back pain	36 (8%)	36 (12%)	0 (0%)*
Maternal brain damage	32 (7%)	17 (6%)	14 (11%)
Emotional distress	31 (7%)	23 (8%)	8 (6%)
Newborn death	27 (6%)	16 (6%)	8 (6%)
Aspiration pneumonitis	20 (5%)	2 (1%)	18 (14%)*

The most common maternal injuries in the obstetric anesthesia files are shown in order of decreasing frequency. Percentages are based on the total files in each group. Some files, especially those with a fatal outcome, had more than one injury and are represented more than once. Cases involving brain damage only include patients who were alive when the file was closed (ASA Closed Claims Project, *n* = 3533)
*In some files the type of anaesthetic was not recorded
**$P \leq 0.01$.

to remember that obstetric and not anaesthetic factors are the commonest cause of post partum neurological deficits (Donaldson 1989).

BLADDER FUNCTION

Difficulty with micturition is common during labour and post partum. Urinary retention most commonly occurs post partum and, if overlooked, can lead to long term sequelae. A study of the effects of epidural analgesia on bladder sensation demonstrated that the bladder takes up to 8 h to regain its sensation after an epidural top-up and if a post partum diuresis occurs during this time the woman might be susceptible to overdistension, which can result in permanent detrusor damage (Khullar & Cardozo 1993). The effect of low dose local anaesthetic/opioid infusions on bladder function has not yet been studied.

Care of the bladder following delivery requires vigilance and is the responsibility of all those involved in the mother's care, midwife, anaesthetist and obstetrician. Mothers at increased risk of developing urinary retention include those who have had a prolonged labour, a difficult delivery, epidural analgesia or a caesarean section. Following caesarean section, a urinary catheter should remain in situ until the regional block has completely resolved. Postpartum mothers who have had a vaginal delivery should void at least 200 ml urine at more than two hourly intervals. Frequent small volumes of urine indicates incomplete emptying. If a woman is unable to void after delivery, she should not be left more than 6–8 h before a catheter is passed to avoid overdistension of the bladder. If a second catheterisation is required, it may be advisable to leave an indwelling catheter in position for 24–48 h. If after this time voiding is still unsatisfactory, a urological opinion should be sought.

Epidural analgesia is the only technique, currently available, which can successfully relieve the pain of labour. The benefits of the technique far outweigh the documented side effects and complications.

References

Beilin Y, Rosenblatt M A, Bodian C A, Laquay-Aroesty M M, Berustein H H 1996 Information and concerns about obstetric anesthesia: a survey of 320 mothers. Int J Obstet Anesth 5: 145–151

Blanch R, Eisenach J C, Tuttle R, Dewan D M 1994 Previous wet tap does not reduce success rate of labor epidural analgesia. Anesth Analg 79: 291–294

Borum S E, McLeshey C H, Williamson J B, Harris F S, Knight A B 1995 Epidural abscess after obstetric epidural analgesia. Anesthesiology 82: 1523–1526

Bourne T M, de Melo A E, Bastianpillai B A, May A E 1997 A survey of how British obstetric anaesthetists test regional anaesthesia before caesarean section. Anaesthesia 52: 901–903

Bromage P R 1994 Neurologic complications of labor, delivery and regional anesthesia. In: Chestnut D H (ed) Obstetric Anesthesia, Principles and Practical. St Louis: Mosby

Capogna G, Alahunta S, Cellano D et al 1996 Maternal expectations and experiences of labour pain and analgesia; a multicentre study of nulliparous women. Int J Obstet Anesth 5: 229–235

Carli F, Creagh-Barry P, Gordon H, Logue M M, Dore C J 1993 Does epidural analgesia influence the mode of delivery in primiparae managed actively. Int J Obstet Anesth 2: 15–20

Cassio M, Heath G 1996 Meningitis following a combined spinal-epidural technique in a labouring term parturient. Can J Anaesth 43: 399–402

Chadwick HS 1996 An analysis of obstetric cases from the American Society of Anesthesiologists closed claim project database. Int J Obstet Anesth 5: 258–263
Chamberlain G, Wraight A, Steer P 1993 Pain and its Relief in Childbirth: Report of the 1990 NBT Survey. Edinburgh: Churchill Livingstone
Cheek T G, Samuels P, Tobin M, Gutsche B B 1996 Normal saline IV, load decreases uterine activity in labor. Br J Anaesth 77: 632–635
Chestnut D H, Vandewalker G E, Owen C L, Bates J N, Choi W W 1987 The influence of continuous bupivacaine analgesia on the second stage of labour and the method of delivery in nulliparous women. Anesthesiology 66: 774–780
Collis R E, Davies D W L, Aveling W 1995 Randomised comparison of combined spinal-epidural and standard epidural analgesia in labour. Lancet 345: 1413–1416
Donaldson J O 1989 Neurology of Pregnancy. 2nd edn. London: Saunders
HMSO 1993 Changing Childbirth London: HMSO
Holdcroft A, Gibbard F B, Hargrove R L, Hawkins D F, Dellaportas C I 1995 Neurological complications associated with pregnancy. Br J Anaesth 75: 522–526
Harding S A, Collis R E, Morgan B M 1994 Meningitis after combined spinal-epidural anaesthesia in obstetrics. Br J Anaesth 73: 545–547
Igarashi T, Hirabagashi Y, Shimizu R et al 1996 Inflammatory changes after extradural anaesthesia may affect the spread of local anaesthetic within the extradural space. Br J Anaesth 77: 345–351
Khullar V, Cardozo L D 1993 Bladder sensation after epidural analgesia. Neurourol Urodyn 12: 424–425
Lindler C, Leeberger W, Siegmund M, Schneider M 1996 Extra dural abscess complicating lumbar extradural anaesthesia and analgesia in an obstetric patient. Acta Anaesthesiol Scand 40: 858–861
Lindt B, Hoel T M 1989 Alleviation of labor pain in Norway. Acta Obstet Gynecol Scand 68: 125
MacArthur C, Lewis M, Knox E G 1993 Evaluation of obstetric analgesia and anaesthesia; long-term maternal recollections. Int J Obstet Anaesth 2: 3–11
Melzack R 1984 The myth of painless childbirth. Pain 19: 321–327
Miller A C 1997 The effects of epidural analgesia on uterine activity and labor. Int J Obstet Anaesth 6: 2–18
Neuhoff D, Burke M S, Porreco R P 1989 Caesarean birth for failed progress in labor. Obstet Gynecol 73: 915–920
Noble A W, Morrison C M, Brockway M S, Mclure J H 1991 Adrenaline, fentanyl or fentanyl and adrenaline as adjuncts for extradural anaesthesia in elective caesarean section. Br J Anaesth 66: 645–650
Paech M J 1991 The King Edward Memorial Hospital 1000 Mother Survey of pain relief in labor. Anaesth Intens Care 19: 393–399
Ramin S M, Gambling D R, Lucas M J, Sharma S K, Sidawi J E, Levens R J 1995 Randomised trial of epidural versus intravenous analgesia during labor. Obstet Gynecol 86: 783–789
Robson M, Boylan P, McParland P, McQuillan C, O'Neill M 1993a Epidural analgesia need not influence the spontaneous vaginal delivery rate (Abstract). Am J Obstet Gynecol 168: 364 (A240)
Robson M, McQuillan C, Stronge J M 1993b Elective forceps delivery not indicated (Letter). BMJ 306: 1339
Russell I F 1995 Levels of anaesthesia and intraoperative pain at caesarean section under regional block. Int J Obstet Anaesth 4: 71–77
Russell R, Quinlan J, Reynolds F 1995 Motor block during epidural infusions for nulliparous women in labour. Int J Obstet Anesth 4: 82–88
Scott D B, Tunstall M E 1995 Serious complications associated with epidural/spinal blockade in obstetrics. Int J Obstet Anesth 4: 133–139
Swan H D, Borshoff D C 1994 Informed consent – recall of risk information following epidural analgesia in labour. Anaesth Intens Care 22: 139–141
Thorp J A, Hu D H, Albin R M et al 1993 The effect of intrapartum epidural analgesia on nulliparous labour; a randomised controlled prospective trial. Am J Obstet Gynecol 169: 851–858
Yentis S M 1997 Time to abandon loss of resistance to air. Anaesthesia 52: 184

Maurizio Renna

Acute pain in adults: a survey of techniques

Significant progress has been made in the last 25 years in our understanding of acute pain after surgery. Anaesthetists have today a much wider choice of techniques for relieving postoperative pain but, despite that, optimal analgesia is not always achieved. In this chapter some of the most relevant of these techniques will be reviewed.

PATIENT CONTROLLED ANALGESIA

Since the introduction of the Cardiff Palliator in 1976, there has been an enormous development in the technology associated with patient controlled devices for delivering analgesic drugs intravenously. Patient controlled analgesia (PCA) is commonly associated with the use of such devices, although some authors extend the concept of PCA to any analgesic drug administered by any route on immediate patient demand.

The class of drugs most frequently used with PCA pumps is opioids. Only one study has compared a non-steroidal anti-inflammatory drug, ketorolac, with morphine (Cepeda et al 1995). However, it remains unclear what the optimal PCA opioid is or even if such a thing as 'optimal PCA opioid' exists. The selection criteria for the use of a certain PCA narcotic are largely empirical and the number of controlled trials comparing various opioids is surprisingly low.

The question of comparison is relevant in that equi-analgesic doses of different opioids might have different effects on certain functions, cognitive performance for instance (Rapp et al 1996). However, no matter which opioid is selected, the great advantage of the concept of PCA is that it is a goal directed therapy, the goal being patient satisfaction, in which the patient himself/herself decides when the goal has been reached. By doing so the

Dr Maurizio Renna MD, Consultant Anaesthetist, Department of Anaesthetics, Ealing Hospital NHS Trust, Uxbridge Road, Southall, Middlesex UB1 3HW, UK

problem of the nurse/doctor's lack of 'objective' criteria for assessing pain and administering an analgesic drug is overcome.

In theory, self administration of small doses of opioid should allow perfect titration of the drug and keep its plasma levels within the 'therapeutic window' for that particular narcotic. If plasma levels are too low, the patient will experience pain and will self-administer a bolus of narcotic; if plasma levels are too high, the patient will be sedated and won't give himself/herself an overdose. This simple 'PCA paradigm' explains why this technique has always been considered intrinsically safe. Clinical practice suggests that this is not always the case, intravenous PCA being not 100% efficacious or safe. However, we will now briefly look at some of the most relevant issues concerning this useful technique.

FEATURES

There are several PCA devices available for use at present. Standard programming features that should be available in every modern PCA infusion pump include:

Bolus dose

The amount of drug delivered every time a patient presses a button connected to the machine.

Lock out time

The time interval in which the machine is not delivering a bolus dose even if the patient presses the button.

Loading dose

The dose administered as 'one off' to make the patient comfortable immediately after surgery, for instance, or for breakthrough pain.

Basal rate

The hourly background infusion rate administered continuously by the machine.

Four hour (or 1 hour) limit

This is the maximum amount of drug that the machine would deliver during 4 h (or 1 h).

Not all these features are commonly used in clinical practice. Background infusion is not a popular choice in view of enhanced risk of respiratory depression. A 4 h limit could give nurses a false sense of security about the risk of overdose, whereas it is well known that doses which are analgesic for certain individuals could lead to respiratory depression in others. A certain loading dose may be too small or too high for a particular patient at a particular time, so it seems more practical to administer small incremental i.v. doses until the patient is comfortable. The other controls are set differently according to the opioid chosen. Commonly selected choices are listed in Table 10.1.

Unfortunately, only a few controlled studies have compared various settings, finding surprisingly little difference in patient satisfaction (Ginsberg

Table 10.1 Commonly selected choices

Drug	Bolus dose	Lock out time
Morphine	0.5–3 mg	5–15 min
Diamorphine	0.5–1.5 mg	5–15 min
Fentanyl	10–25 μg	4–10 min
Pethidine	10–30 mg	5–12 min
Methadone	0.5–2.5 mg	8–20 min

et al 1995, Woodhouse et al 1996). The same could be said for comparisons between different opioids (Ginsberg et al 1995, Rapp et al 1996, Woodhouse et al 1996). When the PCA pump is programmed, the selected bolus will remain constant until the pump is re-programmed. One paper (Owen et al 1995) has reported preliminary data on the use of a computer controlled device that enables patients to select a different bolus dose according to the intensity of pain experienced at a certain moment. This is an interesting idea, although it needs further evaluation.

INDICATIONS

PCA is indicated for surgery requiring a significant amount of analgesia in the postoperative period. Sickle cell disease related pain is also increasingly treated with PCA, with good results. Clinical experience suggests that PCA is best used when the natural history of pain is self-limiting and benign. In a chronic pain scenario, other techniques and modalities of drug administration seem more suitable.

CONTRAINDICATIONS

There are very few contraindications for the use of PCA. Patient's inability to understand and comply with the technique is probably the most relevant. Psychiatric patients and very young children (below 4 years old) are not suitable candidates for PCA. Care must also be taken when dealing with patients with chronic obstructive airway disease, in view of their notorious sensitivity to opioids. Old age, as well as paediatric age, is not a contraindication to the use of the technique (Egbert et al 1993, Doyle et al 1993).

SAFETY

The notion that PCAs are intrinsically safe is probably not entirely true. Several case reports have recently appeared (Etches 1994, Looi-Lyons et al 1996) highlighting the danger of respiratory depression even in the presence of good nursing, monitoring and care. It is difficult to determine the incidence of serious respiratory depression (respiratory rate below 8) in the absence of misprogramming of the device or equipment malfunction. It was 0.2% in a retrospective series of 1600 patients (Etches 1994) but larger prospective studies are needed.

Our experience at Ealing Hospital, London, confirms that respiratory depression can occur in the presence of optimal nursing care. Contributing factors can be identified, namely long acting opioids administered in theatre, presence of an adjuvant analgesic technique, excessive enthusiasm in the prescription of PCA for minor operations requiring minimal postoperative analgesia. Indeed, pain counteracts the negative effects of opioids on the ventilatory function; prescribing a PCA narcotic in the absence of pain can lead to disasters.

SIDE EFFECTS

We are all familiar with the side effects of opioids, i.e. nausea, vomiting, pruritus, urinary retention and ileus. Nausea in particular can be very distressing for some patients, who prefer to self administer lower doses and feel some pain rather than taking higher doses and feeling sick. Antiemetic drugs should be prescribed accordingly. Some studies have looked at adding an antiemetic to the analgesic solution, but the usefulness of the technique has not been definitely proven yet. However, the overall incidence of side effects associated with PCA does not seem to be higher than what is seen with other ways of administration of the same opioid.

MONITORING

In view of the risks of respiratory depression discussed earlier, a good deal of monitoring care is mandatory. Clear guidelines on nursing observation must be in place to make sure that no episodes of respiratory depression go undetected with potentially fatal consequences. Our policy at Ealing is that observations must be done after surgery every 15 min in the recovery area for the first 2 h, then hourly in the wards until the next morning. At that stage, the Acute Pain Team re-assesses the situation and, if clinically indicated, orders 2 hourly observations thereafter. These include determination of blood pressure, heart rate, respiratory rate, pain score, sedation score, nausea score and itching plus records of the amount of drug used, number of attempts and amount left in the syringe. In the absence of a good level of nursing monitoring, the possible risks associated with the use of PCA must be carefully weighted against its benefits.

EFFICACY

How well does intravenous PCA work? Unfortunately, not many studies have tried to answer this question. Intravenous PCA has been compared with epidural infusions of the same or sometimes of a different opioid, with the overall impression that epidural infusions are associated with lower pain scores (Joshi et al 1995, Eriksson et al 1997). This does not mean that they are ultimately better, because frequently patient satisfaction is equal or higher with i.v. PCA (Harrison et al 1988). A possible explanation is that with i.v. PCA, patients feel in control of their analgesia, which puts them in a better psychological attitude to tolerate higher levels of pain. However, more data and better designed controlled studies are needed.

OTHER ROUTES

Patient controlled epidural analgesia (PCEA)

In this modality, the patient self-administers a bolus of opioid via an epidural catheter. PCEA tries to combine the advantages of epidural infusions with the flexibility of i.v. PCA. Labour pain seems to be a perfect field for the application of PCEA and indeed much work has been done with controversial results. For example, it is unclear whether adding a background infusion is beneficial or not, nor does consensus exist regarding optimal settings of bolus doses, lock out time or choice of opioid. The same considerations apply to the non-obstetric population in which PCEA administration of several opioids, alone or in combination with bupivacaine, has been studied. Unfortunately, in most studies, the initial settings of the PCEA pump are based on clinical experience and not controlled data. Therefore, it is very difficult to compare results from different papers. We still lack clear data about the optimal dose and lock out time for each individual opioid. One study (Ngan-Kee et al 1996) evaluated 5 doses of PCEA pethidine after caesarean section showing that 25 mg is the best choice as a bolus, higher doses being associated with the same degree of analgesia but higher incidence of side effects. More work like this is needed before we can take full advantage of the potentials of this promising technique.

Other modalities

It is worth mentioning that PCA has been used via the oral route (PCORA) (Striebel et al 1996a), the nasal route (PCINA) (Striebel et al 1996b) and the subcutaneous route (Bruera et al 1991).

In summary, intravenous PCA is a very effective technique for post-operative pain relief. It is associated with great patient satisfaction and its safety profile is good, although not perfect as initially believed. Indeed, care must be taken when PCA is administered in conjunction with other analgesic techniques or after minor operations. Good levels of nursing observations are required. Other modalities of PCA have been explored, particularly via the epidural route, but controversy still exists regarding their use in clinical practice.

EPIDURAL ANALGESIA

Epidurals, together with PCAs, are the most widely used postoperative analgesic technique after major surgery. Many patients have been treated with this excellent type of pain relief but, despite that, controversy still exists with regard to the optimal clinical management of epidurals. I will now briefly discuss some of the most controversial issues involved.

CHOICE OF OPIOID

Since the discovery of the opioid receptors in the spinal cord, opioids have been extensively used for epidural administration. Morphine was the first to be considered, but practically all other narcotic drugs have been studied at some point. It has been traditionally taught that the best characteristic which would explain the behaviour of an epidural opioid as an analgesic is lipophilicity (Sjostrom et al 1987). Lipid solubility of an opioid is revealed by its partition coefficient between water and fat at a given pH. A drug with low partition coefficient, i.e. morphine (1), will be described as hydrophilic whereas a drug with high partition coefficient, i.e. fentanyl (950), will be considered lipophilic.

An hydrophilic opioid, once injected in to the epidural space, is not absorbed by fat or blood vessels near the site of injection, but slowly penetrates the dura mater, entering the CSF. Once there, it will be subject to low vascular uptake, therefore, maintaining high concentration for a relatively long time. Consequently, the drug will follow the hydrodynamics of the CSF spreading within it, acting on opioid receptors at various levels of the spinal cord and the CNS. This would lead to analgesia in spinal dermatomes distant from the injection site, but also to the possibility of late onset of the well known side effects of opioids (respiratory depression, nausea, vomiting, itching, urinary retention).

A lipophilic opioid, injected epidurally, shows a different kind of behaviour. It will be avidly absorbed by epidural fat and blood vessels, entering the systemic circulation and leaving only small amounts of the drug for migration across the dura. Once in the CSF, it will be subject to a relatively large vascular uptake leading to rapid clearance from the receptors in the spinal cord. Rapid clearance of fentanyl from the CSF means less chance of rostral migration and, therefore, less chance of fentanyl related side effects, particularly respiratory depression. Adding adrenaline to a bolus injection (Robertson et al 1985) or an infusion (Baron et al 1996) of epidural fentanyl resulted in longer lasting analgesia and lower plasma levels of opiate, indicating adrenaline induced reduction in vascular uptake of fentanyl.

The above pharmacokinetic considerations had led some authors to recommend the use of lipophilic epidural opioids for surgery in dermatomes near the site of injection, whereas hydrophilic opioids should be used where the surgical incision is large and/or distant from the site of injection (VadeBoncouer & Ferrante 1993).

With regard to this recommendation, there is certainly general agreement about the use of an hydrophilic opioid like morphine and its mechanism of action. Indeed:

(i) epidural morphine provides analgesia of better quality and longer duration than the same dose injected intravenously or intramuscularly (Cousins & Mather 1984);

(ii) plasma levels of morphine are poorly correlated with the extent of analgesia both after intravenous and epidural administration (Eriksson et al 1997); and

(iii) morphine concentrations in the CSF are 100–200 times higher than in plasma after administration of a single dose epidurally (Nordberg et al 1984).

The above are just some of the observations which strongly suggest the spinal mechanism of action for morphine, which makes it a logical choice for epidural use. Matters are much more controversial, however, where we consider lipophilic opioids. Several papers have suggested that the same dose is required to achieve analgesia whether the lipophilic narcotic is administered by the intravenous or the epidural route. In a double blind crossover study, Glass et al (1991) could not demonstrate any difference between intravenous and epidural fentanyl after lower abdominal surgery. Epidural and intravenous fentanyl were equivalent in 20 patients undergoing knee surgery (Loper et al 1990), with similar plasma levels in both groups. Sandler (1992) compared lumbar epidural and intravenous infusions of fentanyl in post thoracotomy patients obtaining similar clinical and pharmacokynetic data. Other studies support the same opinion. Finally, McQuay (1994), in the *Textbook of Pain*, states that 'lipophilic opioids...may be a poor choice for epidural use;...they have low spinal potency and substantial systemic analgesic effect makes it difficult to determine any spinal action'. However, other authors have recently challenged the notion that a lipophilic opioid injected epidurally gives analgesia only because of systemic absorption.

Pharmacokinetic observations of sufentanil, which is about twice as lipophilic as fentanyl, have shown that after epidural administration sufentanil concentrations in CSF by far exceed those after intravenous administration, suggesting a spinal site of action (Hansdottir et al 1995). Moreover, CSF concentrations of the drug are higher near the site of injection and the gradient is maintained even after prolonged infusions (Hansdottir et al 1996), indicating a segmental distribution of analgesia.

The Scandinavian author's theory is that plasma concentrations of sufentanil, although contributing to analgesia after epidural administration, do not reflect the concentration at the receptor site. CSF concentration is probably a better indicator of receptor activity. Epidural sufentanil analgesia is more likely to be related to specific activity at spinal opiate receptors.

Clearly, the notion of CSF/plasma concentration ratio is of paramount importance but only a few studies, possibly for ethical reasons, have managed to measure CSF as well as plasma concentrations of lipophilic opioids after epidural administration.

Summarising, whereas general consensus exists about morphine being a very good choice of epidural use, the controversy over the use of epidural lipophilic opioids is far from being resolved. Further studies are needed to answer questions as to the best choice of type and dose of narcotic. Based on the limited data available, it seems inappropriate to recommend the withdrawal of lipophilic epidural opioids from clinical practice.

ADDITION OF A LOCAL ANAESTHETIC

Several animal studies have conclusively proven that local anaesthetics and opioids have a synergistic effect at a spinal cord level. Subthreshold doses of either drug, combined with equally ineffective doses of the other, result in spinal analgesia (Vercauteren et al 1992).

Clinical practice in humans has suggested that a combination of a local anaesthetic and an opioid results in profound postoperative analgesia and this has been confirmed by several studies. However, the desire to avoid unwanted side effects, coupled with the demonstration of synergism in animals has led to the search of the minimum effective combination dose. Bupivacaine has been the most widely used local anaesthetic, as lignocaine is associated with high incidence of tachyphylaxis while chlorprocaine antagonises opioid induced analgesia.

Bupivacaine has been used in combination with opioids for postoperative analgesia in concentrations as low as 0.015% (Cohen et al 1996), but evidence that such a low concentration adds on to the analgesic effect of the opioid is missing. A concentration of 0.1–0.125% in combination with an opioid is quite commonly used by most acute pain services, but results from different studies give a contradictory picture.

Epidural infusions of morphine alone compared with morphine plus 0.1% bupivacaine showed no difference in analgesia for patients after thoracotomy (Logas et al 1987). A similar lack of beneficial effect was seen with a combination of fentanyl plus bupivacaine 0.1% compared with fentanyl alone (Badner & Komar 1992), although the same authors using the same protocol found bupivacaine 0.125% plus fentanyl better than fentanyl alone (Badner & Komar 1994).

All these studies assessed pain at rest, whereas it is commonly believed that the combination of bupivacaine plus opioid is more effective when testing pain levels during mobilisation or coughing (Cullen et al 1985). Indeed, pain on movement was significantly reduced by a mixture of 0.1% bupivacaine plus fentanyl versus fentanyl alone in patients with epidurals for abdominal surgery (Paech et al 1994), but this was not confirmed by another study (Salomaki et al 1995).

Various factors should be considered when assessing the use of epidurals in postoperative pain, i.e. catheter location, type of surgery, type of pain component measured, use of concomitant drugs, type of analgesic mixture used and total dose of bupivacaine administered. Lack of uniformity in study protocols has led to contradictory results and substantial work is still required to clarify this matter.

Summarising, bupivacaine has been widely used in combination with opioids for the treatment of postoperative pain with epidural infusions. Concentrations of 0.25% are certainly effective but at the expense of significant side effects (sensory and motor block, lack of mobilisation, and hypotension). Lower concentrations are associated with minimal side effects but controversy exists on their efficacy, in combination with an opioid, when compared to the effect of the opioid alone.

ROPIVACAINE

Ropivacaine is not a new local anaesthetic, since it has been known about for some years. However, it has become available for clinical use only recently. Ropivacaine is a less toxic compound than bupivacaine after i.v. administration in human volunteers. It is less lipophilic and has higher clearance than bupivacaine. The sensory block provided by ropivacaine is similar to that produced by equivalent doses of bupivacaine, whereas the motor block is less pronounced and shorter in duration. This characteristic, together with a more favourable toxicity profile, allows ropivacaine to be used in higher concentrations than bupivacaine. The greater sensory motor separation of the block produced by ropivacaine has led the manufacturer to introduce on the market pre-loaded bags of 0.2% ropivacaine, intended for epidural use in labour pain and in postoperative analgesia. However, limited data are available about the use of epidural ropivacaine in the postoperative setting (Erichsen et al 1996) and trials are in progress.

POSITION OF CATHETER

This is also an area in which much controversy exists. The problem could be posed in the following way: is there an advantage in positioning thoracic as opposed to lumbar epidural catheters for postoperative pain management after thoracic and upper abdominal surgery?

The question is relevant in view of the technical difficulties, and possible complications, associated with thoracic epidural catheterisation, although a recent series of over 4,000 patients shows a very low incidence of complications (Giebler et al 1997) following thoracic epidurals. In order to answer to that, we must go back to the previously discussed issue of the choice between hydrophilic and lipophilic opioids. Epidural infusions of morphine (partition coefficients = 1, very hydrophilic) and diamorphine (partition coefficient = 10, relatively hydrophilic) can be used for treating pain in dermatomes far from the catheter side because the drugs will spread evenly in the CSF (Sullivan et al 1987). Consequently, thoracic epidurals offer no advantage over lumbar epidurals when morphine is used to treat postoperative pain after thoracic or upper abdominal surgery. Moreover, care must be taken when giving a bolus of morphine via a thoracic epidural catheter, because an excessive dose of opioids could reach the brain stem leading to respiratory depression (Cousins & Mather 1984).

With lipophilic opioids like fentanyl (partition coefficient = 950) or sufentanil (partition coefficient = 1750) the situation is very different. The use of lumbar epidural fentanyl cannot be recommended for the treatment of pain in dermatomes distant from the insertion point of the catheter. There is clear evidence that any analgesic effect would be obtained by a systemic absorption, with plasma levels similar to equally analgesic intravenous doses (Sandler et al 1992). As far as sufentanil is concerned, the volume in which the opiate is diluted might be of relevance as it appears that the same dose of sufentanil gives better epidural analgesia if it is diluted in a higher, rather than in a lower, volume. Thus, it seems reasonable to recommend the use of a lipophilic opioid only if administered by an epidural catheter located at the interspace crossed by the middle dermatome of the surgical incision.

Going back to our original question, it would seem more appropriate to use thoracic epidurals when fentanyl is used to treat postoperative pain after upper abdominal or thoracic surgery. However, the argument is still debated with studies in favour (Chisakuta et al 1995, Salomaki et al 1991) or against (Bouchard & Drolet 1995) this hypothesis.

ADDING OTHER DRUGS

Clonidine

Clonidine is a selective α_2-agonist. It has an analgesic effect mediated both by opioid independent and opioid dependent mechanisms. There is good evidence of synergism between opioids and clonidine at the spinal cord level.

Studies on epidural co-administration of opioids and clonidine (in doses of 3–5 mcg/kg) have shown longer lasting analgesia and ultimately a sparing effect on opioid consumption. Clonidine can cause hypotension by central vasomotor effects, but this is usually minimised by maintaining good intravascular volume.

Adrenaline

When added to sufentanil (Klepper et al 1987) or morphine (Bromage et al 1982) adrenaline shows an opioid-sparing effect which is also seen with fentanyl given as a bolus (Robertson et al 1985) or by infusion (Baron et al 1996). Its mechanism of action is thought to be related to reduction in the vascular uptake of the opioid. Another possibility is synergistic interaction with opioids due to the intrinsic α_2-agonist properties of adrenaline. Interestingly, it seems that a higher incidence of pruritus occurs when adrenaline is added to fentanyl but the mechanism is unknown (Baron et al 1996). Larger studies are required to assess the safety of adrenaline-opioid epidural infusion in the daily clinical practice of an acute pain service.

Steroids

Epidural steroids are not beneficial as adjuvant drugs for postoperative pain relief. Their efficacy in the treatment of sciatic pain has been recently evaluated in a meta-analysis by Watts et al (1995). Epidural steroids are more effective than placebo both in the short-term (58% vs 40%) and in the long-term (51% vs 41%). See also McQuay et al (1996).

REGIONAL TECHNIQUES

Better expertise in the field of clinical management of pain, together with increased availability of acute pain services, has made possible the use of continuous neural blockade techniques as methods for postoperative pain relief. In the brief discussion that follows, no detailed description of such techniques will be given as this goes beyond the scope of this chapter, but the attention will be focused on their clinical relevance in the day-to-day management of acute pain problems.

BRACHIAL PLEXUS ANALGESIA

The brachial plexus is formed by the spinal nerves of C5, C6, C7, C8 and T1. In its route from the vertebrae to the ipsilateral column, the plexus lies within a sheath that extends well beyond the axilla. Velamentous septae can be demonstrated within the sheath but they are usually incomplete and do not form a barrier to the spread of a solution injected inside the sheath. Continuous brachial plexus blockade techniques are employed by inserting a catheter into the sheath. Repeated bolus injections or a continuous infusion of a local anaesthetic solution can then be administered directly in to the nerve sheath.

Indications for the use of continuous brachial plexus blockade are:

(i) pain relief after interventions on the upper limb; and

(ii) sympathectomy of the upper limb, resulting in increased blood flow which could be useful after trauma or procedures like digit re-implantation.

The brachial plexus can be blocked at various levels:

Axilliary approach. Technically easier and devoid of the risk of pneumothorax, and not suitable for upper arm and shoulder pain because the musculocutaneous and the axillary nerves leave the neuromuscular bundle more proximally and are usually missed at this level. Moreover, there is increased risk of catheter dislodgement with upper limb movements.

Infraclavicular approach. It is associated with a lower risk of dislodgement than other approaches, but it is more difficult to perform. A pneumothorax, although rare, can occur.

Supraclavicular approach. It has a higher risk of side effects, i.e. pneumothorax, Horner's syndrome, phrenic and vagus nerve blockade.

Subclavian perivascular approach. Lower risk of pneumothorax, but it is more difficult to thread a catheter into the neurovascular bundle.

Interscalene approach. Ideal in obese patients but perpendicular to the direction of the brachial plexus. It is, therefore, difficult to advance the catheter into the sheath. Side effects are rare but serious, i.e. subarachnoid and epidural injection, intravascular injection into a vertebral artery or phrenic nerve block.

Continuous brachial plexus blockade can be achieved by repeated bolus injections or continuous infusion of the chosen local anaesthetic solution. Bupivacaine has been the most widely used. Several studies report optimal analgesia with an infusion of 0.25% bupivacaine at 8–10 ml/h. Recent work from Japan reports the use of butorphanol, alone and in combination with mepivacaine, for continuous infusion into the brachial plexus (Wajima et al 1995). Preliminary data showed better analgesia with the opioid + local anaesthetic mixture, although larger studies are needed to assess the clinical relevance of this technique.

FEMORAL NERVE BLOCK

The femoral nerve arises from the nerve roots of L2, L3, and L4. It is one of the three major branches of the lumbar plexus, the others being the obturator and the lateral femoral cutaneous nerve. It lies in the femoral sheath lateral to the femoral artery and under the inguinal ligament. It supplies with motor fibres the quadriceps femoris and with sensory fibres part of the knee joint and the medial aspect of the leg. Femoral nerve block is normally used intraoperatively in association with a sciatic nerve block, for operations on the lower leg, or with a general anaesthetic with interventions on the leg and/or knee. Indeed, a femoral block alone cannot be used as a sole anaesthetic for knee surgery because sensory fibres to the knee arise from the lateral femoral cutaneous, the obturator and the sciatic nerve. However, a technique combining i.v. PCA in association with a continuous infusion of local anaesthetic (usually bupivacaine 0.25% at 8–10 ml/h in the normal adult) via a catheter in to the femoral sheath is becoming increasingly popular after knee surgery, as it theoretically decreases the amount of PCA opioid required for optimal analgesia.

Although in theory the argument is sound, a controlled study (Hirst et al 1996) has failed to show any decrease in opioid requirements in patients treated with the association femoral block plus PCA as opposed to PCA alone. One aspect to consider is that catheters can easily be dislodged from the femoral sheath and this may affect the efficacy of a postoperative analgesic infusion. Larger numbers of patients need to be studied for a better assessment of continuous femoral nerve block as a method for postoperative pain relief.

INTRAPLEURAL ANALGESIA

First described in 1984 by Reiestad, intrapleural regional analgesia consists of the installation of local anaesthetic in the space between the parietal and visceral pleura. This is usually performed by an epidural catheter positioned in the above space through a Touhy needle. This technique is becoming increasingly popular in the treatment of postoperative pain after unilateral surgery involving thoracic dermatomes, i.e. cholecystectomy, splenectomy, nephrectomy, breast surgery and chest wall operations. It has been used in thoracotomies, although with controversial results. It has also been used for treating pain after rib fractures and to decrease the pain associated with removal of chest tubes after pneumothorax.

How can analgesia be achieved with intrapleural injection of local anaesthetic? Studies on animals and cadavers have shown that fluid injected in to the intrapleural space diffuses through the parietal pleura into the subpleural and then the paravertebral space, where the intercostal nerves are only covered by parietal pleura. It is suggested that local anaesthetics follow the same route, producing analgesia through intercostal nerve blockade. In other words, the intrapleural space would function as a means of drug access to the intercostal nerves. This mechanism of action is based on local anaesthetic diffusion through the parietal pleura. Indeed, the anatomical and physiological characteristics of the parietal pleura make it suitable for fluid transport, much more so than the visceral pleura (McKenzie & Mathe 1996).

Bupivacaine has been the most widely used local anaesthetic for intrapleural analgesia. A dose of 20 ml of 0.25% in a normal adult provides analgesia lasting for 3–5 h after cholecystectomy, whereas doubling the concentration doesn't seem to add on the duration of analgesia (Brismar et al 1987). Lignocaine and etidocaine have also been used satisfactorily. The latter, in particular, seems an appropriate choice for intrapleural use in view of its rapid plasma clearance coupled with significant uptake in to the lung parenchyma, which decreases its systemic toxicity. Indeed, absorption into the systemic circulation leading to local anaesthetic toxicity is a possible complication of the technique and co-administration of adrenaline seems advantageous. Other complications include:

Pneumothorax. In about 2% of cases, usually small and self absorbing but to be treated when associated with clinical symptoms.

Horner's syndrome. Due to extensive sympathectomy; it is more likely to occur if the patient is in the Trendelenburg position during the procedure.

Pleural effusion. Rare and usually not significant.

Contraindications for the technique are all pleural pathologies, pneumonia, lung malignancy and lung-pleural adhesions. Indications to intrapleural analgesia, as previously mentioned, include unilateral surgical procedures or traumatic injuries involving thoracic dermatomes. Bilateral catheters are necessary for mid-line surgical procedures and are associated with a very high incidence of local anaesthetic toxicity.

Controversy exists regarding the optimum use of intrapleural regional analgesia after thoracotomy. High incidence of inadequate analgesia has been reported (Ferrante et al 1991) and this has been related to a number of possible causes, including rapid absorption in to the systemic circulation through depleuralised areas, sequestration of the local anaesthetic by restricted motion of operated lung and loss of local anaesthetic through chest drainage. Interestingly in a double blind study, Brockmeier (1994) showed no difference in analgesia provided by intrapleural analgesia versus thoracic epidural infusion after thoracotomy when drainage tubes were clamped during the injection of the intrapleural bolus and for 15 min afterwards. However, despite increasing interest in this technique, intrapleural regional analgesia has not yet gained widespread popularity amongst the clinicians who deal with postoperative pain. Lack of familiarity with the technique coupled with the availability of well-established alternative means of analgesia have limited the use of this procedure. In particular, concerns are raised about the possible side effects of intrapleural analgesia, which must be carefully weighted with the advantages associated with it.

INTERCOSTAL BLOCK

Intercostal nerve blockade using intermittent injections of local anaesthetic has been known for many years as an effective method of pain relief in the thoracic area. However, the need for multiple injections in order to provide long lasting analgesia has limited the use of this procedure. In 1981, O'Kelly and Garry described a technique for continuous intercostal analgesia with repeated injections or infusion of local anaesthetic via an epidural catheter located in the intercostal space. Analgesia can be achieved in several thoracic dermatomes because the local anaesthetic solution from the injection site diffuses in to the subpleural space and from there into the adjacent intercostal spaces. Spread of solution has also been demonstrated into the paravertebral and the epidural space. This technique has been used in various clinical circumstances, but only a few controlled studies are available.

Intercostal 0.5% bupivacaine achieved similar analgesia after thoracotomy to that provided by 0.3 mg intramuscular buprenorphine 3 times daily (Deneuville et al 1993). A comparison with lumbar epidural morphine showed that continuous infusion of 0.5% intercostal bupivacaine provided similar pain relief after thoracotomy (Richardson et al 1993), although this study is to be criticised because the epidural regimen used was sub-optimal whereas the dose of bupivacaine was above the toxic threshold. Consequently, the clinical relevance of continuous intercostal block for postoperative pain relief is yet to be determined and consideration must be given to the significant incidence of side effects, especially pneumothorax, associated with this technique.

SUBCUTANEOUS INFUSIONS

It has been recently shown that, despite what was originally believed, subcutaneous administration of morphine results in reliable absorption of the drug (Semple et al 1997). The subcutaneous route has been used for some time for opioid administration in cancer patients, but potential advantages of this technique could be exploited in the postoperative setting as well. For instance, it is not always possible to insert separate cannulas for i.v. fluids and analgesia infusions in infants; anti-reflux valves, very useful in adults, may be dangerous in this population. Indeed diamorphine was equally effective after i.v. or subcutaneous administration in children after abdominal surgery (Semple et al 1996). Subcutaneous morphine has been compared with the extradural route giving good analgesia in adults (Hindsholm et al 1993) and mention deserves the use of subcutaneous low dose ketamine for acute musculo-skeletal trauma (Gurnani et al 1996). It is important to stress that the presence of an intravenous cannula during a postoperative opioid infusion, whatever the route of administration, is a mandatory basic safety requirement which must be applied in all circumstances. However, infusions via the subcutaneous route represent a useful alternative mode of opioid administration which deserves more investigation.

References

Badner N H, Komar W E 1992 Bupivacaine 0.1% does not improve postoperative epidural fentanyl analgesia after abdominal or thoracic surgery. Can J Anaesth 39: 330–336

Badner N H, Bhandari R, Komar W E 1994 Bupivacaine 0.125% improves continuous postoperative epidural fentanyl analgesia after abdominal or thoracic surgery. Can J Anaesth 41: 387–392

Baron C M, Kowalski S E, Greengrass R et al 1996 Epinephrine decreases postoperative requirements for continuous thoracic epidural fentanyl infusions. Anesth Analg 82: 760–765

Bouchard F, Drolet P 1995 Thoracic versus lumbar administration of fentanyl using patient-controlled epidural after thoracotomy. Reg Anesth 20: 385–388

Brismar B, Petterson N, Tokics L 1987 Postoperative analgesia with intrapleural administration of bupivacaine-adrenaline. Acta Anaesthesiol Scand 31: 515–518

Brockmeier V, Moen H, Karlsson B R et al 1994 Interpleural or thoracic epidural analgesia for pain after thoracotomy. A double blind study. Acta Anaesthesiol Scand 38: 317–321

Bromage P R, Camporesi E M, Durant P A, Neilsen C H 1982 Influence of epinephrine as an adjuvant to epidural morphine. Anesthesiology 58: 257–262

Bruera E, MacMillan K, Hanson J, MacDonald R N 1991 The Edmonton injector: a simple device for patient controlled subcutaneous analgesia. Pain 44: 167-169

Cepeda M S, Vargas L, Ortegon G, Sanchez M A, Carr D B 1995 Comparative analgesic effect of patient-controlled analgesia with ketorolac versus morphine after elective intraabdominal operations. Anesth Analg 80: 1150–1153

Chisakuta A M, George K A, Hawthorne C T 1995 Postoperative epidural infusion of a mixture of bupivacaine 0.2% with fentanyl for upper abdominal surgery. A comparison of thoracic and lumbar routes. Anaesthesia 50: 72–75

Cohen S, Amar D, Pantuck C B et al 1996 Epidural analgesia for labour and delivery: fentanyl or sufentanil. Can J Anaesth 43: 341–346

Cousins M J, Mather L E 1984 Intrathecal and epidural administration of opioids. Anesthesiology 61: 276–310

Cullen M L, Staren E D, El-Ganzouri A et al 1985 Continuous epidural infusion for analgesia after major abdominal operations: a randomized, prospective, double-blind study. Surgery 98: 718–727

Deneuville M, Bisserier A, Regnard J F et al 1993 Continuous intercostal analgesia with 0.5% bupivacaine after thoracotomy: a randomized study. Ann Thorac Surg 55: 381–385

Doyle E, Harper I, Morton N S 1993 Patient-controlled analgesia with low dose background infusions after lower abdominal surgery in children. Br J Anaesth 71: 818–822

Egbert A M, Lampros L L, Parks L L 1993 Effects of patient controlled analgesia on postoperative anxiety in elderly men. Am J Crit Care 2: 118–124

Erichsen C J, Sjovall J, Kehlet H, Hedlund C, Arvidsson T 1996 Pharmacokinetics and analgesic effect of ropivacaine during continuous epidural infusion for postoperative pain relief. Anesthesiology 84: 834–842

Eriksson-Mjoberg M, Svensson J O, Almkvist O, Olund A, Gustafsson L 1997 Extradural morphine gives better pain relief than patient-controlled i.v. morphine after hysterectomy. Br J Anaesth 78: 10–16

Etches R C 1994 Respiratory depression associated with patient controlled analgesia: a review of eight cases. Can J Anaesth 41: 125–132

Ferrante F M, Chan V W S, Arthur G R, Rocco A G 1991 Interpleural analgesia after thoracotomy. Anesth Analg 72: 105–109

Giebler R M, Scherer R U, Peters J 1997 Incidence of neurologic complications related to thoracic epidural catheterization. Anesthesiology 86: 55-63

Ginsberg B, Gil K M, Muir M et al 1995 The influence of lockout intervals and drug selection on patient-controlled analgesia following gynaecological surgery. Pain 62: 95–100

Glass P S A, Estok P, Ginsberg B, Goldberg J S, Sladen R N 1991 Use of patient-controlled analgesia to compare the efficacy of epidural and intravenous fentanyl administration. Anesth Analg 72: 345–351

Gurnani A, Sharma P K, Rautela R S, Bhattacharya A 1996 Analgesia for acute musculoskeletal trauma: low dose subcutaneous infusion of ketamine. Anaesth Intensive Care 24: 32–36

Hansdottir V, Woestenborghs R, Nordberg G 1995 The cerebrospinal fluid and plasma pharmacokinetics of sufentanil after thoracic or lumbar epidural administration. Anesth Analg 80: 72

Hansdottir V, Woestenborghs R, Nordberg G 1996 The pharmacokinetics of continuous epidural sufentanil and bupivacaine after thoracotomy. Anesth Analg 83: 401–406

Harrison D M, Sinatra R, Morgese L, Chung J H 1988 Epidural narcotic and patient-controlled analgesia for post-cesarean section pain relief. Anesthesiology 68: 454–459

Hindsholm K B, Bredhal C, Jensen M K et al 1993 Continuous subcutaneous infusion of morphine – an alternative to extradural morphine for postoperative pain relief. Br J Anaesth 71: 580–582

Hirst G C, Lang S A, Dust W N, Cassidy J D, Yip R W 1996 Femoral nerve block. Single injection versus continuous infusion for total knee arthroplasty. Reg Anesth 21: 292–297

Joshi G P, McCarrol S M, O'Rourke K 1995 Postoperative analgesia after lumbar laminectomy: epidural fentanyl infusion versus patient-controlled intravenous morphine. Anesth Analg 80: 511–514

Klepper I D, Sherril D L, Boetger C L, Bromage P R 1987 Analgesic and respiratory effects of extradural sufentanil in volunteers and the influence of adrenaline as an adjuvant. Br J Anaesth 59: 1147–1156

Logas W G, El-Baz N, El-Ganzouri A 1987 Continuous thoracic epidural analgesia for postoperative pain relief following thoracotomy: a randomized prospective study. Anesthesiology 67: 787–791

Looi-Lyons L C, Chung F F, Chan V W, McQuestion M 1996 Respiratory depression: an adverse outcome during patient controlled analgesia therapy. J Clin Anesth 8: 151–156

Loper K A, Ready L B, Downey M et al 1990 Epidural and intravenous fentanyl infusions are clinically equivalent after knee surgery. Anesth Analg 70: 72–75

McKenzie A G, Mathe S 1996 Interpleural local anaesthesia: anatomical basis for mechanism of action. Br J Anaesth 76: 297–299

McQuay H J 1994 Epidural Analgesics. In: Textbook of pain. 3rd edn. Edinburgh: Churchill Livingstone, 1025–1034

McQuay H J, Moore A 1996 Epidural steroids for sciatica. Anaesth Intensive Care 24: 284–285

Ngan-Kee W D, Lam K K, Chen P P, Gin T 1996 Epidural meperidine after cesarean section. A dose-response study. Anesthesiology 85: 289–294

Nordberg G, Hedner T, Mellstrand T 1983 Pharmacokinetic aspects of epidural morphine analgesia. Anesthesiology 58: 545–551

O'Kelly E, Garry B 1981 Continuous pain relief for multiple fractured ribs. Br J Anaesth 53: 989–991

Owen H, Plummer J, Ilsley A et al 1995 Variable-dose patient-controlled analgesia. A preliminary report. Anaesthesia 50: 855–857

Paech M J, Westmore M D 1994 Postoperative epidural fentanyl infusion – is the addition of 0.1% bupivacaine of benefit? Anaesth Intensive Care 22: 9–14

Rapp S E, Egan K J, Ross B K et al 1996 A multidimensional comparison of morphine and hydromorphone patient-controlled analgesia. Anesth Analg 82: 1043–1048

Richardson J, Sabanathan S, Eng J et al 1993 Continuous intercostal nerve block versus epidural morphine for postthoracotomy analgesia. Ann Thorac Surg 55: 377–380

Robertson K, Douglas J M, McMorland G H 1985 Epidural fentanyl with and without epinephrine for post-cesarian section analgesia. Can Anaesth Soc J 32: 502–505

Salomaki T, Laitinen J, Nuutinen L 1991 A randomized double-blind comparison of epidural versus intravenous fentanyl infusion for analgesia after thoracotomy. Anesthesiology 75: 790–795

Salomaki T, Laitinen J O, Vainionpaa V, Nuutinen L S 1995 0.1% bupivacaine does not reduce the requirement for epidural fentanyl infusion after major abdominal surgery. Reg Anesth 20: 435–443

Sandler A, Stringer D, Panos L et al 1992 A randomized, double-blind comparison of lumbar epidural and intravenous fentanyl infusions for postthoracotomy pain relief. Anesthesiology 77: 626–634

Semple D, Aldridge L A, Doyle B 1996 Comparison of i.v. and s.c. diamorphine infusions for the treatment of acute pain in children. Br J Anaesth 76: 310–312

Semple T J, Upton R N, Macintyre P E, Runciman W B, Mather L E 1997 Morphine blood concentrations in elderly postoperative patients following administration via an indwelling subcutaneous cannula. Anaesthesia 52: 318–323

Sjostrom S, Hartvig P, Persson M P 1987 Pharmacokinetics of epidural morphine and meperidine in humans. Anesthesiology 67: 877–881

Striebel H W, Romer M, Kopf A, Schwagmeier R 1996a Patient controlled oral analgesia with morphine. Can J Anaesth 43: 749–753

Striebel HW, Oelmann T, Spies C, Rieger A, Schwagmeier R 1996b Patient-controlled intranasal analgesia: a method for non invasive postoperative pain management. Anesth Analg 83: 548–551

Sullivan S P, Cherry D A 1987 Pain from an invasive facial tumor relieved by lumbar epidural morphine. Anesth Analg 66: 777–780

VadeBoncouer T R, Ferrante F M 1993 Epidural and subarachnoid opioids. In: Postoperative Pain Management. New York: Churchill Livingstone, 279–303

Vercauteren M, Meert T, Boersma F 1992 Spinal sufentanil in rats. Part II: effect of adding bupivacaine to epidural sufentanil. Acta Anaesthesiol Scand 36: 245–249

Wajima Z, Shitara T, Nakajima Y et al 1995 Comparison of continuous brachial plexus infusion of butorphanol, mepivacaine and mepivacaine-butorphanol mixtures for postoperative analgesia. Br J Anaesth 75: 548–551

Watts R W, Silagy C A 1995 A meta-analysis on the efficacy of epidural corticosteroids in the treatment of sciatica. Anaesth Intensive Care 23: 564–569

Woodhouse A, Hobbes A F, Mather L E, Gibson M 1996 A comparison of morphine, pethidine and fentanyl in the postsurgical patient-controlled analgesia environment. Pain 64 : 115–121

Rajesh Munglani

Advances in chronic pain therapy with special reference to low back pain

Scenario 1

A patient has clear symptoms of a prolapsed intervertebral disc with leg weakness and pain. This is confirmed by clinical examination and a MRI scan. There is initially a good response to discectomy, however, after 1–2 months the pain begins to return. The repeat MRI shows no further prolapse or scarring and the patient does not understand why he is in pain again. The persistent unexplained pain and inability of the surgeons to offer any further treatment leads to fear of movement (in case he does any more damage to his back) and development of chronic disability. Loss of self esteem, secondary depression, loss of income and strain on family relationships rapidly follow . . .

Scenario 2

A previously fit young man develops back pain a day or so after playing squash. There are no symptoms or signs of nerve root compression and MRI scans are not helpful. The pain seems undulating in nature and increasing amounts of time are taken off work; suggestions are made that he may be a malingerer. Physiotherapy may aggravate the pain, the lack of explanation for the pain makes the patient aggressive towards the medical profession. Loss of self esteem, secondary depression, loss of income and strain on family relationships rapidly follow . . .

In the past two decades, our understanding of the mechanisms of chronic pain have advanced tremendously. In particular, there is clear evidence for the role of the spinal cord and spinal cord structures in both initiation and maintenance

Dr Rajesh Munglani DCH FRCA, John Farman Professor at the Royal College of Anaesthetists; Lecturer and Consultant, University Department of Anaesthesia, Addenbrookes Hospital, Hills Road, Cambridge CB2 2QQ, UK

of chronic pain. They not only give good explanations for the scenarios outlined above but also provide a better scientific foundation for chronic pain therapy.

The literature is vast and in this article I will focus on those mechanisms which may help us understand chronic low back pain. For a more complete introduction, I suggest the reader refer to a previous chapter in this series (Munglani et al 1996d). To save on space, I have deliberately cited review papers rather than original references in this present article and apologise in advance to those authors who have, therefore, not been directly cited. If no reference is apparent, then it is because it has been previously mentioned in the above chapter.

Long lasting changes in the spinal cord following peripheral inflammation or nerve injury

Damage to a peripheral nerve (such as compression of a nerve root by a prolapsing disc) or peripheral tissue inflammation (e.g. in arthritis) leads to an initiation of a cascade of molecular events within the peripheral nerve and also the spinal cord

Tissue inflammation is known to sensitise peripheral nerves so that they respond much more dramatically to stimulation. This partly explains, for example, the painful joint movement associated with arthritis. However, it is also well recognised that inflammation or nerve injury produces dramatic changes in the spinal cord (see Fig. 11.1). These events involve the release of neurotransmitters, such as glutamate, substance P, neurokinin A and calcitonin gene-related peptide. This is followed by activation of certain receptors, such as the NMDA channel, which initiate a further cascade of events within neurones. This includes activation of second messengers (including calcium, prostaglandins and nitric oxide) and also expression of particular genes, such as *c-fos*. The amount of protein product of the *c-fos* gene in the spinal cord seems to correlate with both the magnitude of the initial stimulus yet also mediates some of the adaptive responses of the spinal cord (see later).

There are also changes within the spinal cord neurones of levels of certain neuropeptides. The levels of GABA, a profoundly inhibitory neuropeptide, drop within the spinal cord and, in addition, there is an increase in the number of excitable nerves due to production of excessive novel sodium channels on nerves mediated by both nerve injury and/or the availability of growth factors, such as NGF. Furthermore, after peripheral nerve injury, the levels of a neuropeptide called cholecystokinin (CCK) with anti-opioid actions rise dramatically within the spinal cord. Events such as these lead to a general state of dis-inhibition within the spinal cord which then becomes much more receptive to incoming stimuli. This can be shown, for example, by the enhanced expression of *Fos* in the spinal cord after peripheral nerve stimulation in models of chronic pain (see references in Munglani & Hunt 1995a,b; Munglani et al 1996b, 1997; Hudspith & Munglani 1997).

Both nerve injury and inflammatory pain also cause other profound changes within the spinal cord. For example, large diameter primary afferent neurones, which normally are associated with transmission of non-noxious stimuli, now start to express substance P (SP) (Noguchi et al 1995, Neumann et al 1996). SP is usually only associated with small diameter neurones that give rise to C-fibres which transmit pain and temperature. The exact significance of this phenotypic switch by large diameter fibres is not known but it has been suggested that, since SP expression and release is usually involved in transduction of noxious information, it may be that the usual light touch and proprioceptive information that is usually carried by these Aβ fibres maybe misinterpreted by the spinal cord and brain. Structural changes also occur with nerve injury causing the formation of novel contacts with other neurones within the spinal cord. This sprouting of Aβ nerve fibres from deeper laminae of the spinal cord into the more superficial laminae associated with C-fibre input has also been suggested to form the basis of chronic pain and allodynia in particular (Woolf et al 1992). There is evidence that, gradually, this central sprouting of Aβ fibres seems to recede with time (Woolf et al 1995). Again the significance of these observations to the development and resolution of hyperalgesia is not certain, but certainly illustrates the remarkable plasticity of spinal cord systems.

Neuropathic pain is associated with the loss of opiate sensitivity

Nerve injury in particular, induces a number of changes which diminish the action of opioids. Rather perversely, nerve injury not only causes a loss of

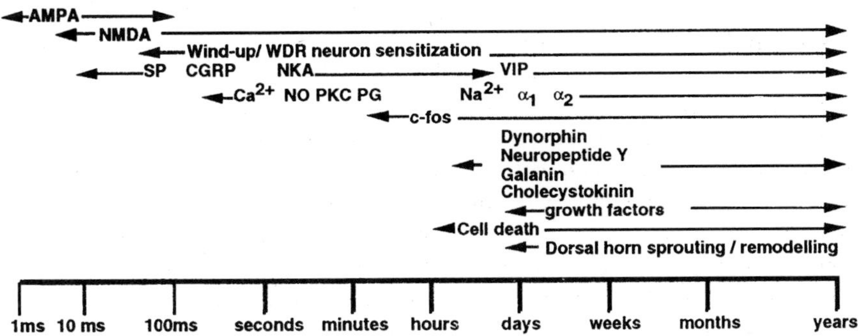

Fig 11.1 This schematic diagram outlines the cascade of some of molecular events which may occur in the spinal cord following peripheral nerve injury or stimulation. Some of the changes only occur in certain situations. However, many changes are common to both pain states, e.g. the activation of the NMDA channel, increase in intracellular Ca^{2+}, involvement and upregulation of neuronal nitric oxide synthase, and increase in *c-fos*. These changes in ion channel function, second messengers, immediate early genes such as *c-fos* and neuropeptides may then be followed by more permanent changes in the nervous system consisting of changes in synaptic efficacy of pre-existing synapses, nerve sprouting and formation of novel synapses via growth factors. These latter changes may be the basis of pain memories in the spinal cord and brain. Particular changes may be prominent in certain conditions, e.g. changes in adrenoreceptor ($\alpha_{1,2}$) function may contribute to sympathetically maintained pain. There is some evidence that inhibiting the earlier events may delay and perhaps prevent some of the later events, i.e. prevent the formation of long-term changes which are associated with persistent pain. From Munglani & Hunt (1995), Munglani et al (1996a,b) and Wilcox (1991).

Abbreviations: AMPA, α-amino-3-hydroxy-5-methyl-isoxazole; NMDA, N-methyl-D-aspartate; SP' substance P; CGRP, calcitonin gene-related peptide; NKA, neurokinin A; NO, nitric oxide; PKC, protein kinase C; PG, prostaglandins; VIP, vasoactive intestinal polypeptide.

opioid receptors, causing a reduction in sensitivity to opioids, it also causes the de novo production of cholecystokinin and other neuropeptides within the spinal cord which are known to antagonise the actions of opioids (Hokfelt et al 1994). This reduction in opioid sensitivity may apply to both endogenously produced and exogenously administered opiates. It has been shown recently that activation of the NMDA receptor not only plays a fundamental role in initiating and maintaining chronic pain, but it also causes tolerance to develop at the opioid receptor (Mao et al 1995). Thus chronic pain has to be managed in a radically different way to acute postoperative pain where, for example, opioids are the main stay of treatment. Opioids do have some effect in chronic pain but it is likely to be mediated in the brain rather than spinally (see references in Roud Mayne et al 1996).

Neuropathic pain may be associated with involvement of the sympathetic nervous systems

Peripheral nerve injury has been associated with sprouting of sympathetic fibres in the DRGs which may excite sensory neurones (Chung et al 1993, McLachlan et al 1993). Furthermore, in the periphery, it has been shown that nerve injury causes the expression of adrenergic receptors which make the peripheral nerve sensitive to peripheral sympathetic stimulation including that of circulating noradrenaline. These two possible sites of sympatho-somatic nervous interaction should make one suspect the involvement of the sympathetic nervous system in pain, especially after obvious nerve injury. The role of the sympathetic nervous system in back pain is being increasingly recognised despite often little or no evidence of the autonomic signs traditionally associated with sympathetic contributions to pain states, such as swelling, colour and temperature changes of the affected part (see below).

These events outlined above have profound functional implications leading to long lasting changes in the processing of information entering the spinal cord

The activation of the NMDA receptor and second messengers and changes in levels of neuropeptides have functional implications. They lead to the heightened response of the nervous system to further peripheral stimulation giving rise to **allodynia** (the interpretation of previously innocuous sensation as if it was noxious) and **hyperalgesia** (a heightened response to noxious stimulation). The general name given to this heightened response of the spinal cord is **central sensitisation**. The cascade of events initiated by a single insult or stimulation of a peripheral nerve may go on for weeks or even months after the initial event. It has been shown that even if a peripheral nerve injury has resolved, the changes associated with it in the spinal cord in expression of neuropeptides and *c-fos* for example may continue to persist (Munglani et al 1996a,b, 1997). These permanent plastic changes may be akin to a memory trace and fundamentally, and perhaps permanently, alter the way the nervous system handles information.

These mechanisms outlined above may explain the persistence or recurrence of pain seen in Scenario 1. The exact importance of any particular event will vary with the specific disease but may also vary between patients. If the spinal cord does show some permanent alterations in the way it processes information, then perhaps at some point in the natural history of the disease the best way to modify the perception of pain is to concentrate on cortical mechanisms which have a powerful influence at the level of the spinal cord as well as in the brain, for example by the use of antidepressents and pain management programmes.

Can we prevent the development of chronic pain and the cascade of spinal cord events occurring after neuronal injury or stimulation by conventional anaesthesia and analgesia?

Much has been written about pre-emptive analgesia in the possible prevention of short term hyperalgesia and perhaps long term pain states. Many studies have examined efficacy of various anaesthetic agents given around the time of formalin administration in inhibiting the subsequent pain related behaviour known as the phase 2 formalin response. The phase 2 formalin response consists of complex pain related behaviour, including licking of and flinching with the affected paw, which occurs 10–60 min after the administration of the formalin. This latter phase of pain behaviour can be distinguished pharmacologically from the first phase of paw flinching that immediately follows formalin injection into the paw, in that activation of spinal cord NMDA receptor is critical to the second phase, but not first phase of flinching. In contrast, the first phase occurs within the first 5 min of formalin administration and has been shown to be sensitive to AMPA antagonists. The activation of the NMDA receptor has, in other studies, also been shown to mediate sensitisation of individual spinal cord neurones (including 'windup') and also to mediate enhancement of spinal cord reflexes (see Munglani et al 1996d).

Unfortunately, only in some of these studies does conventional anaesthesia suppress phase 2 flinching with pre-emptive treatment (O'Conner & Abram 1995). Often the effect is weak, for example even 2.5% isoflurane only reduced phase 2 flinching by 35% when given pre-emptively (and, incidentally, in this study the addition of nitrous oxide to the isoflurane abolished this benefit) whilst intrathecal morphine did reduce flinching by 80% (Abram & Yaksh 1993). Even pre-emptive high dose systemic opioids did not reduce phase 2 flinching (Abram & Olson 1994). Other authors have shown that pre-emptive propofol does not reduce phase 2 flinching (Goto et al 1994, Gilron & Coderre 1996). Barbiturates show variable efficacy in inhibiting spinal cord sensitisation (Cleland et al 1994, Goto et al 1994, Gilron & Coderre 1996). Abram and Yaksh (1993) also point out that many of the studies that examined C-fibre induced spinal sensitisation were carried out under surgical plane of anaesthesia (see Dickenson & Sullivan 1987).

Clinical studies show that a simple noxious stimulus evoked reflex in volunteers could be inhibited by 0.25–0.5% end-tidal isoflurane. However, repetition (5 times at 2 Hz) of the same nociceptive stimulus caused facilitation of the nociceptive reflex and required 1–1.5% isoflurane to suppress it (and the authors point out that this dose is similar to the MAC of isoflurane). The authors then suggest that even this higher dose of isoflurane alone would not be adequate for inhibiting surgically evoked excitability seen in actual operations (Petersen-Felix et al 1996). We can conclude that clinically accepted doses of anaesthetics alone have only moderate ability, at best, to: (i) inhibit primary afferent input, (ii) prevent the development of spinal cord sensitisation and (iii) modify short and long term pain perception. However, conventional anaesthetics do show some analgesic effects, including NMDA receptor blocking activity, but this is unlikely to be contributing to their anaesthetic effect (Little 1996).

By using immediate early gene expression (such as that of *c-fos*) as endpoint, it is clear that noxious stimulation still enters the spinal cord during seemingly adequate anaesthesia (see references in Munglani et al 1996). It is not surprising that clinical studies of pre-emptive analgesia show so little effect (Richmond et al 1993, Woolf & Chong 1993). It has been demonstrated previously that radically different outcomes in terms of long-term pain behaviour (and indeed modification of long term spinal cord changes) can be produced experimentally with different adjuncts to isoflurane anaesthesia (α_2 agonists, NMDA antagonists, peripheral blocks with local anaesthetic, but interestingly enough not μ agonists) despite similar lack of responsiveness during anaesthesia. Interestingly, the ability to suppress short and long term *Fos* expression by these adjuncts parallels these behavioural outcomes (see references in Yamamoto et al 1993, Munglani et al 1995, 1996a,b, 1997).

Can we not produce profound inhibition of noxious primary afferent input by the use of spinal anaesthesia?

Unfortunately, neurophysiological studies show that intrathecal local anaesthesia, and even intrathecal morphine, as well as causing some suppression of primary afferent input also seem to cause some excitation at low doses, or even after larger doses have been given (Wisenfeld-Hallin et al 1991, Luo & Wisenfeld-Hallin 1995). Analysis of the spinal cord after intrathecal local anaesthesia actually shows **increased** *Fos* expression after these manoeuvres, which may represent the excitation seen in the neurophysiological studies (Nivarthi et al 1996). Long term behavioural studies following intrathecal local anaesthesia show it to be less effective in preventing development of chronic pain related behaviour than local anaesthetic on the sciatic nerve (Luo & Wisenfeld-Hallin 1995). Up until recently, the clinical evidence for poor perioperative pain control associated with the subsequent development of chronic pain has been patchy but has been reported recently after thoracotomy (Katz et al 1996).

In summary, then, we can not use lack of behavioural responses at the time of conventional anaesthesia and analgesia as an index of prevention of primary afferent input and its consequences. As Abram and Olsen (1994) have previously written: 'there is a dichotomy between behavioural response to a noxious stimulus and the development of enhanced responsiveness'. Indeed, the anaesthetised state, as defined by loss of consciousness or lack of motor response, may be disassociated from the processes leading to post injury facilitation (Abram & Yaksh 1993, Goto et al 1996). The electrophysiological and immediate early gene studies mentioned above suggest we need to radically rethink what our goals are for anaesthesia and the perioperative period and how we are to achieve them.

Why do nerve blocks cause a reduction in intensity of the pain?

The molecular and behavioural changes produced within the central nervous system, once initiated, may be maintained by further input from the periphery (Chi at al 1993a,b). However, this input does not have to be abnormal in nature, input from surrounding undamaged nerves may be enough (Kingery et al 1993, see references in Munglani et al 1996d). It has also has been shown clinically by Gracely et al (1992) that peripheral blocks could bring about general decreases in pain perception over large areas of the body. These findings suggest that peripheral nerve activity entering the spinal cord will continue to maintain central sensitisation and has implications for why nerve denervation procedures may work in so many patients, regardless of whether the nerve traffic is abnormal or not. However, what is even more interesting is the prolonged action of these nerve blocks, outlasting the known action of the local anaesthetic (Arner et al 1990). Nerve blockade, as performed in many chronic pain clinics, may play a helpful role by producing a global reduction in nerve traffic into the spinal cord, allowing the system to 'wind-down' again. The mechanisms underlying wind-down as distinct to wind-up are even less well understood than those which underlie wind-up and sensitisation, but the work of Randic et al (1993) has thrown some light on this. They have shown that a particular level of nerve stimulation into the spinal cord can cause either long term sensitisation or adaptation depending on the electrical potential of the receiving neurone. A few millivolts either way will cause a profound change in the response of the system. Thus, a concept whereby a nerve block with a simple local anaesthetic may flip a system from a hypersensitivity to adaptation may be cautiously suggested. In addition to the possible mechanism postulated above, the administration of epidural steroids (Koes et al 1995), NMDA antagonists and α_2 agonists, for example, help to antagonise the actions of upregulated spinal cord second messengers (such as the spinal cord prostaglandins) and so help to reduce further the level of central sensitisation.

Why doesn't everybody get chronic pain?

The degree of pain experienced after tissue trauma and nerve injury is likely to be the net result of opposing adaptive changes and maladaptive changes within the nervous system

In the period immediately after an acute inflammatory injury, it can be shown that the administration of intrathecal antisense *c-fos* causes enhanced hyperalgesia behaviour, suppresses the production of *Fos* protein and also suppresses production of the opioid peptide, dynorphin (Hunter et al 1995). Thus, *Fos* expression must, at least in part, mediate some of the analgesic responses of the spinal cord acutely. In fact infusions of antisense *c-fos* in normal animals brings about a progressive increase in mechanical hypersensitivity indicating that *Fos* protein is likely to have a low-level, but fundamental, role in normal sensory transduction (Malan et al 1995). This is despite the fact that in the spinal cord of naive (i.e. unstimulated) animals, most groups report no *Fos* expression (Hunt et al 1987).

Some of the neuropeptide changes described are also adaptive. It has also been shown that both after nerve injury and in inflammatory models of pain, levels of analgesic peptides, such as NPY, rise within the spinal cord and DRG (Wakisaka et al 1991, 1992, Munglani et al 1995a,b, 1996c). In inflammatory models, the levels of GABA rise whilst after nerve injury there are decreases in the level of neuropeptides such as SP and CGRP associated with primary afferent transmission. It has been also shown that, in the long term, even when the peripheral nerve lesion has healed, these neuropeptide changes continue to persist (Munglani et al 1996). The possible significance of these persistent neuropeptide changes as an adaptive process is discussed below.

Surpraspinal as well as spinal adaptive responses exist

As well as local spinal cord responses seen above, there are also supraspinal attempts to activate noradrenergic and serotonergic descending inhibitory controls within the spinal cord. These descending systems supply a tonic inhibition which inhibits primary afferent input. Spinalisation of an animal receiving noxious primary afferent input causes enhanced *Fos* expression in the spinal cord, indicating increased primary afferent input reaches the cord and an enhanced local attempt to deal with it (Ren & Ruda 1996). We can suggest the relative balance between adaptive and sensitisation mechanisms will determine the possible development to chronic pain and there is also some evidence that there is genetic component to this (Devor & Raber 1991).

Chronic pain may represent a failure of supraspinal and spinal cord adaptive responses

Recent work in a rat model of neuropathic pain has shown that the hyperalgesia disappears well before the peripheral nerve injury has resolved (as determined by electron microscopy; see references in Munglani et al 1996). It has also been shown that the application of colchicine (a fast axonal transport blocker) proximal to the site of nerve injury (i.e. applying it between the site of nerve injury and the spinal cord) causes the temporary resolution of the pain state (Yamamoto & Yaksh 1993). The implication of this study are that, in this model of neuropathic pain, a peripherally produced factor, probably a cytokine, from the site of nerve injury and transported into the spinal cord is responsible for the maintenance of the pain state. As the animals continued to move their legs normally, the temporary resolution of hyperalgesia is not due to blockade of nerve activity, since, unlike local anaesthetics, colchicine does not block nerve conduction. If then, as mentioned earlier, the nerve injury resolves much later than the disappearance of the hyperalgesia, one can, therefore, postulate that central mechanisms within the spinal cord may play a part both in modifying the effects of the nerve injury initially and perhaps in bringing about resolution of the hyperalgesia in the long term after nerve injury. The failure of such adaptive mechanisms may underlie the development of chronic pain and is suggested by some recent findings (Zimmerman 1991, Cougon et al 1997). Interestingly Boden et al (1990a,b) have shown that if one does MRI of the lumbar spine on the general population one can show that approximately 30% of subjects have a surgically treatable condition. This observation may represent failure of the technique of MRI or else that the presence of a nociceptive source may not always translate into pain at the cognitive level and, perhaps, that the level of activity of adaptive mechanisms within the nervous system may be important in determining the final clinical picture.

Not all pathology that lead to the development of chronic low back pain can be seen on an MRI scan

Non-neuropathic causes of back pain: the precision diagnosis of mechanical low back pain

> 'Whatever it is that causes pain in the back must have a nerve supply'
> Bogduk 1983

In the preceding paragraphs I have suggested how tissue trauma or nerve injury may give rise to long lasting pathological changes within the spinal cord. The work of Mixter and Barr in the 1930s focused the medical community's attention on disc prolapse causing nerve compression as a source of back pain (Mixter & Barr 1934). However, it had been suggested previously that other spinal structures apart from the spinal cord itself may give rise to back pain and referred pain down the leg (Goldwait 1911, and see references in North et al 1994). In Scenario 2, a case of someone with back pain, little or no demonstrable nerve pathology is given. To understand non-neuropathic causes of one must first understand the nerve supply of spinal structures (Table 11.1). It is clear from provocation studies that spinal cord structures, that were previously shown not to give rise to pain, will do so after moderate degrees of injury. All the structures outlined in Table 11.1 can be shown to give rise to pain. However, the two main causes of non-neuropathic pain are lumbar zygopophysial joint arthritis or facet joint and internal disc disruption (IDD). IDD is not the same as disc protrusion. Disc protrusion can be seen on an MRI scan. In contrast, IDD does not show up well on MRI scans and can be demonstrated best by disc stimulation and CT discography. There is good correlation between degree of annular disruption seen on CT discography and pain experienced by disc stimulation. The patients who are shown to have facet and IDD include some of those that have been diagnosed previously to

Table 11.1 Innervation of the lumbar spinal structures

Structure	Nerves
Lumbar disc	Sinuvertebral nerve Ventral rami, gray rami communicantes
Posterior longitudinal ligament	Sinuvertebral nerve
Anterior longitudinal ligament	Gray rami communicantes
Iliocostalis lumborum and longissimus thoracis	Lateral and intermediate branches of the dorsal rami
Facet joints, multifidus, interspinous ligament	Medial branch of the dorsal rami

Note well the innervation of spinal structures by sympathetic fibres. The sinuvertebral nerves have both a somatic and sympathetic component (Bogduk 1983).

Table 11.2 Causes of spinal pain found in patients referred to an Australian specialist pain clinic where no other cause was found for the pain (data from Bogduk 1996)

Type of spinal pain	Type of lesion	Percentage of patients
Low back pain	Lumbar internal disc disruption causing pain	39%
	Sacroiliac joint pain	12%
	Lumbar zygopophysial joint pain	15–40%
Neck pain	Cervical zygopophysial joint pain	50%

By testing for these conditions one can clarify 50% of neck pain and 60% of non-specific low back pain. The low back pain group described above probably comprises about 85% of low back pain patients seen. The table excludes those patients where another reason for back pain was found including (Deyo 1995): disc herniation requiring surgery (2%); vertebral compression (4%); spondylolisthesis (3%); spinal stenosis, spinal malignancy (0.7%); spondylitis (0.03%); infection (0.001%), etc., as well as non-spinal causes including multi-system inflammatory disease.

have non-specific mechanical low back and neck pains (Table 11.2) (Bogduk & Marsland 1988, Bogduk 1992, Bogduk & Aprill 1993, Barnsley et al 1994, Moneta et al 1994, Schwarzer et al 1994a,b, 1995a–d, Bogduk 1996).

Does precision diagnosis of spinal pain (as detailed above) help in the treatment of these patients?

There is both good and bad news about mechanical low back pain. The good news is that whatever one does after an **acute** episode of low back pain, the patient is likely to get better. The recent Clinical Standards Advisory Group (CSAG) document on low back pain detailed the evidence for management of acute low back pain, including the following treatments: (i) bed rest for less than 2 days; (ii) a trial of a strong non steroidal; (iii) a trial of an antidepressant, such as amitryptiline; and (iv) some sort of physical therapy (Meade et al 1986, Spitzer & Leblanc 1987, Rosen 1994, Fordyce 1995, Frost et al 1995). With regard to regular exercise, it has been specifically shown not reduce the frequency of future attacks of low back pain but does reduce the impact of each attack on the patient's lifestyle and promotes quicker recovery. However, exercise involving pronounced flexion or extension of the lumbar spine can aggravate both disc and facet joint derived pain, an observation supported by stress studies in cadaveric spines (Adams 1996). However, it must be made clear that there is very little evidence that any of the treatments (i–iv) outlined above have any effect in reducing long term morbidity. It is likely that they only shorten the severity of the acute attack without changing the vast numbers of patients who end up with chronic intractable back pain.

So the bad news about low back pain is that even if one appropriately treats the early stages, there is little evidence that one changes the long term outcome, i.e. there is still an intractable core of disabled patients at 6 months for which, so far, there has been little treatment as judged by randomised controlled trials (Nachemson 1992). The studies show that if a patient has not gone back to work 12 months, it is likely they will never return. Even outcome after spinal surgery is not much better (Young 1996).

Within this gloomy outlook, however, one or two bright lights have appeared. Firstly, as listed in Table 11.2, up to 40% of patients who were diagnosed as having nonspecific low back pain have facet joint derived pain. If one selects those who respond to diagnostic injections of the facet joint, and permanently thermocoagulates the tiny nerves that supply them, one can produce quite remarkable reductions in pain scores and, móre importantly, marked reduction in disability. About 50% of patients responding to diagnostic blockade will gain some benefit from the more permanent procedure. These improvements are sustained with a duration of years in randomised controlled trials. What is also remarkable is that the dramatic responses seen in these later studies apply to patients with spinal pain referred to the head and neck regions including whiplash, and post laminectomy back and leg pain (Mehta & Sluijter 1979, Ignelzi & Cummings 1980, Bogduk & Marsland 1988, Silvers 1990, Bogduk & Aprill 1993, Gallagher et al 1994, North et al 1994, Schwarzer et al 1994a,b, Gallagher et al 1994, Lord et al 1996). Reasons for the involvement of these joints in both post laminectomy and mechanical pain are given below. In fact there is more evidence presently for this thermocoagulation procedure as a treatment of chronic low back pain than virtually any other treatment in carefully selected populations of patients.

As well as allowing quite specific, potentially dramatic and efficacious treatment in the long term in a proportion of patients, precision diagnosis is useful medico-legally and to reassure patients that they do have a real cause for their pain, for example in cases of whiplash, though care must be taken in interpreting the results of blocks (Bogduk & Aprill 1993, Schwarzer et al 1994a,b, Sethna & Berde 1995). As has been stated previously by Bogduk (1996), if at all possible, patients should be allowed the dignity of a diagnosis.

Why should these facet joints give rise to so much pain and disability in mechanical and post laminectomy low back pain?

Surprising as it may seem, once arthritis has developed in the facet joints, up to 47% of a person's weight may go through the facet joints (Yang & King 1984,

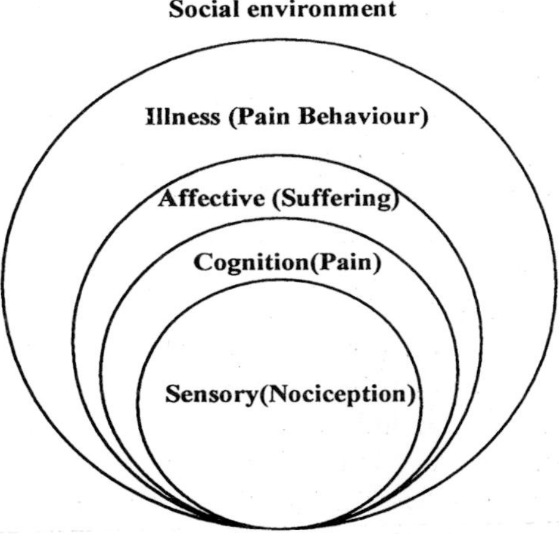

Fig. 11.2 The consequences of pain are manifest at many different levels. Once it has become established, the treatment of nociceptive input alone may not lead to resolution of the other levels. Modified from Loeser (1980) and Waddell (1987).

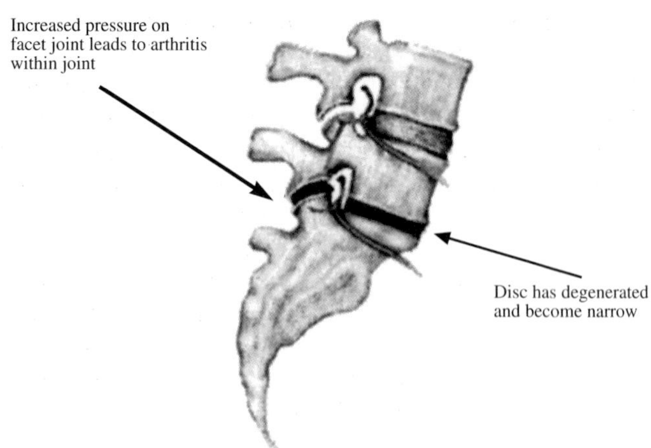

Fig. 11.3 Disc degeneration leading to increased facet joint loading. Loss of disc height is not uncommon even in young patients and may be associated with smoking (which reduces disc nutrition). Note how the spinal nerve gives rise to posterior branches including a branch to the facet joint before supplying the leg. The pain from the facet joint may be referred down dermtomal distribution of the spinal nerve as well as causing local pain and muscle spasm.

Lewinnek & Warfield 1986). Disc degeneration causes further loading of the joints and pain (Fig. 11.3). Patients often complain of diurnal variation in pain. This is because disc height decreases through the day and, therefore, facet joint loading increases (Fig. 11.4; Adams 1996). After surgery, the mechanical disruption and loss of disc height (perhaps secondary to discectomy) may lead to increase loading of the facet joints.

Why should lumbar facet joint pain radiate down the leg?

The facet joint is supplied by the posterior rami of the same nerve that innervates the leg. Sensation from the facet joint does not normally reach

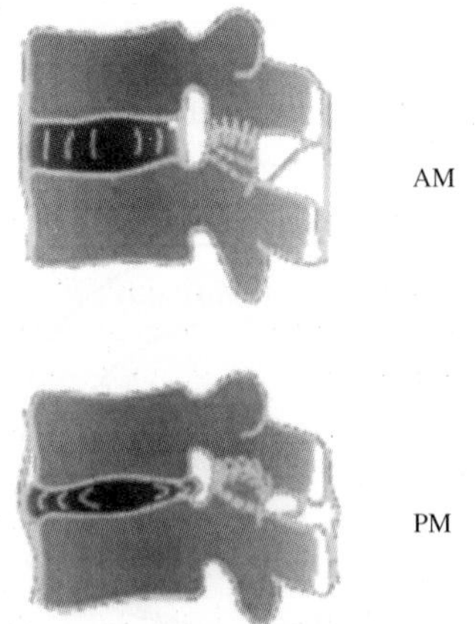

Fig. 11.4 Diurnal changes in vertebral disc height leading to: (i) increased loading of facet joints; (ii) compressive forces in annulus fibrosis; and (iii) slack intravertebral ligaments. This may explain diurnal variation in pain (adapted from Adams 1996).

conscious experience and it is easy to envisage a situation in which pain from the (facet) joint is referred to somatosensory areas that do reach conscious experience, i.e. down the legs. This mechanism is supported by electrophysiological (Gillette et al 1993) and clinical studies (Mooney & Robertson 1976, McCall et al 1979) In cases of mechanical low back pain, the referred pain to the buttock and legs is described as toothache-like or cramping. In post laminectomy conditions, pain from the facet joints may be perceived as sharp and tingling, very much like the pain from original disc prolapse despite the fact the disc has now been removed. This altered perception and mingling of pain experiences is classically seen in chronic pain and is due to some of the mechanisms alluded to in Figure 11.1. Pain from the cervical facet joints is referred to the occipital region, over the shoulders and between the shoulder blades Bogduk & Marsland 1988; Fukui et al 1996a,b).

Are there any other treatment options if one does not respond to facet joint blocks? A possible role for the sympathetic system

What happens if patients are not fortunate enough to fall into the category of those amenable to denervation of the facet joints? It is likely that the pain may be arising from the disc itself, the ligaments or other structures. There are case reports suggesting that thermocoagulation of the inner nucleus pulposus of the disc causes reduction in pain intensity. The reasons for this result are unclear and have not been shown in randomised controlled trials yet (Kleef et al 1996).

Another possible treatment lies with interruption of the sympathetic innervation of the discs and other structures. Some authors have suggested that the sympathetic outflow arising at L2 supplies the discs and other spinal structures and may be effectively blocked by a lumbar sympathetic block (LSB) at this level (Takahashi et al 1996). Again in a series of case reports LSB may treat discogenic pain (Nakamura et al 1996). Obviously, lumbar epidurals may have sympatholytic effect. Interest in this approach is heightened as LSB can be made permanent and indeed there have been many advocates of sympathetic blockade in backpain, e.g Sluijter (1988) has previously advocated thermocoagulation of specific communicating rami (which have a sympathetic component; see Table 11.1) for disc pain arising form specific sites (see also references in Stolker et al 1994).

Specific treatment of the muscle spasm in low back pain

An alternative approach to the problem of intractable back pain is not to concentrate on the source of pain but the **consequence** of the spinal pain, i.e. the muscle spasm (especially that in the back) that may secondarily result. The first attempts at denervation of the facet joints actually involved the use of a scalpel producing incisions paraspinally through the muscles. Rees, the surgeon who performed this manoeuvre, claimed a success rate of 99.8% (Rees 1971). It was subsequently shown that the scalpel blade could not have reached the posterior rami that supply the facets, however, what may have happened is that the spasm in the muscle bulk may have been reduced by this myofasciotomy. A procedure known as intramuscular stimulation (IMS, a modified form of acupuncture) which is said, amongst other effects, to desensitise muscles so that they tend not to go into spasm so easily, has been shown to produce long lasting reductions in pain scores in back pain patients (Gunn et al 1980, Gunn 1989a,b). Physical therapists also are said to reduce muscle tension and their surface stimulation can easily be envisaged to be akin to the invasive IMS in producing relief in muscle spasm. Certainly, some trials of physical therapy, such as osteopathy, chiropractice and physiotherapy, show a benefit in a proportion of back patients especially early on in back pain (references given previously).

The basis of chronic pain therapy has to be enhancement of the adaptive mechanisms and opposition of those mechanisms which lead to central sensitisation

Multiple therapies may be needed to treat chronic pain

From Figure 11.1 it can be seen that there may be many points in the cascade where we may intervene and some of these are listed in Table 11.3. Chekov wrote in the play *The Cherry Orchard* that 'when a lot of remedies are suggested for a disease, that means it can't be cured'.

The multitude of therapies suggested by Figure 11.1 and listed in Table 11.2 suggest precisely this. But, in addition, this panoply of treatments offered also reflect the complexity of the system we are dealing with. Most of present day therapies will not cure chronic pain but will reduced pain perception and reduce physical and social disability (Fig. 11.2). The mechanisms leading to 'wind-down' and **reduction** of central sensitisation are very poorly understood, but the use of NMDA antagonists, such as ketamine – a recent introduction to the pain clinic armamentarium, may be useful. Nerve blocks provide a therapeutic window encouraging adaptation of the nervous system to a lower intensity of pain produced by afferent blockade (Ossipov et al 1995) and allowing a reduction of secondary muscle spasm. In addition, they allow time to introduce other therapies, such as antidepressants which enhance endogenous pain control mechanisms, oral sodium channel blockade which controls hyperexcitable nerves, and enhancers of GABA activity [particularly Gabapentin a novel anticonvulsant with an uncertain mode of action with good tolerability (Rosner et al 1996)]. Max (1994) and McQuay et al (1996a,b) have demonstrated the efficacy of both antidepressants and anticonvulsants in chronic pain.

The treatment of pain at many levels; cognitive and behavioural approaches to back pain

As implied in the first half of this chapter, as well as treatment of the pain itself, treatment at the cognitive, affective and perhaps the social level may also be required to reduce overall levels of disability (Fig. 11.2). The powerful nature of the cognitive in both promoting and reducing the effect of original nociceptive problem is clear from studies which show that, for example, there is reduced incidence of whiplash syndrome in subjects after rear end car collisions in Lithuania where whiplash syndrome is not well known, and no insurance benefit is available for it. Does that mean that a set of symptoms is

Table 11.3 Pharmacological treatments for chronic pain arising from Figure 11.1

Tackykinin release, such as of substance P, NKA	NK1/2 antagonists in phase 1–2 trials
NMDA activation	NMDA antagonists such as **ketamine infusion**
Sensitisation of spinal cord neurones	NMDA antagonists such as **ketamine infusion** ***epidural steroids*** GM1 gangliosides. ***NSAIDS***
Loss of spinal cord inhibition	***GABA agonists; some anticonvulsants. Enhancement of endogenous noradrenergic and sertonergic inhibitory mechanisms with; some antidepressants.*** **(TENS)**
Changes in neuropeptides NPY, galanin, VIP CCK_b	Novel therapies; some in phase 1–2 trials
Nerve sprouting in spinal cord and cell death	?? Neurotrophins NMDA antagonists and cytokines
Hyper-excitable, ectopic, sodium channel production	**Sodium channel blockers, lignocaine infusions; oral sodium channel blockers** ***some anticonvulsants***
Peripheral and sympathetic maintenance of central sensitisation	**Peripheral and axial nerve blocks (+ *steroids*), guanethidine blocks α_1 receptors antagonists and α_1 receptor agonist.** ***NSAIDS***

Those treatments indicated in bold are available from pain clinics, those in italic have been shown to have a significant medium term impact (6 months at least) in either randomised control trials or in meta-analysis.

entirely dependent on the social and financial circumstances? In another study, it was shown that it was impossible for subjects to fake a whiplash response (Wallis & Bogduk 1996). Furthermore, recent and accumulating evidence shows that patients in pain have very different central representation patterns as shown by PET scanning. Perhaps the physical manifestations on the one hand and the cognitive and behavioural disturbances on the other are two sides of the same coin (see Hsieh et al 1995 and references within). The polarisation of pain management specialists into those seeking the nociceptive source and those concentrating on the cognitive issues was well seen in the intense discussions that followed the publication of the document *Back Pain in the Work Place* by Fordyce (1995). This latter publication highlighted the behavioural reinforcement and medicalisation of back pain. Western style medical insurance and invalidity benefit may be leading to the almost exponential rise in back pain related disability. In that document, data were summarised which showed that sickness rates from back pain are linked to levels of disability benefit available in that country (Fig. 11.5). The extreme view (which is predominant in the report by Fordyce) is that we have created an intractable disease out of what should be a self-limiting condition. In the same document, chapter 8 consists of suggestions to counteract this problem, some of which are summarised in Box A below.

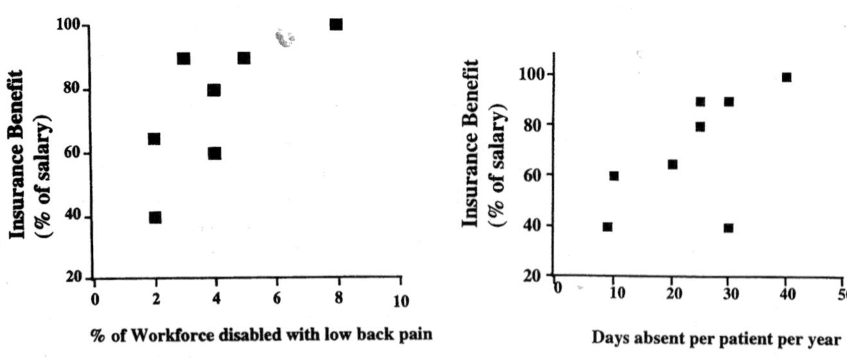

Fig. 11.5 Relationship between disability and days absent due to back pain on the one hand and insurance benefit on the other. Graphs plotted from summarised data from many papers cited in Fordyce (1996). Where more than one level of benefit was given, a simple mean figure was calculated.

The treatment of the cognitive and behavioural aspects is as important as localisation and treatment of a nociceptive source and its consequences (Fig. 11.2). The failure to address issues such as these explains why apparent relief of chronic pain is not translated into improved quality of life and a patient who has been off work for more than 12 months is unlikely to return if left untreated

Box A Suggestions for preventing chronicity

- Incentives to health care providers and disability recipients need to be arranged such that they do not promote more enduring disability.
- Medical benefits should be separated from disability benefits.
- Non specific low back pain should be regarded as activity intolerance.
- The intervention of either primary care physicians or specialists have at best only a modest relevance to the problem
- Treatment should not be pain complaint contingent. Pain complaints are not a reliable index of a medical problem.
- The evidence suggests that the first 6 weeks are crucial in preventing chronicity. Invalidity benefit starts at 28 weeks and by this stage there is a high risk of continued chronic pain and disability.
- The need for development of a back pain service. Fordyce and his colleagues recommend a consultant be in charge of this service which provides diagnostic triage, and have access to physical therapy and pain control, rehabilitation and counselling services.

(Fordyce 1995)

Box B Practical points and guidelines for referral of patients with low back pain to a pain clinic

- Exclude causes that require initial referral to a neurosurgeon or rheumatologist, e.g. prolapsed intervertebral disc, spinal stenosis, multisystem inflammatory disorder. Beware of back pain in the extremes of age – these are likely to have a diagnosable cause. Referrals after treatment, e.g. for persistent post laminectomy pain, should be done early to help prevent secondary disability.
- The 1 year prevalence of low back pain in the general population is 30–60%.
- Back pain is the most common cause of activity limitation in persons less than 45 years of age.
- If no obvious treatable cause has been found, the natural history is for resolution and most episodes resolve in 10–30 days. The only treatments that have been shown to be of significant benefit in the acute phase are: (i) bed rest less than 3 days, (ii) NSAIDS, (iii) antidepressant therapy and (iv) some sort of gentle physiotherapy.
- 2–7% of people develop chronic low back pain.
- 1–3% of people require surgery.
- Referral to a pain clinic is appropriate when the rheumatologists or neurosurgeons have ascertained that a diagnosis has been made (even if it is of non-specific low back pain) and no other therapy is appropriate and the pain has become a predominant cause of the disability. This may occur at about 3 months after the first episode. Referral for post back surgery pain should be made at an earlier stage
- The treatment approach should include the nociceptive level and also at the cognitive, behavioural and social levels of pain

(see references in Rosen 1994, Fordyce 1995). Randomised controlled trials into effects of pain management programmes (PMPs) tend to show increased quality of life and reduction of consumption of healthcare resources certainly at 6 months post treatment and even years afterwards. PMPs address the pain at a number of levels, cognitive and behavioural and one may even suggest at the nociceptive level perhaps by enhancement of descending inhibitory controls. What exactly that is in a PMP which has such profound effects is not certain, but certainly effectiveness does seem to be linked to the number of hours of patient–healthcare professional contact (Moffett et al 1986, Harkapaa et al 1990 Bendix et al 1995).

Practical points and guidelines for referral of patients with low back pain to a pain clinic

It is not my intention to give a detailed account of the diagnosis and management of back pain. But see Box B (above) for a few pointers which may be useful (Andersson 1995).

Chronic pain can be a symptom of underlying disease but is also now recognised that it may become a disease in itself

In summary, we should recognise that: (i) a nociceptive source may have initiated, and perhaps be contributing to, the maintenance of this pain state and (ii) that psychosocial factors influence the outcome of most disease processes. Evidence based medicine suggests that we should treat: (i) the nociceptive source if identifiable, e.g. pain from spinal column structures, and be open to the results of new research in this field and (ii) the psychosocial elements with, for example, pain management programmes. We should emphasise human illness as a global entity rather than simply concentrating on one particular aspect or another of the disease (adapted from Waddell 1987).

References

Abram S, Olson E 1994 Systemic opioids do not suppress spinal sensitization after subcutaneous formalin in rats. Anesthesiology 80: 1114–1119

Abram S E, Yaksh T L 1993 Morphine but not inhalational anesthesia blocks post injury facilitation. Anesthesiology 78: 713–721

Adams M A 1996 Biomechanics of low back pain. Pain Rev 3: 15–30

Andersson G B J 1995 Epidemiology. In: Weistein J N, Rydevik B L, Sonntag V K H (eds) Essentials of the spine. New York: Raven, 1–10

Arner S, Lindbolm U, Meyerson B A, Molander C 1990 Prolonged relief of neuralgias after regional anaesthetic blocks. A call for further experimental and sytematic clinical studies. Pain 43: 287–297

Barnsley L, Lord S, Bogduk N 1994 Whiplash syndrome. Pain 58: 283–307

Bendix A F, Bendix T, Ostenfeld S, Bush E, Andersen A 1995 Active treatment programs for patients with chronic low back pain: a prospective, randomized, observer-blinded study. Eur Spine J 4: 148-152

Boden S D, Davis D O, Dina T S, Patronas N J, Wiesel S W 1990a Abnormal magnetic resonance scans of the lumbar spine in asymptomatic subjects. A prospective investigation. J Bone Joint Surg [Am] 72: 403–408

Boden S D, McCowin P R, Davis D O, Dina T S, Mark A S, Wiesel S W 1990b Abnormal magnetic resonance scans of the cervical spine in asymptomatic subjects. A prospective investigation. J Bone Joint Surg [Am] 72: 1178–1184

Bogduk N 1983 The innervation of the lumbar spine. Spine 8: 286–293

Bogduk N 1992 The causes of low back pain. Med J Aust 156: 151–153

Bogduk N 1996 Precision diagnosis of spinal pain. In: Campbell J N (ed) Pain 1996 – an updated review. Seattle: IASP 313–323

Bogduk N, Aprill C 1993 On the nature of neck pain, discography and cervical zygapophysial joint blocks. Pain 54: 213–217

Bogduk N, Marsland A 1988 The cervical zygapophysial joints as a source of neck pain. Spine 13: 610–617

Chi S I, Levine J D, Basbaum A I 1993a Effects of injury discharge on the persistent expression of spinal cord fos-like immunoreactivity produced by sciatic nerve transection in the rat. Brain Res 617: 220–224

Chi S I, Levine J D, Basbaum A I 1993b Peripheral and central contributions to the persistent expression of spinal cord fos-like immunoreactivity produced by sciatic nerve transection in the rat. Brain Res 617: 225–237

Chung K, Kim H J K, Park M J, Chung J M 1993 Abnormalities of sympathetic innervation in the area of an injured peripheral nerve in a rat model of neuropathic pain. Neurosci Lett 162: 85–88

Cleland C L, Lim F Y, Gebhart G F 1994 Pentobarbital prevents the development of C-fiber-induced hyperalgesia in the rat. Pain 57: 31–43

Cougnon N, Hudspith MJ, Munglani R 1997 The therapeutic potential of NPY in central nervous disorders with special reference to pain and sympathetically maintained pain. Exp Opin Invest Drugs 6(6): 759–769

Deyo R A 1995 Understanding the accuracy of diagnostic tests. In: Weistein J N, Rydevik B L, Sonntag V K H (eds) Essentials of the spine. New York: Raven, 55–71

Devor M, Raber P 1991 Experimental evidence of a genetic predisposition to neuropathic pain. Eur J Pain 12: 65–68

Dickenson A, Sullivan A 1987 Subcutaneous formalin-induced activity of dorsal horn neurones in the rat: differential response to an intrathecal opiate administered pre or post formalin. Pain 30: 349–360

Fordyce W E 1995 Backpain in the workplace. Seattle, IASP

Frost H, Klaber Moffett J A, Moser J S, Fairbank J C T 1995 Randomised controlled trial for evaluation of fitness programme for patients with chronic low back pain. BMJ 310: 151–154

Fukui S, Ohseto K, Shiotani M et al 1996a Cervical zygapophyseal joint pain patterns – pain distribution determined by electrical stimulation of the cervical dorsal rami. Pain Clin 9: 285–293

Fukui S, Ohseto K, Shiotani M et al 1996b Patterns of cervical zygapophyseal joint pain. Pain Clin 9: 275–283

Gallagher J, Petriccione Di Vadi P L, Wedley J R et al 1994 Radiofrequency facet joint denervation in the treatment of low back pain: a prospective controlled double-blind study to assess its efficacy. Pain Clin 7: 193–198

Gillette R G, Kramis R C, Roberts W J 1993 Characterisation of spinal somatosensory neurons having receptive fields in lumbar tissues of cats. Pain 54: 85–98

Gilron I, Coderre T J 1996 Pre-emptive analgesic effect of steroid anaesthesia with alphaxalone in the rat formalin test. Anesthesiology 84: 572–579

Goldwait J E 1911 The lumbosacral articulation: an explanation of many cases of lumbago, sciatica and paraplegia. Boston Med Surg J 164: 365–372

Goto T, Marota J J A, Crosby G 1994 Pentobarbitone, but not propofol, produces pre-emptive analgesia in the rat formalin model. Br J Anaesth 72: 662–667

Goto T, Marota J J A, Crosby G. 1996 Volatile agents antagonize nitrous oxide and morphine induced analgesia in the rat. Br J Anaesth 76: 702–706

Gracely R H, Lynch S A, Bennett G J 1992 Painful neuropathy: altered central processing maintained dynamically by peripheral input. Pain 51: 175–194

Gunn C C 1989a The Gunn approach to the treatment of chronic pain. New York: Churchill Livingstone

Gunn C C 1989b Neuropathic pain: a new theory for chronic pain of intrinsic origin. Ann R Coll Phys Surg Can 22: 327–330

Gunn C C, Milbrandt W E, Little A S, Mason K E 1980 Dry needling of muscle motor points for chronic low-back pain. A randomized clinical trial with long-term follow-up. Spine 5: 279–291

Harkapaa K, Mellin G, Jarvikoski A, Hurri H 1990 A controlled study on the outcome of inpatient and outpatient treatment of low back pain. Part III. Long-term follow-up of pain, disability, and compliance. Scand J Rehabil Med 22: 181–188

Hokfelt T, Zhang X, Wiesenfeld-Hallin Z 1994 Messenger plasticity in primary sensory neurons following axotomy and its functional implications. Trends Neurosci 17: 22–30

Hsieh J C, Belfrage M, Stone-Elander S, Hansson P, Ingvar M 1995 Central representation of chronic ongoing neuropathic pain studied by positron emission tomography. Pain 63: 225–236

Hudspith M J, Munglani R 1997 Enhanced spinal cord Fos expression following thermal injury in the mononeuropathic rat. Br J Anaesth 78: 469

Hunt S P, Pini A, Evan G 1987 Induction of c-fos like protein in spinal cord neurons following sensory stimulation. Nature 328: 632–634

Hunter J, Woodburn V L, Durieux C, Pettersson E, Poat J, Hughes J 1995 *c-fos* antisense oligodeoxynucleotide increases formalin-induced nociception and regulates preprodynorhin expression. Neuroscience 65: 485–492

Ignelzi R J, Cummings T W 1980 A statistical analysis of percutaneous radiofrequency lesions in the treatment of chronic low back pain and sciatica. Pain 8: 181–187

Indahl A, Velund L, Reikerås O 1995 Good prognosis for low back pain when left untampered: a randomized clinical trial. Spine 20: 473–477
Katz J, Jackson M, Kavanagh B P Sandler A N 1996 Acute pain after surgery predicts long term post thoracotomy pain. Clin J Pain 12: 50–55
Kingery W S, Castellote J M, Wang E E 1993 A loose ligature induced mononeuropathy produces hyperalgesia mediated by both the injured sciatic nerve and the adjacent saphenous nerve. Pain 55: 297–304
Kleef M, Barendse G A, Wilmnik J T et al 1996 Percutaneous intradiscal radio-frequency thermocoagulation in chronic non-specific low back pain. Pain Clin 9: 259–268
Koes B W, Scholten R, Mens J M A, Bouter L M 1995 Efficacy of epidural steroid injections for low-back pain and sciatica: a systematic review of randomized clinical trials. Pain 63: 279–288
Lewinnek G E, Warfield C A 1986 Facet joint degeneration as a cause of low back pain. Clin Orthop 213: 216–222
Little H J 1996 How has molecular pharmacology contributed to our understanding of the mechanism(s) of general anaesthesia? Pharmacol Ther 69: 37–58
Loeser JD 1980 Low back pain. Res Publ Assoc Res Nerv Ment Dis 58: 363–377
Lord S M, Barnsley L, Wallis B J, McDonald G J Bogduk N 1996 Percutaneous radio-frequency neurotomy for chronic cervical zygopophyseal joint pain. N Engl J Med 335: 1721–1726
Luo C, Wiesenfeld-Hallin Z 1995 Effects of intrathecal local anaesthetics on spinal excitability and the development of autotomy. Pain 63: 173–179
Malan T P, Mata H, Kovelowski C J, Porreca F 1995 Basal c-fos expression regulates tactile sensitivity in rats. Anesthesiology 83: A769
Mao J, Price D D, Mayer D J 1995 Mechanisms of hyperalgesia and morphine tolerance: a current view of their possible interactions. Pain 62: 259–274
Max M 1994 Antidepressant as analgesics. In: Fields H L, Liebskind J C (eds) Pharmacological approaches to the treatment of chronic pain: new concepts and critical issues. Seattle, IASP, 1
McCall I W, Park W M, O'Brien J 1979 Induced pain referral from posterior elements in normal subjects. Spine 4: 441–446
McLachlan E M, Janig W, Devor M, Michaelis M 1993 Peripheral nerve injury triggers noradrenergic sprouting within dorsal root ganglia. Nature 363: 543–545
McQuay H J, Caroll D, Jadad A R, Wiffen P J, Moore R A 1996a Anticonvulsant drugs for the management of pain: a systematic review. BMJ 311: 1047–1052
McQuay H J, Tramer M, Nye A, Caroll D, Wiffen P J, Moore R A 1996b A systematic review of antidepressants in neuropathic pain. Pain 68: 217–227
Meade T W, Browne W, Mellows S et al 1986 Comparison of chiropractic and hospital outpatient management of low back pain: a feasibility study. J Epidemiol Community Health 40: 12–17
Mehta M, Sluijter M E 1979 The treatment of chronic back pain. A preliminary survey of the effect of radiofrequency denervation of the posterior vertebral joints. Anaesthesia 34: 768–775
Mixter W J, Barr J S 1934 Rupture of the intervertebral disc with involvement of the spinal canal. N Engl J Med 211: 210–215
Moffett J A K, Chase S M, Portek I, Ennis J R 1986 A controlled, prospective study to evaluate the effectiveness of a back school in the relief of chronic low back pain. Spine 11: 120–122
Moneta G B, Videman T, Kaivanto K et al 1994. Reported pain during lumbar discography as a function of anular ruptures and disc degeneration: a re-analysis of 833 discograms. Spine 19: 1968–1974
Mooney V, Robertson J 1976 The facet syndrome. Clin Orthop 115: 149–156
Munglani R, Bond A, Smith G et al 1995a Changes in neuronal markers in a mononeuropathic rat model: relationship between neuropeptide Y, pre-emptive drug treatment and long term mechanical hyperalgesia. Pain 63: 21–31
Munglani R, Fleming B, Hunt S P 1996a General anaesthesia – what do we achieve? Br J Anaesth 77: 300–301
Munglani R, Fleming B, Hunt S P 1996b Remembrance of times past: the role of c-fos in pain. Br J Anaesth 76: 1–4
Munglani R, Fleming B. Smith G D et al 1997 Effect of pre-emptive NMDA antagonist treatment on long term Fos expression and hyperalgesia in a model of chronic neuropathic pain. Submitted

Munglani R, Harrison S, Smith G et al 1995b Effect of different pre-emptive treatments on long-term neuropeptide expression in the dorsal root ganglia in a model of neuropathic pain. Br J Anaesth 74: 482P

Munglani R, Harrison S, Smith G et al 1996c Neuropeptide changes persist in spinal cord despite resolving hyperalgesia in a rat model of mononeuropathy. Brain Res 743; 102–108

Munglani R, Hunt S 1995a Proto-oncogenes: basic concepts and stimulation induced changes in the spinal cord. In: Wiesenfeld-Hallin S, Sharma H S, Nyberg F (eds) Neuropeptides in the spinal cord. Fundamental and clinical aspects. Amsterdam: Elsevier, 104: 283–298

Munglani R, Hunt S P 1995b Molecular biology of pain. Br J Anaesth 75: 186–192

Munglani R, Hunt S, Jones J G 1996d Spinal cord and chronic pain. In: Kaufman L, Ginsburg R (eds) Anaesthesia Review. Edinburgh:Churchill Livingstone, 12: 53–76

Munglani R, Jones J G, Hunt S 1993 Pre-emptive analgesia – use of immediate early gene expression as markers of neuronal stimulation. Br J Anaesth 73: 458

Munglani R, Hudspith M, Hunt S P 1996e Therapeutic potential of NPY. Drugs 52: 371–389

Nachemson A L 1992 Newest knowledge of low back pain: a critical look. Clin Orthop 279: 8–20

Nakamura S I, Takahashi K, Takahashi Y, Yamagata M, Moriya H 1996 The afferent pathways of discogenic low-back pain. Evaluation of L2 spinal nerve infiltration. J Bone Joint Surg [Br] 78: 606–612

Neumann S, Doubell T P, Leslie T, Woolf C J 1996 Inflammatory pain hypersensitivity mediated by phenotypic switch in myelinated primary sensory neurons. Nature 384: 360–364

Nivarthi R N, Grant G J, Turndorf H, Basinath M 1996 Spinal anaesthesia by local anaesthetics stimulates the enzyme protein kinase C and induces the expression of an immediate early oncogene, c-fos. Anesth Analg 83: 542–547

Noguchi K, Kawai Y, Fukuoka T, Senba E, Miki K 1995 Substance P induced by peripheral nerve injury in primary afferent sensory neurons and its effect on dorsal column nucleus neurons. J Neurosci 15: 7633–7643

North R B, Han M, Zahurak M, Kidd D H 1994 Radiofrequency lumbar facet denervation: analysis of prognostic factors. Pain 57: 77-83

O'Conner T, Abram S E 1995 Inhibition of nociception induced spinal sensitization by anesthetic agents. Anesthesiology 82: 259–266

Ossipov M H, Lopez Y, Nichols M L, Porreca F 1995 The loss of antinociceptive efficacy of spinal morphine in rats with nerve ligation injury is prevented by reducing spinal afferent drive. Neurosci Lett 199: 87–90

Petersen-Felix S, Arendt-Nielsen L, Bak P, Fischer M, Bjerring P, Zbinden A M 1996 The effects of isoflurane on repeated nociceptive stimuli (central temporal summation). Pain 64: 277-281

Randic M, Jiang M C, Cerne R 1993 Long term potentiation and long term depression of primary afferent neurotransmission in the rat spinal cord. J Neurosci 13: 5228–5241

Rees W E S 1971 Multiple bilateral subcutaneous rhiizolysis of segemental nerves in the treatment of the intervertebral disc syndrome. Ann Gen Practice 26: 126–127

Ren K, Ruda M A 1996 Descending modulation of Fos expression after persistent peripheral stimulation. Neuroreport 7: 2186–2190

Richmond C E, Bromley L M, Woolf C J 1993 Preoperative morphine pre-empts postoperative pain. Lancet 342: 73–75

Rosen M 1994 The Clinical Standards Advisory Group (CSAG) Report on back pain. London: HMSO

Rosner H, Rubin L, Kestenbaum A 1996 Gabapentin adjunctive therapy in neuropathic pain states. Am J Pain 12: 56–58

Roud Mayne C, Hudspith M J, Munglani R 1996 Epidural morphine and post-hepetic neuralgia (letter). Anaesthesia 51:1190

Schwarzer A C, Aprill C N, Derby R, Fortin J, Kine G, Bogduk N 1994a The false positive rate of uncontrolled diagnostic blocks of the lumbar zygopophysial joints. Pain 58: 195–200

Schwarzer A C, Aprill C N, Derby R, Fortin J, Kine G, Bogduk N 1994b The relative contributions of the disc and zygapophyseal joint in chronic low back pain. Spine 19: 801–806

Schwarzer A C, Aprill C N, Derby R, Fortin J, Kine G, Bogduk N 1995a The prevalence and clinical features of internal disc disruption in patients with chronic low back pain. Spine 20: 1878–1883

Schwarzer A C, Wang S C, Bogduk N, McNaught P J, Laurent R 1995b Prevalence and clinical features of lumbar zygapophysial joint pain: a study in an Australian population with chronic low back pain. Ann Rheum Dis 54: 100–106

Schwarzer A C, Wang S C, Odriscoll D, Harrington T, Bogduk N, Laurent R 1995c The ability of computed tomography to identify a painful zygapophysial joint in patients with chronic low back pain. Spine 20: 907–912

Schwarzer A C, Aprill C N, Bogduk N 1995d The sacroiliac joint in chronic low back pain. Spine 20: 31–37

Sethna N, Berde C B 1995 Diagnostic blocks: caveats and pitfalls in interpretation. IASP Newsletter: 3–5

Silvers H R 1990 Lumbar percutaneous facet rhizotomy. Spine 15: 36–40

Sluijter M E 1988 The use of radiofrequency lesions for pain relief in failed back patients. Int Disability Studies 10: 37–43

Spitzer W, Leblanc F E A 1987 Scientific approach and management of activity related spinal disorders. Spine 11: S1-S59

Stolker R J, Vervest A C M, Groen G J 1994 The management of chronic spinal pain by blockades: a review. Pain 58: 1–20

Takahashi H, Yanagida H, Morita S 1996 Analysis of the underlying mechanism of sympathetically maintained pain in the back and leg due to lumbar impairment: pain relieving effect of lumbar chemical sympathetectomy. Pain Clin 9: 251–258

Waddell G 1987 A new clinical model for the treatment of low-back pain. Spine 12: 632–644

Wakisaka S, Kajander K C, Bennett C J 1992 Effects of peripheral nerve injuries and tissue inflammation on the levels of neuropeptide Y-like immunoreactivity in rat primary afferent neurons. Brain Res 598: 349–352

Wakisaka S, Kajander K C, Bennett G J 1991 Increased neuropeptide Y (NPY)-like immunoreactivity in rat sensory neurons following peripheral axotomy. Neurosci Lett 124: 200–203

Wallis B J, Bogduk N 1996 Faking a profile: can naive subjects stimulate whiplash responses? Pain 66: 223–227

Wiesenfeld-Hallin Z, Xu X-J, Hakanson R, Fenf D M, Folkers K 1991 Low dose intrathecal morphine facilitates the spinal flexor reflex by releasing different neuropeptides in rats with intact and sectioned peripheral nerves. Brain Res 551: 157–162

Wilcox G L 1991 Excitatory neurotransmitters and pain. In: Bond M R, Charlton J E, Woolf C J (eds) Proceedings of the VIth World Conference on Pain. Amsterdam: Elsevier, 97–118

Woolf C J, Chong M S 1993 Preemptive analgesia – treating postoperative pain by preventing the establishment of central sensitization. Anesth Analg 77: 362–379

Woolf, C. J., P. Shortland and R. E. Coggeshall (1992). Peripheral nerve injury triggers central sprouting of myelinated afferents. Nature 355 75-78.

Woolf C J, Shortland P, Reynolds M, Ridings J, Doubell T, Coggeshall R E 1995 Reorganization of central terminals of myelinated primary afferents in the rat dorsal horn following peripheral axotomy. J Comp Neurol 360: 121–134

Yamamoto T, Shimoyama N, Mizuguchi T 1993 Role of the injury discharge in the development of thermal hyperaesthesia after sciatic nerve constriction in the rat. Anesthesiology 79: 993–1002

Yamamoto T, Yaksh T L 1993 Effects of colchicine applied to the peripheral nerve on thermal hyperalgesia evoked with chronic nerve constriction. Pain 55: 227–233

Yang K H, King A I 1984 Mechanism of facet load transmission as a hypothesis for low-back pain. Spine 9: 557–565

Young R B 1996 Preoperative and intraoperative predictors of lumbosacral surgery outcome: a literature review. Pain Rev 3: 203–219

Zimmerman M 1991 Central nervous system mechanisms modulating pain-related information: do they become deficient after lesions of the peripheral or central nervous system? In: Casey K L (ed) Pain and central nervous system disease:the central pain syndromes. New York: Raven, 183–199

Leon Kaufman

12

Update – 1

ABDOMINAL ANAESTHESIA

Nimmo & Drummond (1996) studied respiratory mechanics after abdominal surgery and found there were two abnormal patterns of respiration associated with airway obstruction. One pattern was an increase in abdominal pressure at the onset of respiration with a lag in abdominal movement. The second pattern was a decrease in abdominal pressure and the abdominal wall moved inwards at the onset of inspiration. Both patterns of respiration were associated with activation of the abdominal muscles during expiration. Drummond et al (1996) also used thoracic impedance for measuring chest wall movement in postoperative patients and found difficulty in correlating results due to transient respiratory obstruction.

It is known that hypoxaemia may occur following major abdominal surgery and it is recognised that oxygen is of value for a few days to prevent postoperative hypoxaemia. Mynster et al (1996) also found that the oxygen saturation was significantly higher during sitting and standing when compared with patients in the supine position, for up to four days following laparotomy. They stress the importance of early mobilisation following major surgery.

Powell et al (1996) have outlined the effects of hypoxaemia on the cardiovascular and neurological systems and made the following recommendations:

1. Oxygen saturation should be monitored in all patients breathing room air in the recovery area. Inspired oxygen concentration should always be recorded.

Leon Kaufman MD FRCA, 145 Harley Street, London W1N 2DE, UK

2. Certain patients are liable to develop persistent hypoxaemia, postoperatively, and require prolonged monitoring and oxygen supplements. These include obese patients; patients who have undergone upper abdominal surgery or thoracotomy; patients receiving opioids; patients with acute or chronic airways disease.

3. Other patients may be at risk of hypoxaemia due to hypovolaemia, hypotension, anaemia, myocardial ischaemia, cerebrovascular ischaemia, increased oxygen consumption and sickle cell disease.

4. Oxygen should be administered until the SpO_2 is > 93% while breathing air, or has returned to the pre-operative value.

5. Care should be exerted with patients with chronic obstructive airways disease, who rely on hypoxic ventilatory drive. Caution should be taken with the administration of oxygen and frequent measurements should be made of arterial oxygen tension.

The development of neurones affecting the gastrointestinal system are reviewed by Goyal & Hirano (1996) and there is more to the control of bowel function beyond the autonomic nervous system. It has now been found that enteric neurones resemble more the central nervous system and the gut has 'a brain of its own'.

The maintenance of mesenteric blood flow is of importance during major abdominal surgery as it can affect the dehiscence of the intestinal anastomosis. O'Beirne & Bellamy (1996) found that the blood flow was significantly greater with desflurane when compared with isoflurane, but Zwijsen et al (1996) considered that surgical stimulation was a major factor as anaesthetic drugs appear to have little influence: they compared the effects of total intravenous anaesthesia with inhalation anaesthesia.

Postoperative infection following colorectal surgery may be associated with blood transfusion. Jensen et al (1996) recommend the use of leucocyte-depleted blood in all patients undergoing colorectal surgery, especially those who are on immuno-suppressant drugs. The leucocytes appear to produce immuno-suppression, as well as potentiating the action of drugs in patients with inflammatory bowel disease.

Kurz et al (1996) advocated normothermia during major abdominal surgery. In a study of over 200 patients they found that hypothermia delayed healing and predisposed to wound infection. Wound infection was also commoner in smokers (see also Mortensen & Garrard 1996). In addition, attempts have been made to maintain body temperature by heating blankets and heating coils with intravenous therapy. Duthie (1996) has drawn attention to the fact that intravenous amino acids prevent postoperative hypothermia.

It is also known that hypothermia may affect platelet function and coagulation, increasing blood loss and the need for transfusion, in patients undergoing hip surgery (Schmied et al 1996). It is also worthy of note that the use of the plasma expander Haemaccel increases bleeding time and the need for volume replacement in patients suffering from trauma (Evans et al 1996). Further complication of hypothermia is postoperative shivering, which may be related more to peripheral than core temperature. Shivering leads to hypoxaemia, lactic acidosis and hypercarbia and may be prevented by the use of space blankets and can be treated by intravenous pethidine or doxapram (Crossley 1995).

It is also of note that a cold environment has effects on the myocardium leading to increased myocardial oxygen demand, increased cardiac work and impaired coronary blood flow. Pulmonary vasoconstriction may give rise to pulmonary oedema (Wilmshurst 1994).

Bardram et al (1995) have attempted to provide 'stress-free' conditions for colonic resection for malignancy in high-risk patients by combination of laparoscopic surgery, epidural analgesia, oral nutrition and mobilisation. Mertes et al (1996) have studied the effects of continuous intravenous clonidine, an α_2-adrenergic agonist, and found it appeared to attenuate the endocrine response to surgery, either by inhibiting sympathetic nervous system activity or by stimulating the release of growth hormone. The end result is inhibition of nitrogen loss which occurred postoperatively.

Finn et al (1996) studied the profound loss of body protein in critically ill patients having major trauma or severe sepsis. They found that intracellular water decreased by 15–20%, total body protein by 15% and total body potassium by 20%. The loss of protein and potassium is accompanied by progressive cellular dehydration. In fact, the protein loss is triggered and maintained by reduction in cell volume due to loss of intracellular water. They suggest there may be a place for glutamine, which causes cell swelling, to be used in the treatment of the initial dehydration.

Although laparoscopic cholecystectomy may be more prolonged procedure than the open operation, Karayiannakis et al (1996) found that pulmonary function was less impaired following the laparoscopic technique. Gasless laparoscopy, involving a mechanical abdominal wall lift, leads to a more rapid recovery than with conventional carbon dioxide pneumo-peritoneum (Koivusalo et al 1996).

There is a high density of 5-HT_3 receptors in the nerve terminals of the vagus in the intestinal mucosa and on vagal afferent nerves located in the brain stem vomiting system. Gan & Mythen (1995) have suggested that hypoperfusion of the intestinal mucosa may be a cause of postoperative nausea and vomiting. 5-HT_3 antagonists are often administered for their anti-emetic effects, but they can cause adverse reactions such as headache and gastrointestinal symptoms and also hypersensitivity reactions (Kataja & de Bruijn 1996).

Pope (1994) has drawn attention to the laryngeal complications of acid reflux disorders. The gastric contents may irritate the larynx resulting in hoarseness, persistent nonproductive cough and the need to clear the throat. Endoscopy may show erythema or white plaques on the posterior larynx and there may even be ulceration or polyp formation on the vocal cords. It has been suggested that the acid laryngitis may result in bronchial symptoms due to vagal stimulation. The act of swallowing, as a protective effect on the upper respiratory tract, is outlined in detail by Nishino (1993).

Finucane & Bynum (1996) have investigated the risk of aspiration pneumonia in patients with neurogenic dysphagia. They suggest, initially, that all patients who are conscious should be hand fed. Tube feeding should be reserved for those patients who have had recurrent pneumonia, who find coughing during meals uncomfortable and who are acutely ill with impaired consciousness. Nakagawa et al (1995) measured substance P in the sputum of elderly patients with aspiration pneumonia and found that substance P was markedly reduced and may be an indicator of increased aspiration pneumonia in the elderly.

References

Bardram L, Funch-Jensen P, Jensen P et al 1995 Recovery after laparoscopic colonic surgery with epidural analgesia, and early oral nutrition and mobilisation. Lancet 345: 763–764

Crossley A W A 1995 Postoperative shivering: the influence of body temperature. BMJ 311: 764–765

Drummond G B, Nimmo A F, Elton R A 1996 Thoracic impedance used for measuring chest wall movement in postoperative patients. Br J Anaesth 77: 327–332

Duthie D J R 1996 Aminoacid infusions to prevent postoperative hypothermia. Lancet 347: 1199

Evans P A, Garnett M, Boffard K, Kirkman E, Jacobson B F 1996 Evaluation of the effect of colloid (Haemaccel) on the bleeding time in the trauma patient. J R Soc Med 89: 101–104

Finn P J, Plank L D, Clark M A et al 1996 Progressive cellular dehydration and proteolysis in critically ill patients. Lancet 347: 654–656

Finucane T E, Bynum J P W 1996 Use of tube feeding to prevent aspiration pneumonia. Lancet 348: 1421–1424

Gan T J, Mythen M G 1995 Does peroperative gut-mucosa hypoperfusion cause postoperative nausea and vomiting? Lancet 345: 1123–1124

Goyal R K, Hirano I 1996 The enteric nervous system. N Engl J Med 334: 1106–1115

Jensen L S, Kissmeyer-Nielsen P, Wolff B, Qvist N 1996 Randomised comparison of leucocyte-depleted versus buffy-coat-poor blood transfusion and complications after colorectal surgery. Lancet 348: 841–845

Karayiannakis A J, Makri G G, Mantzioka A et al 1996 Postoperative pulmonary function after laparoscopic and open cholecystectomy. Br J Anaesth 77: 448

Kataja V, de Bruijn K 1996 Hypersensitivity reactions associated with 5-hydroxytryptamine$_3$-receptor antagonists: a class effect? Lancet 347: 584–585

Koivusalo, A-M, Kellokumpu I, Lindgren L 1996 Gasless laparoscopic cholecystectomy: comparison of postoperative recovery with conventional technique. Br J Anaesth 77: 576–580

Kurz A, Sessler D I, Lenhardt R 1996 Perioperative normothermia to reduce the incidence of surgical-wound infection and shorten hospitalization. N Engl J Med 334: 1209–1215

Mertes N, Coeters C, Kuhmann M, Zander J F 1996 Postoperative α_2-adrenergic stimulation attenuates protein catabolism. Anesth Analg 82: 258–263

Mortensen N, Garrard C S 1996 Colorectal surgery comes in from the cold. N Engl J Med 334: 1263

Mynster T, Jensen L M, Jensen F G et al 1996 The effect of posture on late postoperative oxygenation. Anaesthesia 51: 225–227

Nakagawa T, Ohrui T, Sekizawa K 1995 Sputum substance P in aspiration pneumonia. Lancet 345: 1447

Nimmo A F, Drummond G B 1996 Respiratory mechanics after abdominal surgery measured with continuous analysis of pressure, flow and volume signals. Br J Anaesth 77: 317–326

Nishino T 1993 Swallowing as a protective reflex for the upper respiratory tract. Anesthesiology 79: 588–601

O'Beirne H, Bellamy M C 1996 Effects of desflurane and isoflurane on splanchnic microcirculation during surgery. Br J Anaesth 76: 592P

Pope C E 1994 Acid-reflux disorders. N Engl J Med 331: 656–660

Powell J F, Menon D K, Jones J G 1996 The effects of hypoxaemia and recommendations for postoperative oxygen therapy. Anaesthesia 51: 796–772

Schmied H, Kurz A, Sessler D I et al 1996 Mild hypothermia increases blood loss and transfusion requirements during total hip arthroplasty. Lancet 347: 289–292

Wilmshurst P 1994 Temperature and cardiovascular mortality. BMJ 309: 1029–1030.
Zwijsen J H M, Bovill J G, Geelkerken R H et al 1996 Comparison of sufentanil/propofol versus isoflurane/nitrous oxide anaesthesia on mesenteric blood flow. Anaesthesia 51: 1060–1063

MUSCLE RELAXANTS

See also chapter by Hunter. Magnesium sulphate has been used for its antiarrhythmic and antihypertensive effects and it has been shown that it may prolong the neuromuscular blockade produced by vecuronium (Fuchs-Buder & Tassonyi 1996). The mode of action is believed to be due to a reduction in the release of acetylcholine at the neuromuscular junction.

Sekerci & Tulunay (1996) have drawn attention to the possibility that calcium channel blockers may potentiate the action of neuromuscular blocking agents and reversal with neostigmine may be ineffectual.

BOTULINUM TOXIN

Botulinum toxin prevents the presynaptic release of acetylcholine and is now being used routinely for blepharospasm, torticollis, facial spasms and squint. It also appears to have a place in the management of cerebral palsy (Neville 1994), anal fissure (Gui et al 1994, Jost & Schimrigk 1995) as well as achalasia (Pasricha et al 1995, Cohen & Parkman 1995).

Tacrine was initially introduced to potentiate the action of succinylcholine, but now may have a place in the management of Alzheimer's disease (Davis & Powchik 1995).

MYASTHENIA GRAVIS

Drachman (1994) has outlined in detail many of the aspects of myasthenia gravis, including the clinical features and the abnormality at the neuromuscular junction which consists of a decrease in the number of acetylcholine receptors. It is accepted that 80–90% of patients with myasthenia gravis have serum antibodies to the acetylcholine receptor, but the concentration of the antibody does not correlate with the severity of the disease. Treatment consists of anti-cholinesterase agents: the most widely used is pyridostigmine (mestinon). It is also agreed that patients with generalised myasthenia, between the ages of puberty and 60 years, should have a thymectomy. Immunosuppressive treatment may also be used, including prednisone, azathioprine and cyclosporin. Plasmapheresis removes antibodies and produces short-term clinical improvement. In some cases immunoglobulin may be effective. Attempts were made to suppress the B cells which produce the antibodies, as well as targeting the T cells.

ORGANOPHOSPHATE PESTICIDES

These inhibit neuromuscular cholinesterase leading to symptoms related to the autonomic nervous system (abdominal cramps, nausea and diarrhoea, salivation, miosis) and the central nervous system (dizziness, anxiety and confusion). Symptoms last until further cholinesterase is synthesised. It appears also that organophosphates inhibit a further enzyme leading to peripheral neuropathy 10–14 days after exposure (Steenland 1996).

Organophosphorous compounds are present in many pesticides and recently a study has shown that long-term exposure to organophosphates in sheep dip lead to subtle nervous system changes and a predisposition to psychiatric disorders (Stephens et al 1995).

References

Cohen S, Parkman H P 1995 Treatment of achalasia – from whalebone to botulinum toxin. N Engl J Med 332: 815–816

Davis K L, Powchik P 1995 Tacrine. Lancet 345: 625–630

Drachman D B 1994 Myasthenia gravis. N Engl J Med 330: 1797–1810

Fuchs-Buder T, Tassonyi E 1996 Magnesium sulphate enhances residual neuromuscular block induced by vecuronium. Br J Anaesth 76: 565–566

Gui D, Cassetta E, Anastasio G et al 1994 Botulinum toxin for chronic anal fissure. Lancet 344: 1127–1128

Jost W H, Schimrigk K 1995 Botulinum toxin in therapy of anal fissure. Lancet 345: 188–189

Neville B 1994 Botulinum toxin in the cerebral palsies. BMJ 309: 1526–1527

Pasricha P J, Ravich W J, Hendrix T R et al 1995 Intrasphincteric botulinum toxin for the treatment of achalasia. N Engl J Med 322: 774–778

Sekerci S, Tulunay M 1996 Interactions of calcium channel blockers with non-depolarising muscle relaxants in vivo. Anaesthesia 51: 140–144

Steenland K 1996 Chronic neurological effects of organophosphate pesticides. BMJ 312: 1312–1313

Stephens R, Spurgeon A, Calvert I A et al 1995 Neuropsychological effects of long-term exposure to organophosphates in sheep dip. Lancet 345: 1135–1139

PHAEOCHROMOCYTOMA AND β-BLOCKERS

Having mastered the intricacies of the β_1 and β_2-adrenoceptors, readers will be disheartened to learn of a further sub-type of receptor, β_3, which is involved in lipolytic and thermic responses in brown and white adipose tissue. Receptors are seen in the viscera, including the gall bladder and colon and in addition they appear to be present in skeletal muscle and myocardium. β_3-Agonists may have a place in the management of diabetes and obesity and possibly irritable bowel syndrome (Lipworth 1996).

Reference

Lipworth B J 1996 Clinical pharmacology of β_3-adrenoceptors. Br J Clin Pharmacol 42: 291–300

RESUSCITATION AND INTENSIVE CARE

It is generally accepted that results of cardiac arrest out of the hospital environment carry a high mortality. Grubb et al (1995) found that the most important factor determining outcome was the skill of the resuscitator. Ambulance technicians using basic techniques and semi-automatic defibrillators were more successful than paramedics in resuscitation (Guly et al 1995).

Chronic memory impairment is not uncommon following cardiac arrest outside hospital, especially when related to the duration of the cardiac arrest (Grubb et al 1996a).

A recent study by Cobbe et al (1996) reported an improvement in survival from out-of-hospital cardiac arrest. Of initial survivors, 40% were discharged home without major neurological disability. On the other hand, Schindler et al (1996) found that in out-of-hospital cardiac arrest the prognosis was poor for children in whom resuscitation lasted more than 20 min and who required more than 2 doses of adrenaline.

Charlton (1996) has reviewed the criteria for diagnosing death which in hospital, apart from clinical examination, depends on the absence of electrical activity in the heart and brain. It is conceded that these criteria are not absolute and it may be difficult to determine the actual moment of death, which is not an event but a process. In the patient's own home, the diagnosis is more difficult, but should include the absence of responsiveness at body temperature over 35°C, absence of depressive drugs, absence of spontaneous movements, apnoea, absence of reflexes (including corneal, gag and vestibulo-ocular reflexes) and fixed dilated pupils.

Accidental hypothermia is discussed in detail by Danzl & Pozos (1994) and Larach (1995) and is defined as a core temperature below 35°C. If cooling occurs rapidly without hypoxaemia to less than 32°C before the onset of cardiac arrest, ischaemia of vital organs may not occur. There have been reports of successful resuscitation after cardiac arrest lasting over 4 h, with temperatures as low as 17.5°C in which there was no neurological deficit. Re-warming strategies are discussed including external warming, internal warming, extracorporeal shunt re-warming and cardiopulmonary bypass. Passive rewarming is not recommended. Patients should be intubated and ventilated, although this may precipitate an attack of ventricular fibrillation. Other arrhythmias may occur and these readily respond to bretylium. Low doses of catecholamines are only indicated in those who have a lower blood pressure than expected and who are not responding to intravenous therapy.

The prognostic value of measurements of serum albumin has been assessed by McCluskey et al (1996). They found that serum albumin, on admission to intensive care units, was lower in non-survivors than survivors, but the admission serum albumin was an insensitive prognostic indicator. Serum albumin after 24 h was as accurate as APACHE II (Acute Physiology and Chronic Health Evaluation) in correctly classifying patients as to outcome.

Childs & Mercer (1996) have reported one patient who emerged from permanent vegetative state following trauma. She was treated with bromocriptine and dextroamphetamine and was able to follow commands and write. However, she still required long-term nursing care (see also Ramsay 1996, Grubb et al 1996b, Andrews et al 1996, Powner et al 1996).

Parr et al (1996) have drawn attention to cardiogenic shock complicating subarachnoid haemorrhage. Cardiac arrhythmias and pulmonary oedema are not uncommon with abnormal ST segments or T waves.

Parr et al (1996) describe five cases of profound myocardial dysfunction which responded to intense and aggressive treatment which included inotropes and intra-aortic balloon counter-pulsation as well as mechanical ventilation. The inotropes used were adrenaline and dobutamine.

Day et al (1996) questioned the use of adrenaline in septicaemia from infections, such as malaria, in view of the fact that, in large doses, it causes lactic acidosis whereas dopamine has the opposite effect reducing plasma lactic concentration, while increasing arterial pH and base excess. Wray & Coakley (1996) have reported a case of septic shock unresponsive to noradrenaline, but in whom an infusion of angiotensin II was effective.

The timing of intravenous therapy for hypotensive patients has been questioned by Bickell et al (1994) and in fact they found that delaying the administration of fluids until operation improves the outcome. This view is shared by Dalton (1995) in view of the possibility that, by raising the blood pressure, one would increase the bleeding in patients suffering from haemorrhagic shock, but Jacobs (1994) expresses caution in the interpretation of the results and advises further clinical trials. On the other hand, Wardrop et al (1995) maintain that critically ill patients are often short of blood, but the guidelines for transfusion are not clear cut due to a variety of clinical problems. It has been suggested that a haemoglobin concentration less than 70 g/l justified transfusion, but the haemoglobin concentration or packed cell volume gave insufficient information regarding the need for transfusion. Under-transfusion may increase the duration the patient requires respiratory support and inadequate organ perfusion leads to cardiac, pulmonary and renal impairment as well as multiple organ failure (see Blood transfusion).

The tumour necrosis factor ligand and receptor families are reviewed by Bazzoni & Beutler (1996). It was shown many years ago that tumour necrosis factor (TNF) was able to kill tumour cells and had the ability to produce pro-inflammatory effects and hence was a mediator of endotoxic shock. Fisher et al (1996) have evaluated the efficacy of a dimeric form of type II tumour necrosis factor which is linked with the Fc portion of human immunoglobulin GI (TNFR:Fc) in man with septic shock. In animals, it provides protection against Gram-positive and Gram-negative bacterial sepsis but, in man, it does not reduce the morbidity and in higher doses in fact increases mortality.

Multiple organ failure has been discussed in a Symposium edited by Bion & Strunin (1996).

References

Andrews K, Murphy L, Munday R, Littlewood C 1996 Misdiagnosis of the vegetative state: retrospective study in a rehabilitation unit. BMJ 313: 13–16

Bazzoni F, Beutler B 1996 The tumor necrosis factor ligand and receptor families. N Engl J Med 334: 1717–1725

Bickell W H, Wall M J, Pepe P E et al 1994 Immediate versus delayed fluid resuscitation for hypotensive patients with penetrating torso injuries. N Engl J Med 331: 1105–1109

Bion J, Strunin L (Eds) 1996 Multiple organ failure: from basic science to prevention. Br J Anaesth 77: 1–127

Charlton R 1996 Diagnosing death. BMJ 313: 956–957

Childs N L, Mercer W N 1996 Late improvement in consciousness after post-traumatic vegetative state. N Engl J Med 334: 24–25

Cobbe S M, Dalziel K, Ford I, Marsden A K 1996 Survival of 1476 patients initially resuscitated from out of hospital cardiac arrest. BMJ 312: 1633–1637

Dalton A M 1995 Prehospital intravenous fluid replacement in trauma: an outmoded concept? J R Soc Med 88: 213P–216P

Danzl D F, Pozos R S 1994 Accidental hypothermia. N Engl J Med 331: 1756-1760

Day N P J, Phu N H, Bethell D P et al 1996 The effects of dopamine and adrenaline infusions on acid-base balance and systemic haemodynamics in severe infection. Lancet 348: 219–223
Fisher C J, Agosti J M, Opal S M et al 1996 Treatment of septic shock with the tumor necrosis factor receptor:Fc fusion protein. N Engl J Med 334: 1697–1702
Grubb N R, Elton R A, Fox K A A 1995 In-hospital mortality after out-of-hospital cardiac arrest. Lancet 346: 417–421
Grubb N R, O'Carroll R, Cobbe S M et al 1996a Chronic memory impairment after cardiac arrest outside hospital. BMJ 313: 143–146
Grubb A, Walsh P, Lambe N et al 1996b Survey of British clinicians's views on management of patients in persistent vegetative state. Lancet 348: 35–40
Guly U M, Mitchell R G, Cook R et al 1995 Paramedics and technicians are equally successful at managing cardiac arrest outside hospital. BMJ 310: 1091–1094
Jacobs L M 1994 Timing of fluid resuscitation in trauma. N Engl J Med 331: 1153–1154
Larach M G 1995 Accidental hypothermia. Lancet 345: 493–498
McCluskey A, Thomas A N, Bowles B J M, Kishen R 1996 The prognostic value of serial measurements of serum albumin concentration in patients admitted to intensive care units. Anaesthesia 51: 724–727
Parr M J A, Finfer S R, Morgan M K 1996 Reversible cardiogenic shock complicating subarachnoid haemorrhage. BMJ 313: 681–683
Powner D J, Ackerman B M, Grenvik A 1996 Medical diagnosis of death in adults: historical contributions to current controversies. Lancet 348: 1219–1223
Ramsay S 1996 British group presents vegetative-state criteria. Lancet 347: 817
Schindler M, Bohn D, Cox P B et al 1996 Outcome of out-of-hospital cardiac or respiratory arrest in children. N Engl J Med 335: 1473–1479
Wardrop C A J, Holland B M, Jones J G 1995 Consensus on red cell transfusion. BMJ 311: 962–963
Wray G M, Coakley J H 1995 Severe septic shock unresponsive to noradrenaline. Lancet 346: 1604

BLOOD TRANSFUSION

The maintenance of a constant blood volume in health and disease is discussed by McManus et al (1995), especially how a constant volume is maintained by osmotic mechanisms. These mechanisms can be interrupted in treatment of cerebral oedema by the administration of hypertonic solutions and frusemide. Plasma hypertonicity occurs in diabetes mellitus, dehydration, renal failure and sickle cell crisis (HbS can precipitately polymerize resulting in deformation of the red cell). The sickled cells are rigid and occlude the small vessels resulting in thrombosis, ischaemia and pain. Hydroxyurea therapy appears to ameliorate the clinical cause of sickle cell anaemia, but the beneficial effects may not be recognised for several months (Charache et al 1995). However, the long-term effects are still unknown (Schechter & Rodgers 1995).

There are problems with the management of blood loss in Jehovah's Witnesses and even autologous blood is prohibited. Recombinant human erythropoietin can be given to anaemic patients, but is expensive. During operation, intra-operative blood salvage and isovolaemic haemodilution with autotransfusion may be acceptable if the diverted blood is kept in contact with the patient's circulation.

Those who suffer from thalassaemia major will receive regular transfusions and for those whose serum ferritin concentration is below 2500 ng/ml on chelation therapy the prognosis is good (Olivieri et al 1994, see also Dover & Valle 1994).

Wedgwood & Thomas (1996) have assessed acceptable haemoglobin levels in the peri-operative period and made the following recommendations:

1. In fit, healthy individuals who are able to compensate a haemoglobin > 7 g/dl would be acceptable.

2. If there is known or suspected intercurrent disease, including drug therapy, affecting the ability to compensate the level would be > 9.5 g/dl.

3. In individuals with chronic anaemia (with ability to compensate) haemoglobin > 6 g/dl would be acceptable.

4. If there is increased oxygen demand, haemoglobin > 10 g/dl is satisfactory.

They also outline the effect of anaemia on morbidity and mortality, and the physiological implications of haemodilution including reduction in blood viscosity, a reduction in systemic vascular resistance, an increase in venous return, an increase in cardiac output, redistribution of blood flow, increased oxygen extraction, release of oxygen tissues and increase in 2-3-DPG.

The use of autologous blood has its advocates, but Etchason et al (1995) doubt whether the increased protection justifies the increased cost. Recombinant erythropoietin (rhEPO) reduces the homologous blood requirement in autologous blood donors (Biesma et al 1994).

In intensive care units, blood transfusion can cause acute leucocytosis. It is not seen in patients who receive plasma (Fenwick et al 1994). Plasma can cause febrile reactions in patients given platelet concentrates (Heddle et al 1994). The supernatant plasma contains two cytokines, interleukin-1β and interleukin-6, which release pyrogens (Brand 1994).

The use of blood substitutes has been reviewed, in detail, by Dietz et al (1996), including haemoglobin solutions, liposome-encapsulated haemoglobin and perfluorocarbons. The disadvantage of these substitutes are short plasma half-life, low oxygen carrying capacity and the possibilities of side effects such as vasoconstriction and hypertension (Busuttil & Copplestone 1995). There is also the possibility of increased susceptibility to bacterial infection (Griffiths et al 1995).

Regarding gelatin based plasma expanders, Lorenz et al (1994) comment on the dangers of histamine release and they advocated the use of antihistamines prior to the administration of gelatin plasma expanders.

References

Biesma D H, Marx J J M, Kraaijenhagen R J et al 1994 Lower homologous blood requirement in autologous blood donors after treatment with recombinant human erythropoietin. Lancet 344: 367–370

Brand A 1994 Passenger leukocytes, cytokines, and transfusion reactions. N Engl J Med 331: 670–671

Busuttil D, Copplestone A 1995 Management of blood loss in Jehovah's Witnesses. BMJ 311: 1115–1116

Charache S, Terrin M L, Moore R D et al 1995 Effect of hydroxyurea on the frequency of painful crises in sickle cell anemia. N Engl J Med 332: 1317–1322
Dietz N M, Joyner M J, Warner M A 1996 Blood substitutes: fluids, drugs, or miracle solutions? Anesth Analg 82: 390–405
Dover G J, Valle D 1994 Therapy for β-thalassemia – a paradigm for the treatment of genetic disorders. N Engl J Med 331: 609–610
Etchason J, Petz L, Keeler E et al 1995 The cost effectiveness of preoperative autologous blood donations. N Engl J Med 332: 719–724
Griffiths E, Cortes A, Gilbert N et al 1995 Haemoglobin-based blood substitutes and sepsis. Lancet 345: 158–160
Fenwick J C, Cameron M, Naiman S C et al 1994 Blood transfusion as a cause of leucocytosis in critically ill patients. Lancet 344: 855–856
Heddle N M, Klama L, Singer J et al 1994 The role of the plasma from platelet concentrates in transfusion reactions. N Engl J Med 331: 625–628
Lorenz W, Duda D, Dick W et al 1994 Incidence and clinical importance of perioperative histamine release: randomised study of volume loading and antihistamine after injection of anaesthesia. Lancet 343: 933–940
McManus M L, Churchwell K B, Strange K 1995 Regulation of cell volume in health and disease. N Engl J Med 333: 1260–1266
Olivieri N F, Nathan D G, MacMillan J H et al 1994 Survival in medically treated patients with homozygous β-thalassemia. N Engl J Med 331: 574–578
Schechter A N, Rodgers G P 1995 Sickle cell anemia – basic research reaches the clinic. N Engl J Med 332: 1372–1374
Wedgwood J J, Thomas J G 1996 Perioperative haemoglobin: an overview of current opinion regarding the acceptable level of haemoglobin in the perioperative period. Eur J Anaesthesiol 13: 316–324

Leon Kaufman

Update – 2

SPINAL AND EXTRADURAL

Pryle et al (1996) reported a case of spinal subdural haematoma which resulted in permanent neurological damage 8 days following spinal analgesia in a patient taking aspirin. They stated the cardinal features of this complication include localised back pain, with or without root pain and, if symptoms included sensory or motor loss, the condition should be confirmed by MRI scan followed by immediate surgical intervention. An extensive haematomyelia has been reported following spinal analgesia in a patient on heparin (Greaves 1997).

Ketorolac, a NSAID, inhibits platelet function and has the potential to increase bleeding at operation. A single dose of intravenous ketorolac during spinal anaesthesia inhibits platelet function with respect to bleeding time and platelet aggregation, as compared with general anaesthesia (Thwaites et al 1996).

Render (1996) has questioned the accuracy of determining the interspace for epidural analgesia using the line adjoining the iliac crest. This point coincided with the spinous process or the inter space L_{4-5} in only 78.6% of patients. In 3.7% of patients it was as high as L_{3-4}.

A multiplicity of drugs are now being used for spinal and epidural analgesia and Bahar et al (1996) have reported on the promising use of magnesium sulphate in experimental animal studies. The disadvantage is that the duration of motor block exceeded that of the sensory blockade.

Smith et al (1996) have compared the analgesic and side effects of bupivacaine and fentanyl, bupivacaine and diamorphine and pethidine administered via patient-controlled epidural analgesia. It was found that all three solutions produced equivalent analgesia, but pethidine had fewer side effects including motor blockade and pruritus.

Leon Kaufman MD FRCA, 145 Harley Street, London W1N 2DE, UK

Veering et al (1996) have studied the effect of the site of injection of spinal hyperbaric bupivacaine on the spread of analgesia, in particular in elderly patients, in view of the possible association with hypotension. They found there was no significant difference in the spread of analgesia to give motor block or haemodynamic changes whether the injection was given at the $L_{4/5}$ interspace or $L_{3/4}$ interspace.

A disadvantage of spinal anaesthesia is hypotension due to sympathetic blockade. Meyer et al (1996) were able to prevent bilateral sympathetic blockade using a 29-gauge Quincke needle in nearly 70% of patients undergoing unilateral surgery of the lower extremities.

Epidural analgesia is often used for total hip replacement and this has been shown to be associated with a high incidence of urine retention, especially in men, requiring catheterisation (Williams et al 1995).

Repeat epidural analgesia is said to be unreliable compared with the initial epidural analgesia. Igarashi et al (1996) examined the epidural space using a flexible extraduroscope and found that the epidural space was patent in patients with no history of lumbar extradural analgesia, but it was clearly identified in patients who had received epidural analgesia on more than one occasion, because of aseptic inflammatory changes affecting the connective tissue, with adhesions between the dura mater and ligamentum flavum as well as granulation and changes in the ligamentum itself. These changes may affect the spread of analgesia resulting in unilateral or failed blockade.

Removal of the extradural catheter is often left to the nursing staff and there have been reports of difficulty in removing the catheter and breakage of the catheter. Morris et al (1996) investigated the force required to remove the catheter and found that it was greatest in patients when the catheter was inserted in the left lateral position and withdrawn in the sitting position. They recommend that the catheter should be removed in the same position that it was inserted.

Carp et al (1994) have reported favourably on the use of sumatriptan, a serotonin type-1d receptor agonist, in the treatment of postdural puncture headache. The drug is licensed for the treatment of migraine: however, 6 mg of sumatriptan relieved postdural headache within 30 min. However, sumatriptan is not an innocuous drug and is reported to constrict the coronary arteries.

References

Bahar M, Chanimov M, Grinspun E et al 1996 Spinal anaesthesia induced by intrathecal magnesium sulphate. An experimental study in a rat model. Anaesthesia 51: 627–633

Carp H, Singh P J, Vadhera R, Jayaram A 1994 Effects of the serotonin-receptor agonist sumatriptan on postdural puncture headache: report of six cases. Anesth Analg 79: 180–182

Greaves J D 1997 Serious spinal cord injury due to haematomyelia caused by spinal anaesthesia in a patient treated with low-dose heparin. Anaesthesia 52: 150–153

Igarashi T, Hirabayashi Y, Shimizu R et al 1996 Inflammatory changes after extradural anaesthesia may affect the spread of local anaesthetic within the extradural space. Br J Anaesth 77: 347–351

Meyer J, Enk D, Penner M 1996 Unilateral spinal anesthesia using low-flow injection through a 29-gauge Quincke needle. Anesth Analg 82: 1188–1191

Morris G N, Warren B B, Hanson E W et al 1996 Influence of patient position on withdrawal forces during removal of lumbar extradural catheters. Br J Anaesth 77: 419–420

Pryle B J, Carter J A, Cadoux-Hudson T 1996 Delayed paraplegia following spinal anaesthesia. Spinal subdural haematoma following dural puncture with a 25 G pencil point needle at T_{12}–L_1 in a patient taking aspirin. Anaesthesia 51: 263–265
Render C A 1996 The reproducibility of the iliac crest as a marker of lumbar spine level. Anaesthesia 51: 1070–1071
Smith A J, Haynes T K, Roberts D E, Harmer M 1996 A comparison of opioid solutions for patient-controlled epidural analgesia. Anaesthesia 51: 1013–1017
Thwaites B K, Nigus D B, Bouska G W et al 1996 Intravenous ketorolac tromethamine worsens platelet function during knee arthroscopy under spinal anesthesia. Anesth Analg 82: 1176–1181
Veering B Th, Ter Riet P M, Burm A G L et al 1996 Spinal anaesthesia with 0.5% hyperbaric bupivacaine in elderly patients: effect of site of injection on spread of analgesia. Br J Anaesth 77: 343–346
Williams A, Price N, Willett K 1995 Epidural anaesthesia and urinary dysfunction: the risks in total hip replacement. J R Soc Med 88: 699P–701P

COMPLICATIONS

Attention has been drawn by the Committee on Safety of Medicines (1996) to the dangers of an interaction between cisapride, used in the treatment of gastro-oesophageal reflux, and ketoconazole and antibiotics such as erythromycin. The antibiotics inhibit the cytochrome system leading to an increase in cisapride blood levels which can cause cardiac arrhythmias, including prolongation of the QT interval and ventricular fibrillation. Other medications likely to prolong the QT interval are anti-arrhythmic drugs such as quinidine, amiodarone, anti-psychotic agents such as pimozide and thioridazine, anti-malarials and some anti-histamines.

Fortunately, cutaneous allergic reaction to drugs are rare in anaesthesia, although it is estimated that 1 in 1000 hospitalized patients have a serious cutaneous drug reaction (Roujeau & Stern 1994). Serious reactions include Stevens-Johnson syndrome and toxic epidermal necrolysis, which have a high rate of morbidity and mortality, and are induced by drugs such as co-trimoxazole, sulfadoxine and carbamazepine. Barbiturates and allopurinol have also been implicated.

Vale & Proudfoot (1995) have served a timely reminder of the dangers of paracetamol poisoning. Hepatoxicity is unlikely to develop if less than 150 mg of paracetamol per kg have been ingested, which is not an absolute guarantee that symptoms will not develop. It is more likely to develop also in the presence of alcohol. Plasma half-life is a good indicator but tests take time to be performed. Patients at risk are those whose transaminase levels (ALT/AST) are above 1000 IU/l. Treatment involves the use of acetylcysteine. Plasma levels can be estimated from nomograms. Prognosis depends on the extent of liver cell necrosis as evidenced by disturbances of liver function, including problems with coagulation, acid base disturbances, plasma creatinine, hypophosphataemia and phosphaturia as well as serum bilirubin. A high plasma bilirubin usually indicates that patients can survive the early complications of fulminant hepatic failure including cerebral oedema and hypotension.

For the operation of transcervical resection of the endometrium absorption of the irrigation solution can cause hyponatraemia, nausea and cerebral oedema. Istre et al (1994) found that patients could absorb more than 1500 ml of 1.5% glycine.

References

Committee on Safety of Medicines 1996 Cisapride (prepulsid, alimix): interactions with antifungals and antibiotics can lead to ventricular arrhythmias. Current Problems in Pharmacovigilance 22: 1–2
Istre O, Bjoennes J, Naess R et al 1994 Postoperative cerebral oedema after transcervical endometrial resection and uterine irrigation with 1.5% glycine. Lancet 344: 1187–1189
Roujeau J C, Stern R S 1994 Severe adverse cutaneous reactions to drugs. N Engl J Med 331: 1272–1285
Vale J A, Proudfoot A T 1995 Paracetamol (acetaminophen) poisoning. Lancet 346: 547–552

OBSTETRICS

See also Chapter 9 by O'Sullivan.

HYPOXAEMIA

Nocturnal hypoxaemia is known to occur in patients having had abdominal surgery. Bourne et al (1995) have drawn attention to the fact that some pregnant patients suffer from nocturnal hypoxaemia after 35 weeks' gestation. There appears to be some impairment of gas exchange, especially in patients with pre-eclampsia. It is known that PCO_2 is decreased during pregnancy due to direct effect of progesterone on the respiratory centre. CSF concentration of progesterone do not relate directly with enhancement of spinal anaesthesia (Hirabayashi et al 1995).

Porter et al (1996) have assessed the incidence of maternal hypoxaemia during labour in patients who received epidural infusions of bupivacaine, with or without fentanyl. Desaturation was greater in those patients who received fentanyl ($SpO_2 < 90\%$), while during the active phase of second stage of labour it was also more marked in the fentanyl group ($SpO_2 < 95\%$). The degree of maternal hypoxaemia did not appear to affect the fetus, but in high risk patients oxygen therapy would be advisable.

Yun et al (1996) have studied changes in pulmonary function during epidural analgesia for caesarean section. They compared the use of 2% lignocaine with adrenaline and 0.5% bupivacaine and found that 2% lignocaine produced more intense motor blockade resulting in diminution in peak expiratory pressure. They suggest that bupivacaine should be used for patients with pre-existing pulmonary disorders undergoing caesarean section in case reduction in peak expiratory pressure may result in reduced ability to cough effectively.

PRE-ECLAMPSIA

The aetiology of pre-eclampsia is unknown and Schobel et al (1996) have proposed that it is a state of sympathetic over-activity which reverts to normal following delivery. The pathophysiology and management of patients with pre-eclampsia has been outlined in detail by Mushambi et al (1996). It affects all systems of the body, including the cardiovascular and respiratory systems, central nervous system, renal and hepatic systems as well as coagulation, capillary permeability and alterations in colloid, osmotic pressure and intravascular hydrostatic pressure. Anti-platelet therapy, including aspirin, has been advocated in the past but is only advisable in patients who are liable to early onset pre-eclampsia requiring induction of labour before term. Many drugs have been used for the treatment of the hypertension in pregnancy, including methyldopa, β blockers and nifedipine. ACE inhibitors are not recommended because of their effects on the fetus. Labetalol has been advocated but there is also concern about the effects on the fetus. The drug of choice for acute rise in blood pressure is hydralazine and labetalol is a reasonable alternative. Other recommended drugs include diazoxide, sodium nitroprusside and glyceryl trinitrate. For the control of eclampsia itself chlormethiazole has become less popular, and magnesium sulphate appears more efficacious than diazepam and phenytoin (Neilson 1995).

Some patients may develop 'Haemolysis, Elevated Liver enzymes and Low Platelets' (HELLP) syndrome. For the management of labour extradural analgesia is recommended as it not only controls pain, but also controls the blood pressure. Spinal analgesia is not recommended in view of the possibility of profound hypotension. Before embarking on regional analgesia, it is important to check the platelet levels and they should be above 100×10^9 per litre. Orlikowski et al (1996) maintains that haemostasis should be unaffected if the platelet count is $> 75 \times 10^9/l$. For the management of general anaesthesia, it should not be forgotten that laryngeal oedema may be present and there may be marked pressor responses in response to intubation and surgical stimulation.

Hypertension in pregnancy may be due to chronic hypertension, hypertension developing during pregnancy, or pre-eclampsia. Maternal and neonatal outcome in the first two are good, but the potential for morbidity for mother and fetus are high in pre-eclampsia as maternal cardiac output and plasma volume are reduced, while systemic vascular resistance is increased. There is reduced perfusion of the placenta, kidney, liver and brain. Many of the symptoms are due to reduced perfusion rather than hypertension (Sibai 1996). Pre-eclampsia may be recognisable as early as 16–20 weeks and the ratio of urinary secretion of kallikrein to that of creatinine appears to be a predictor (Roberts 1996). Hypertension may be associated with renal insufficiency, due to pre-existing renal disease and, although there is an increase in obstetric complications, as well as hypertension, fetal survival is high (Jones & Hayslett 1996). Pregnancy appears to exacerbate renal disease and this may be due to platelet aggregation, fibrin thrombi and microvascular coagulation leading to further deterioration of kidney function. The production of thromboxane may be increased as well (Epstein 1996).

August et al (1995) demonstrated that the renin-angiotensin system is responsible for maintaining blood pressure in pregnant patients. During pregnancy there is increased vasodilatation, followed by lower blood pressure, resulting in increased renal renin release, followed by increased production of angiotensin II. There may be some disturbance of the renin-angiotensin system in the aetiology of eclampsia which occurs in 1 of 2000 pregnancies in the UK and is associated with a high maternal morbidity and fatality (Douglas & Redman 1994). Liver function is abnormal and is thought to be due to ischaemic injury to the liver, resulting in a rise in aminotransferases. In addition, there may be another phase of the liver injury involving a rise in alkaline phosphatase and γ-glutamyl transferase suggesting cholestasis (Rowan & North 1995). In fact, pre-eclampsia remains the single most common cause of maternal death in the UK and it is possible that the initial rise in blood pressure may be compensatory for fetoplacental hypoxia but, when the compensatory mechanisms fail, multi-system disease occurs. Calcium excretion is reduced, which may also accentuate the blood pressure rise. Most of the cardiovascular changes occur in the second half of pregnancy and are mediated probably by hormones rather than the sympathetic nervous system (Broughton Pipkin 1995).

Knox & Olans (1996) have reviewed the problems of liver disease in pregnancy: this is a rare complication, but can lead to acute fatty degeneration of the liver resulting in jaundice, liver failure and mortality. Liver transplant may be necessary. One of the difficulties is that physiological changes during pregnancy can alter liver function, including a fall in plasma albumin and a rise in alkaline phosphatase due to leakage of placental alkaline phosphatase into maternal blood. However, the transaminases, which are usually normal, may indicate hepatic damage. Cholestatic jaundice may occur due to hyperemesis gravidarum, the effect of drugs or cholestasis associated with pregnancy. During pregnancy, viral hepatitis may occur. The HELLP syndrome may be associated with acute fatty liver of pregnancy, pre-eclampsia or eclampsia. Thrombotic thrombocytopenic purpura and disseminated intravascular coagulation may also occur.

CARDIOVASCULAR DISEASE

Shortness of breath is not uncommon in pregnant patients and Morley & Lim (1995) have warned about the dangers of delay in diagnosing breathlessness during pregnancy, having discovered five patients with severe cardiac disease presenting for the first time during pregnancy.

There are problems with pregnant patients with prosthetic heart valves and it has been shown that warfarin, although crossing the placental barrier, is not associated with any fetal damage. Heparin, which does not cross the placental barrier, was associated with more thrombotic and bleeding complications than warfarin. Bioprosthetic valves deteriorate during pregnancy (Sbarouni & Oakley 1994). Ginsberg & Barron (1994) suggest that these results should be interpreted with caution and that warfarin should not be given between 6–12 weeks of gestation, or close to term to avoid delivery of an anticoagulated fetus. They recommend heparin during these periods and warfarin during the rest of the pregnancy with an INR of 3.0–4.5. A potential danger of long-term heparin is osteoporosis with vertebral body fracture.

NEUROLOGICAL DISORDERS

Reynolds (1995) discussed the maternal sequelae of childbirth, including the neurological complications which could be associated, not only with regional analgesia, but also with childbirth. MacArthur et al (1990, 1992), in retrospective surveys, suggested there was an association between long term backache and epidural analgesia in labour. However, Reynolds and her co-workers, in a prospective study, found that there was no significant increase in long term backache in women who had received epidural analgesia in labour (Russell et al 1996). In their study of nearly 600 patients, of whom 75% responded to a questionnaire, it was found that half of these women suffered from backache during the pregnancy, but forgot about this when questioned retrospectively. Neurological problems can be present during pregnancy and prior to labour, and as advocated in *Anaesthesia Review 13*, a simple neurological examination should be carried out before embarking on epidural analgesia. This may not always be possible due to the rapidly changing situations in obstetrics, but every endeavour should be made to examine patients in early labour.

Forster et al (1996) described a patient who developed a prolapsed intervertebral disc following epidural analgesia during labour. The needle was inserted at the level of $L_{3/4}$ and following delivery the patient was unable to stand and there was a flaccid biparesis. Magnetic resonance imaging (MRI) scan revealed a prolapse at the level of L_5/S_1. The patient was treated conservatively and completely recovered one month later.

SPINAL AND EXTRADURAL ANALGESIA

James et al (1996) studied the effect of positioning of the side eye of the 24 gauge Sprotte spinal needle. They found that if it was directed in a cephalad direction, the onset of sensory block was significantly faster than if it was pointed in other directions. However, there was no difference in the final height of the block, the incidence of hypotension, nausea and vomiting or requirements of ephedrine.

Chung et al (1996) observed the effects of volume on spinal anaesthesia with 0.25% hyperbaric bupivacaine for caesarean section. They found that the frequency of visceral pain and supplementary analgesia was less in the patients who had 3.6–4 ml of the drug, compared with smaller volumes, but there was an incidence of hypotension if the volume exceeded 4 ml.

The effect of spinal anaesthesia is said to be enhanced in pregnant patients. Hirabayashi et al (1996a) investigated the effects of acid/base changes in the CSF and found this had little effect on the spread of anaesthesia, but they did show there were high levels of analgesia in pregnant women during the second and third trimesters compared with non-pregnant patients.

The soft tissue anatomy in the vertebral canal in pregnant women has been studied by Hirabayashi et al (1996b). They found that the extradural venous plexus was engorged, particularly in the supine position. The dura is displaced from the wall of the vertebral canal, in a posterior direction, leading to decrease in the volume of the cerebrospinal fluid in the dural sac. The capacity of the extradural and subarachnoid spaces are thus reduced in late pregnancy and, therefore, extradural analgesia produces a more extensive blockade than in the non-pregnant patient

Scull & Carli (1996) reported cardiac arrest following caesarean section under spinal analgesia with 2 ml of 0.75% hyperbaric bupivacaine and 0.25 mg morphine. It was felt that the cardiac arrest was associated with repositioning the patient as the patient was being transferred to the recovery area and there was a period when monitoring was not in place. They advocated the use of adrenaline to treat the hypotension and bradycardia associated with the spinal blockade.

There has been controversy about the use of vasopressors to maintain arterial blood pressure following spinal anaesthesia for caesarean section. Thomas et al (1996) reported on the favourable use of phenylephrine 100 μg for maintaining maternal blood pressure without detriment to the fetus, although bradycardia, necessitating the use of atropine was a prominent feature.

Hirose et al (1996) found that postoperative pain relief with continuous epidural bupivacaine for 3 days following caesarean section, improved the amount of breast feeding and weight gain of the infant.

References

August P, Mueller F B, Sealey J E, Edersheim T G 1995 Role of renin-angiotensin system in blood pressure regulation in pregnancy. Lancet 345: 896–897
Bourne T, Ogilvy A J, Vickers R, Williamson K 1995 Nocturnal hypoxaemia in late pregnancy. Br J Anaesth 75: 678–682
Broughton Pipkin F 1995 The hypertensive disorders of pregnancy. Br Med J 311: 609-613
Chung C J, Bae S H, Chae K Y, Chin Y J 1996 Spinal anaesthesia with 0.25% hyperbaric bupivacaine for caesarean section: effects of volume. Br J Anaesth 77: 145–149
Douglas K A, Redman C W G 1994 Eclampsia in the United Kingdom. BMJ 309: 1395–1400
Epstein F H 1996 Pregnancy and renal disease. N Engl J Med 335: 277–278
Forster M R, Nimmo G R, Brown A G 1996 Prolapsed intervertebral disc after epidural analgesia in labour. Anaesthesia 51: 773–775.
Ginsberg J S, Barron W M 1994 Pregnancy and prosthetic heart valves. Lancet 344: 1170–1172
Hirabayashi Y, Shimizu R, Saitoh K, Fukuda H 1995 Cerebrospinal fluid progesterone in pregnant women. Br J Anaesth 75: 683–687
Hirabayashi Y, Shimizu R, Saitoh K et al 1996a Acid-base state of cerebrospinal fluid during pregnancy and its effect on spread of spinal anaesthesia. Br J Anaesth 77: 352–355
Hirabayashi Y, Shimizu R, Fukuda H et al 1996b Soft tissue anatomy within the vertebral canal in pregnant women. Br J Anaesth 77: 153–156
Hirose M, Hara Y, Hosokawa T, Tanaka Y 1996 The effect of postoperative analgesia with continuous epidural bupivacaine after cesarean section on the amount of breast feeding and infant weight gain. Anesth Analg 82: 1166–1169
James K S, Stott S M, McGrady E M et al 1996 Spinal anaesthesia for caesarean section: effect of Sprotte needle orientation. Br J Anaesth 77: 150–152
Jones D C, Hayslett J P 1996 Outcome of pregnancy in women with moderate or severe renal insufficiency. N Engl J Med 335: 226–232
Knox T A, Olans L B 1996 Liver disease in pregnancy. N Engl J Med 335: 569–576
MacArthur C, Lewis M, Knox E G et al 1990 Epidural anaesthesia and long term backache after childbirth. BMJ 301: 9–12
MacArthur C, Lewis M, Knox E G 1992 Investigation of long term problems after obstetric epidural analgesia. BMJ 304: 1279–1282
Morley C A, Lim B A 1995 The risks of delay in diagnosis of breathlessness in pregnancy. BMJ 311: 1083–1084
Mushambi M C, Halligan A W, Williamson K 1996 Recent developments in the pathophysiology and management of pre-eclampsia. Br J Anaesth 76: 133–148
Neilson J P 1995 Magnesium sulphate: the drug of choice in eclampsia. BMJ 311: 702–703
Orlikowski C E P, Rocke D A, Murray W B et al 1996 Thrombelastography changes in pre-eclampsia and eclampsia. Br J Anaesth 77: 157–161
Porter J S, Bonello E, Reynolds F 1996 The effect of epidural opioids on maternal oxygenation during labour and delivery. Anaesthesia 51: 899–903
Reynolds F 1995 Maternal sequelae of childbirth. Br J Anaesth 75: 515–517
Roberts J M 1996 Preventing pre-eclampsia. Lancet 348: 281–282
Rowan J A, North R A 1995 Abnormal liver function tests after pre-eclampsia. Lancet 345: 1367
Russell R, Dundas R, Reynolds F 1996 Long term backache after childbirth: prospective search for causative factors. BMJ 312: 1384–1388

Sbarouni E, Oakley C M 1994 Outcome of pregnancy in women with valve prostheses. Br Heart J 71: 196–201
Schobel H P, Fischer T, Heuszer K et al 1996 Preeclampsia – a state of sympathetic overactivity. N Engl J Med 335: 1480–1485
Scull T J, Carli F 1996 Cardiac arrest after caesarean section under subarachnoid block. Br J Anaesth 77: 274–276
Sibai B M 1996 Treatment of hypertension in pregnant women. N Engl J Med 335: 257–265
Thomas D G, Robson S C, Redfern N et al 1996 Randomized trial of bolus phenylephrine or ephedrine for maintenance of arterial pressure during spinal anaesthesia for caesarean section. Br J Anaesth 76: 61–65
Yun E, Topulos G P, Body S C et al 1996 Pulmonary function changes during epidural anesthesia for cesarean delivery. Anesth Analg 82: 750–753

PAIN

The pharmacologic treatment of cancer pain is discussed by Levy (1996) and ranges from NSAIDs, opioids, such as codeine and dihydrocodeine, to morphine and its derivatives. Hanks et al (1996) have reviewed the modes of administration of morphine for cancer pain and the optimal route is orally. Controlled release formulations are available and if patients are unable to tolerate drugs orally the rectal and subcutaneous routes are preferred. If the subcutaneous route is impractical, due to oedema or coagulation disorders, the intravenous route is preferred. With these guidelines, it is suggested that 80% of patients have effective control of chronic cancer pain and the buccal, sublingual and nebuliser routes are not recommended. Long-term morphine treatment for cancer does not appear to affect patients ability to drive safely (Vainio et al 1995). Oral morphine relieves chronic non-cancer pain, but does not result in psychological or functional improvement (Moulin et al 1996).

Attempts have been made to explain the mode of action of intrathecal opioids and the α_2 adrenoceptor appears to be involved in antinociception (Goodchild et al 1996).

Anticonvulsant drugs, such as carbamazepine, are effective in the treatment of trigeminal neuralgia, diabetic neuropathy and the prophylaxis of migraine (McQuay et al 1995).

Dell (1996) has favourably reviewed the results of patient-controlled sedation, but there have been dangers of overdose due to failure in the pump system and the need for anti-syphon valves (Southern & Read 1994, Elcock 1994).

Flurbiprofen is a non-steroidal anti-inflammatory analgesic drug. Lotsch et al (1995) have shown that both the (R)- and (S)-enantiomers are active and since the (R)-enantiomer is less toxic, especially to the gastrointestinal system, the side effects may be avoided by using (R)-flurbiprofen for pain relief.

References

Dell R 1996 A review of patient-controlled sedation. Eur J Anaesthesiol 13: 547–552
Elcock D H 1994 Overdosage during patient controlled analgesia. BMJ 309: 1583
Goodchild C S, Guo Z, Davies A, Gent J P 1996 Antinociceptive actions of intrathecal xylazine: interactions with spinal cord opioid pathways. Br J Anaesth 76: 544–551
Hanks G W, de Conno F, Hanna M et al (Expert Working Group of the European Association for Palliative Care) 1996 Morphine in cancer pain: modes of administration. BMJ 312: 823–826

Levy M H 1996 Pharmacologic treatment of cancer pain. N Engl J Med 335: 1124–1132
Lotsch J, Geisslinger G, Mohammadian P et al 1995 Effects of flurbiprofen enantiomers on pain-related chemosomatosensory evoked potentials in human subjects. Br J Clin Pharmacol 40: 339–346
McQuay H, Carroll D, Jadad A R et al 1995 Anticonvulsant drugs for the management of pain: a systematic review. BMJ 311: 1047–1052
Moulin D E, Iezzi A, Amireh R et al 1996 Randomised trial of oral morphine for chronic non-cancer pain. Lancet 347: 143–147
Southern D A, Read M S 1994 Overdosage of opiate from patient controlled analgesia devices. BMJ 309: 1002
Vainio A, Illila J, Matikainen E et al 1995 Driving ability in cancer patients receiving long-term morphine analgesia. Lancet 346: 667–670

ENDOCRINE SYSTEM

THE HYPOTHALAMIC-PITUITARY-ADRENAL AXIS

Chrousos (1995) has re-iterated details of the hypothalamic-pituitary-adrenal axis and how the system is aroused by stimuli including cytokines produced by immune-mediated inflammatory reactions, such as tumour necrosis factor α, interleukin-1 and interleukin-6. When activated, there are changes in the cardiovascular system, metabolism and also there is inhibition of immune-mediated information (see Saper & Breder 1994 on the neurological basis of fever).

Review articles have recently appeared on hypopituitarism (Vance 1994) and Cushing's syndrome (Orth 1995). The molecular basis of thyroid hormone action has been reviewed by Brent (1994) as well as drugs affecting thyroid function (Surks & Sievert 1995). Thyroxine therapy has been reviewed by Toft (1994) and the management of hyperthyroidism by Franklyn (1994). Details of maternal and fetal thyroid function are outlined by Burrow et al (1994)

ADDISON'S DISEASE

Addison's disease is a rare disorder in which there is destruction of the adrenal cortex and lack of production of glucocorticoids, mineralocorticoid and sex hormones. Most cases are due to autoimmune disease, but may be associated with other immune disorders such as thyroid disease, diabetes, pernicious anaemia, hypoparathyroidism and adrenal failure. Brosnan & Gowing (1996) report two cases who were only diagnosed at autopsy, due to the non-specificity of symptoms. Excessive pigmentation is not a universal feature of the disease, especially if the cause is autoimmune.

Patients with Addison's disease also excrete excessive amounts of sodium and retain potassium and this is due to the absence of aldosterone. The most important regulator of steroid secretion is the renin-angiotensin system and potassium. Corticotrophin also stimulates aldosterone, but this is of short duration. In aldosteronism there is marked hypokalaemia and alkalosis, but hypernatraemia is rare. Most patients with primary aldosteronism have a solitary aldosterone-producing adrenal adenoma (White 1994). High doses of intravenous hydrocortisone, used in the treatment of asthma, may produce clinically significant hypokalaemia (Ramsahoye et al 1995).

ANAESTHESIA AND INTENSIVE CARE

Levy (1996) has questioned the ritual of prescribing regimes for steroid cover for the endocrine response to surgery in patients who have had a history of steroid therapy. He suggests that studies are required, not to establish whether adrenal suppression occurs following prolonged steroid therapy, but whether it matters.

Quiney & Durkin (1995) report a case of acute adrenocortical failure in the intensive care unit, in a patient in whom the initial diagnosis was septic shock which can mask the diagnosis. The clinical features are tachycardia and hypotension, fever, oliguria, confusion and gastrointestinal complaints. The patient responded to a stimulation test with tetracosactrin (see Oelkers 1996). Etomidate is also known to cause diminished cortisol production.

ATRIAL NATRIURETIC HORMONES

Three natriuretic peptides have been identified:

1. *Atrial natriuretic hormone, stored mainly in the right atrium and causes natriuresis and vasodilation.*

2. *B type (brain), stored mainly in cardiac ventricles and causes natriuresis and vasodilation (originally isolated from porcine brain).*

3. *C type natriuretic peptide, stored in the vascular endothelial cells and causes vasodilatation.*

ANP suppresses the renin-angiotensin aldosterone system, prevents renin release, suppresses ACE activity and blocks aldosterone release. Possibilities for its clinical use are in the management of hypertension, heart failure, myocardial ischaemia, chronic renal failure and cor pulmonale (Struthers 1994).

Acute hypoxaemia leads to pulmonary vasoconstriction so that blood is diverted from hypoxic areas of the lung to maintain the ventilation perfusion ratio. This effect is detrimental in prolonged hypoxaemia as seen in chronic obstructive airways disease. Cargill & Lipworth (1995) have studied the effects of atrial natriuretic peptide (ANP) and brain natriuretic peptide (BNP) which both relax the pulmonary vasculature. However, only BNP attenuated the rise in mean pulmonary arterial pressure and total pulmonary resistance in response to acute hypoxaemia.

SOMATOSTATIN

Somatostatin was originally recognised as a hormone inhibiting release of growth hormone and two active compounds have been recognised, somatostatin-14 and somatostatin-28. It affects neurotransmission in the central nervous system and, in addition to regulating growth hormone, it also affects thyrotropin. It is widely released in the gastrointestinal tract and has a modulating role in the endocrine pancreas. Five types of somatostatin receptors have been identified. The use of somatostatin has been limited by the fact that it has to be given intravenously and has short duration of action (half-life 3 min) and this is followed by rebound hypersecretion of growth hormone, insulin and glucagon. Octreotide is a somatostatin analogue which can be given subcutaneously. It is used in the treatment of acromegaly, thyrotropin-secreting pituitary adenomas, corticotropin-secreting pituitary adenomas and pancreatic islet-cell tumours, as well as controlling the symptoms of carcinoid tumours. It has also been used in the treatment of oesophageal varices, pancreatic fistula and pseudocysts, as well as patients with intestinal fistula and radiation colitis. Side effects include nausea, diarrhoea, malabsorption of fat, flatulence, hyperglycaemia and gall stones (Lamberts et al 1996).

Somatostatin decreases splanchnic arterial blood flow, portal flow and gastric mucosal blood flow. It inhibits the secretion of gastric acid and pepsinogen and stimulates the secretion of gastric mucus. It appears to be effective in the treatment of gastrointestinal varices, in the management of enterocutaneous fistulae and secretory diarrhoea associated with short bowel syndrome, ileostomy diarrhoea, idiopathic diarrhoea. Octreotide is much safer than vasopressin because of less cardiovascular effects (Shulkes & Wilson 1994).

AVP

Intra-nasal and oral vasopressin have been licensed for use for nocturnal enuresis, but its use may lead to hyponatraemic convulsions. It is recommended that patients should avoid excessive fluid intake and other drugs which increase secretion of endogenous vasopressin such as tricyclic antidepressants (Committee on Safety of Medicines 1996).

Desmopressin, a synthetic analogue of vasopressin, affects coagulation and fibrinolysis, increases factor VII, von Willebrand factor and tissue plasminogen activator. It is a drug of choice in von Willebrand's disease type I and mild haemophilia A. Hartmann & Reinhart (1995) have drawn attention to the potential dangers of vasopressin in that it may result in acute myocardial infarction.

References

Brent G A 1994 The molecular basis of thyroid hormone action. N Engl J Med 331: 847–860

Brosnan C M, Cowing N F C 1996 Addison's disease. BMJ 312: 1085–1087

Burrow G N, Fisher D A 1994 Maternal and fetal thyroid function. N Engl J Med 331: 1072–1078

Cargill R I, Lipworth B J 1995 Acute effects of ANP and BNP on hypoxic pulmonary vasoconstriction in humans. Br J Clin Pharmacol 40: 585–590

Chrousos G P 1995 The hypothalamic-pituitary-adrenal axis and immune-mediated inflammation. N Engl J Med 332: 1351–1360

Committee on Safety of Medicines 1996 Hyponatraemic convulsions in patients with enuresis treated with vasopressin. Current Problems in Pharmacovigilance 22: 4

Franklyn J A 1994 The management of hyperthyroidism. N Engl J Med 331: 1731–1738

Hartmann S, Reinhart W 1995 Fatal complication of desmopressin. Lancet 345: 1302–1303.

Lamberts S W J, Van der Lely A-J, de Herder W W, Hofland L J 1996 Octreotide. N Engl J Med 334: 246–254

Levy A 1996 Perioperative steroid cover. Lancet 347: 846–847

Oelkers W 1996 Adrenal insufficiency. N Engl J Med 335: 1206–1212
Orth D N 1995 Cushing's Syndrome. N Engl J Med 332: 791–803
Quiney N F, Durkin M A 1995 Adrenocortical failure in intensive care. BMJ 310: 1253–1254
Ramsahoye B H, Davies S V, El-Gaylani N et al 1995 The mineralocorticoid effects of high dose hydrocortisone. BMJ 310: 656–657
Saper C B, Breder C D 1994 The neurologic basis of fever. N Engl J Med 330: 1830–1996
Shulkes A, Wilson J S 1994 Somatostatin in gastroenterology. BMJ 308: 1381–1382
Struthers A D 1994 Ten years of natriuretic peptide research: a new dawn for their diagnostic and therapeutic use? BMJ 308: 1615–1619
Surks M I, Sievert R 1995 Drugs and thyroid function. N Engl J Med 333: 1699–1694
Toft A D 1994 Thyroxine therapy. N Engl J Med 331: 174–180
Vance M L 1994 Hypopituitarism. N Engl J Med 330: 1651–1662
White P C 1994 Disorders of aldosterone biosynthesis and action. N Engl J Med 331: 250-258

Index

A

B

C

D

E

F

G

H

I

K

L

M

N

O

P

Q

R

S

T

U

V

W

X

Y

Z